Quality and Safety for Transformational Nursing:
Core Competencies

Kim Siarkowski Amer, PhD, RN
Associate Professor and Interim Director
School of Nursing
DePaul University
Chicago, Illinois

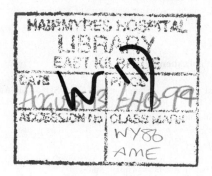
PEARSON

Boston Columbus Indianapolis New York San Francisco Upper Saddle River
Amsterdam Cape Town Dubai London Madrid Milan Munich Paris Montreal Toronto
Delhi Mexico City São Paulo Sydney Hong Kong Seoul Singapore Taipei Tokyo

Editor in Chief: Julie Alexander
Executive Acquisitions Editor: Pamela Fuller
Editorial Project Manager: Maria Reyes
Development Editor: Pamela Lappies
Editorial Assistant: Cynthia Gates
Marketing Manager: Phoenix Harvey
Marketing Manager: Debi Doyle
Production Manager: Debbie Ryan
Art Director/Cover: Jayne Conte

Art Director/Interior: Christopher Weigand
Cover Designer: Suzanne Behnke
Cover Art: Shutterstock
Full-Service Project Management/Composition: Shree
Mohanambal Inbakumar/PreMediaGlobal
Printer/Binder: R. R. Donnelly
Cover Printer: Lehigh-Phoenix Color

Credits and acknowledgments borrowed from other sources and reproduced, with permission, in this textbook appear on the appropriate page within text.

Library of Congress Cataloging-in-Publication Data
Amer, Kim Siarkowski.
Quality and safety for transformational nursing: core competencies / Kim Siarkowski Amer.
    p. ; cm.
Includes bibliographical references and index.
ISBN-13: 978-0-13-272412-8 (alk. paper)
ISBN-10: 0-13-272412-X (alk. paper)
I. Title.
    1. Nursing Process—organization & administration—United States.
2. Clinical Competence—United States. 3. Medical Errors—prevention & control—United States.
4. Patient Safety—United States. 5. Quality of Health Care—United States.
    LC Classification not assigned
610.73—dc23
                                        2012023392

10 9 8 7 6 5 4 3 2 1

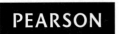

ISBN 10: 0-13-272412-X
ISBN 13: 978-0-13-272412-8

Student Resources

Online Student Resources are **included** with this textbook.
Visit **http://nursing.pearsonhighered.com** for the following assets and activities:

- Learning Outcomes
- Chapter Review Questions
- Case Studies
- Appendix and additional content updates
- Weblinks
- Links to additional nursing resources

Additional resources available. For more information and purchasing options visit nursing.pearsonhighered.com

CLASSROOM

mynursinglab

- MyNursingLab provides you with a one-of-a-kind *guided learning path.* Its proven personalized study plan helps you to *synthesize vast amounts of information* with an engaging **REVIEW**, **REMEMBER**, and **APPLY** approach. Move *from memorization to true understanding* through application with:
  - Even more alternate-item format questions
  - More analysis and application level questions that gauge true understanding
  - An interactive eText (also available via iPad®) with multimedia resources built right in

CLINICAL

Pearson's Nurse's Drug Guide

- Published annually to be your current, comprehensive, and clinically relevant source for drug information

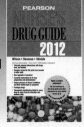

• Your complete mobile solution!

Real Nursing Skills

- Video demonstrations of over 200 clinical nursing skills
- Each skill includes Purpose, Preparation, Procedure, Post-Procedure, Expected and Unexpected Outcomes, Documentation and References and Resources

NCLEX®

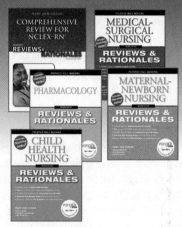

- Concentrated review of core content
- Thousands of practice questions with comprehensive rationales

---

PEARSON

ALWAYS LEARNING

PEARSON NURSING CLASS PREPARATION RESOURCES

New and Unique!

- Use this preparation tool to find animations, videos, images, and other media resources that cross the nursing curriculum! Organized by topic and fully searchable by resource type and key word, this easy-to-use platform allows you to:
  - Search through the media library of assets
  - Upload your own resources
  - Export to PowerPoint™ or HTML pages

Use this tool to find and review other unique instructor resources:

Correlation Guide to Nursing Standards

- Links learning outcomes of core text-books to nursing standards such as the 2010 ANA Scope and Standards of Practice, QSEN Competencies, National Patient Safety Goals, AACN, Essentials of Baccalaureate Education and more!

Pearson Nursing Lecture Series

- Highly visual, fully narrated and animated, these short lectures focus on topics that are traditionally difficult to teach and difficult for students to grasp
- All lectures accompanied by case studies and classroom response questions for greater interactivity within even the largest classroom
- Use as lecture tools, remediation material, homework assignments and more!

MYTEST AND ONLINE TESTING

- Test questions even **more accessible** now with both pencil and paper (MyTest) and online delivery options (Online Testing)
- **NCLEX®-style** questions
- **All New!** Approximately 30% of all questions are in alternative-item format
- **Complete rationales** for correct and incorrect answers mapped to learning outcomes

BOOK-SPECIFIC RESOURCES
Also available to instructors:

- **Instructor's Manual and Resource Guide** outlines chapter content and includes activities
- Comprehensive **PowerPoint™** presentations integrating lecture notes and images
- **Image library**
- **Classroom Response Questions**
- **Online course management systems** complete with instructor tools and student activities

mynursinglab

- **Proven Results:** Pearson's MyLab/Mastering platform has helped millions of students
- Provide your students with a one-of-a-kind guided learning path and personalized study plan! An engaging **REVIEW, REMEMBER,** and **APPLY** approach moves students from memorization to true understanding through application with:
  - Even more alternate-item format questions
  - More analysis and application level questions
  - An interactive eText (also available via iPad®) with multimedia resources built right in
- **Trusted Partner:** A network of customer experience managers and faculty advocates are available to help instructors maximize learning gains with MyNursingLab.

REAL NURSING SIMULATIONS

- 25 simulation scenarios that span the nursing curriculum
- Consistent format includes learning objectives, case flow, set-up instructions, debriefing questions and more!
- Companion online course cartridge with student pre- and post-simulation activities, videos, skill checklists and reflective discussion questions

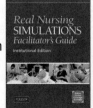

Real Nursing
SIMULATIONS
Facilitator's Guide
Institutional Edition

About the Author

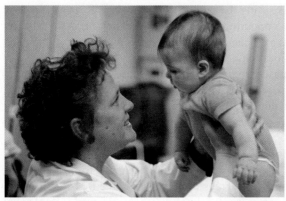

Kim Siarkowski Amer, PhD, RN is a pediatric nurse, associate professor, and interim director of the nursing school at DePaul University. She teaches theory, pediatric nursing, and research. She lives in Chicago, overlooking Lake Michigan.

Shots by Shelley

To My Family
—Lily, Nate, and Mike for their love, humor, support, and encouragement
—And my brother Kevin, my mother Nancy, and my late father Ted for my strong, loving foundation
and
to all the extraordinary nurses who are dedicated to being safe practitioners who deliver quality care despite very challenging situations.
You are the heart and soul of nursing!

Foreword

America's nurses play a central role in ensuring the quality of hospital care. As the primary front line providers, nurses have a unique opportunity to make care safer and more reliable, engage patients and their families, serve as a crucial defense against medical errors, and provide visionary leadership and effective communication.

However, the ability to utilize and master these opportunities has become increasingly challenging. Too often, nurses are overburdened with staffing shortages, communication breakdowns, and system inefficiencies and failures, which ultimately result in compromised care for patients. Nurses must be able to overcome these difficulties in order to continue to provide safe, quality care.

The Robert Wood Johnson Foundation (RWJF) is devoted to studying these problems and implementing programs to help nurses facilitate meaningful changes to hospital work environments. RWJF-funded initiatives, including Transforming Care at the Bedside (TCAB), have created effective models that support nurse-driven solutions that are designed to implement strategies to improve the care nurses provide. The challenges in our healthcare system are significant, but these programs have demonstrated significant progress in improving nurse retention, reducing errors, and improving patient safety.

Quality and Safety for Transformational Nursing: Core Competencies details the models and strategies that have been undertaken to improve the care that nurses provide. The wide range of opinions and methods presented in this book can and should be used by hospitals and healthcare professionals alike to identify problems and implement innovations so that the quality of patient care improves. Uniformity is essential for improving safety, and few other texts consolidate and critique the vast number of efforts in such an effective and instructive way.

The time has come for the United States to be a model not only for the best health care in the world, but also the safest, most efficient, and comprehensive care. To achieve these goals, major structural, philosophical, and behavioral changes are needed within our nation's hospitals, and nurses hold the key.

Nurses are literally on the front lines when it comes to care delivery and at the forefront of the quality-improvement movement in hospitals. We must engage and use nursing resources effectively to safely and consistently provide patients with the care they need, when they need it.

Susan B. Hassmiller PHD, RN, FAAN
Senior Advisor for Nursing
Robert Wood Johnson Foundation

Thank you

Contributors

We extend a heartfelt thanks to our contributors, who gave their time, effort, and expertise so tirelessly to the development and writing of chapters and resources that helped foster our goal of improving the quality of hospital care.

Yvonne Bilak-Krause, MS, RN
Children's Memorial Hospital, Chicago, Illinois
Chapter 8: Transforming Care at the Bedside (TCAB) Experience

Cheryl Carr, MSN, RN, UPMC
Shadyside School of Nursing, Pittsburgh, Pennsylvania
Chapter 5: Quality and Safety Education Strategies

Bernadette Curry, PhD, RN
Molloy College, Rockville Centre, New York
Chapter 12: Future-Focused Quality Nursing

Sherri Ewing, MS, RN
Children's Memorial Hospital, Chicago, Illinois
Chapter 8: Transforming Care at the Bedside (TCAB) Experience

Constance Hill, MSN, RN
Children's Memorial Hospital, Chicago, Illinois
Chapter 8: Transforming Care at the Bedside (TCAB) Experience

Paula Kagan, PhD, RN
Assistant Professor
School of Nursing, DePaul University, Chicago, Illinois
Chapter 4: Power, Empowerment, and Change

Young Me Lee, PhD, RN
Assistant Professor
School of Nursing, DePaul University, Chicago, Illinois
Chapter 10: Person-Centered Care

Mario Ortiz, PhD, RN, PHCNS-BC
Associate Professor and Chair
Duneland Health Council Faculty Scholar
Department of Nursing, Purdue North Central, Westville, Indiana
Chapter 10: Person-Centered Care

Karen Richey, MBA, RN
Children's Memorial Hospital, Chicago, Illinois
Chapter 8: Transforming Care at the Bedside (TCAB) Experience

Matthew Sorenson, PhD, RN
Assistant Professor
School of Nursing, DePaul University, Chicago, Illinois
Chapter 6: Evaluating a Program: Metrics and Stakeholders

Nancy Spector, PhD, RN
Director of Regulatory Innovations
National Council of State Boards of Nursing
Chapter 3: Transition to Practice: An Essential Element of Quality and Safety

Michelle Stephenson, DNP, RN
Children's Memorial Hospital, Chicago, Illinois
Chapter 8: Transforming Care at the Bedside (TCAB) Experience

Deborah Struth, MSN, RN
Associate Director, Quality Improvement and Curriculum
UPMC Shadyside School of Nursing, Pittsburgh, Pennsylvania
Chapter 5: Quality and Safety Education Strategies

Reviewers

Our heartfelt thanks go out to our colleagues from schools of nursing across the country who have given their time generously to help us create this exciting new edition of our book. We have reaped the benefit of your collective experience as nurses and teachers, and we have made many improvements due to your efforts. Among those who gave us their encouragement and comments are:

Gerry Altmiller, EdD, APRN, ACNS-BC
Professor, La Salle University
Philadelphia, Pennsylvania

Cheryl Anema, PhD, RN
Professor, Purdue University–Calumet
Hammond, Indiana

Sharon Beck, PhD, RN
Part-time/Adjunct Instructor, Thomas Edison State College, Drexel University
Trenton, New Jersey

Gail Bromley, PhD, RN
Department Chair, Kent State University
Kent, Ohio

Candace, M. Burns, PhD, ARNP
Professor, University of South Florida College of Nursing
Tampa, Florida

Mary Ann Camann, RN, PhD, PMHCNS-BC
Professor, Kennesaw State University
Kennesaw, Georgia

Candace C. Cherrington, PhD, RN
Associate Professor, Wright State University
Dayton, Ohio

Janet B. Craig, DHA, MBA, RN
Associate Professor, Clemson University
Clemson, South Carolina

Susan B. del Bene, PhD, RN CNS
Associate Professor, Pace University
New York, New York

Denise R. Eccles, RN, MSD/Ed
Professor, Miami Dade College
Miami, Florida

JoAnne Flagg, DNP, CPNP, IBCLC
Assistant Professor, Johns Hopkins University School of Nursing
Baltimore, Maryland

Gloria Fowler, MN, RN
Assistant Professor, University of South Carolina
Columbia, South Carolina

Barbara A. Gilbert, EdD, MSN, RN, CNE
Part-time/Adjunct Instructor, Excelsior College
Albany, New York

Cindy Grandjean, PhD
Graduate Coordinator, The Catholic University of America
Washington, DC

Alice R. Kempe, PhD, CS
Associate Professor, Ursuline College
Pepper Pike, Ohio

Jean M. Klein, PhD, PMHCNS, BC
Associate Professor, Widener University
Chester, Pennsylvania

Tammie Mann McCoy, PhD, RN
Department Chair, Mississippi University for Women
Columbus, Mississippi

Rebecca McMillan, PhD
Professor, Auburn University School of Nursing
Auburn, Alabama

Marylou V. Robinson, PhD, FNP-C
Course Coordinator, University of Colorado
Aurora, Colorado

Cheryl Spencer, PhD, RN
Assistant Professor, Queensborough Community College
Bayside, New York

Sandy Swearingen, PhD, RN
Instructor, University of Central Florida
Orlando, Florida

Lori Thuente, PhD, RN
Instructor, DePaul University
Chicago, Illinois

Diane Whitehead, EdD, RN, ANEF
Department Chair, Nova Southeastern University
Fort Lauderdale, Florida

Becky Wolff, RN, MSN, MA
Assistant Professor, University of South Dakota
Vermillion, South Dakota

Preface

This book began in 2004 when as a nurse faculty member I participated in the safety and quality innovation project called Transforming Care at the Bedside (TCAB). As a pediatric nursing faculty member, I joined the TCAB team at the only pediatric hospital of the 12 medical–surgical hospitals in the project. My role was to disseminate the findings in the TCAB sites. The innovative TCAB project used a rapid-cycle change process that engaged the nurses who provided direct patient care. The nurses were energized by the power of their own ability to influence change.

TCAB was developed in response to severe concerns about safety and quality in hospital settings reported by the Institute of Medicine in 1999. TCAB was funded by the Robert Wood Johnson Foundation (RWJF) and the Institute of Healthcare Improvement (IHI), and the innovations continue to be disseminated in hundreds of hospitals to date. The RWJF web site continues to track the progress of TCAB at rwjf.org.

The TCAB project required that I stretch my mind to learn about "raising the bar," "deep dives," "drilling down for root cause," and "spread." I expanded my knowledge and soaked in the intense energy at the hospital meetings and national conferences. I hope that all who read this book can also expand their knowledge base and become more creative and energized by the possibilities for the power of one nurse in shaping safe, quality nursing care.

The innovative TCAB approaches to creating solutions to the safety crisis in health care are still being integrated into healthcare settings. The philosophy of continuous quality improvement will always remain with me. Taking a more progressive view of problems with the understanding that mistakes are multifaceted and rarely one person's fault is critical for all nurses.

The purpose of this book is to raise awareness in students, nurses, and healthcare providers regarding the threats and risks to safety in hospitals and to provide information about developing core competencies in quality and safety in nursing. The hope is that readers will learn the potential and power within the nurse and collectively the nursing profession to affect change and master the competencies necessary to navigate the complex health system with an emphasis on safe, quality nursing care. While this book's focus is on the education of nurses in practice and in nursing schools, it also applies to all healthcare workers who work alongside nurses. Healthcare providers who are developing plans for improving safety and decreasing adverse events in their setting and students in health care will find it an excellent resource. The primary aim is simple: decrease preventable deaths by taking critical steps needed for establishing quality and safety. Even though this sounds simple, major structural, philosophical, and behavioral changes need to be in place to meet this goal.

The Future of Nursing: Leading Change, Advancing Health (2010) was published with the focus on nursing as the beacon of hope for change in health care and stated the following:

> Nurses are well positioned to help meet the evolving needs of the health care system. They have vital roles to play in achieving patient-centered care; strengthening primary care services; delivering more care in the community; and providing seamless, coordinated care. . . . They must rise to the challenge of providing leadership in rapidly changing care settings and in an evolving health care system (p. 76).

The American Association of Colleges of Nursing (AACN) lists *Basic Organizational and Systems Leadership for Quality Care and Patient Safety* second in the essentials for curriculum in baccalaureate education in nursing. All nursing programs must integrate quality concepts in their programs.

The chapters in this book are developed from AACN, Institute of Medicine recommendations, the Institute for Healthcare Improvement, Robert Wood Johnson Foundation efforts, and pertinent nursing theory and research. All the authors are active scholars and clinicians in nursing practice. This is the first text that combines multiple perspectives aimed at improving safety and providing quality care. QSEN competencies are included with patient-centered care in Chapter 10; teamwork and collaboration are included in Chapters 2 and 9; evidence-based practice is included in Chapters 5, 6 and 1; and quality improvement is included in Chapters 1 and 2. Safety is integrated into all chapters. The QSEN competency of informatics is the focus of Chapter 9.

The first two chapters look at the U.S. healthcare system, safety and quality definitions, and strategies focused on how nurses develop effective changes that improve safety and quality. Chapter 3 includes an excellent model for new nurses with a focus on safety and their mentoring and transition to practice. Chapter 4, on power in nursing, extends the change theme and calls nurses to action to harness the power needed to demand safe nursing care conditions. Chapter 5 includes an overview of Quality and Safety Education in Nursing (QSEN) strategies for practice and teaching. Chapter 6 discusses measuring the safety and quality parameters and provides nursing students and nurses with tools to develop their own safety measures. Chapter 7 looks at interdisciplinary approaches to improving safety, and Chapter 8 describes the TCAB experience and provides examples for projects to improve care. Chapter 9 integrates technology in safety and quality improvement, and addresses the existing technology and recommendations for future technology. Chapter 10 includes the QSEN competency of person-centered care and a cultural competency case study. Chapter 11 addresses the policy and ethical issues related to safety in nursing, and Chapter 12 provides a future-focused care perspective on leadership in safety and quality nursing.

With this new knowledge, future nurses will become part of an ever more valued and trusted profession. Nurses will be the heart of the quality care transformation.

Acknowledgments

Thank you to Pam Fuller and Pearson for giving me this excellent opportunity to work with a great team, and to Pamela Lappies for her stellar and steadfast attention to all levels of creative and formatting editing. To Rina Ranalli, I thank you for being a most loyal creative editor, muse, and friend. You were there from the beginning, and I so appreciate you. Thanks to Adam Michael Boise, Anja Ensio, Ashley Gier, and Kathryn Owen for their scholarly contributions and research. Thanks also to Theresa Auer and Ashley Gier for their meticulous reference checks and glossary development. And to all the reviewers, I thank you for taking your precious time to improve the text. To all the contributors, I offer my grateful thanks for your patience and care to detail. Without your expertise and effort, this book could not have come into being.

Detailed Contents

CHAPTER 1

RISK AND THREATS TO SAFE QUALITY CARE IN HOSPITAL SETTINGS

Kim Siarkowski Amer

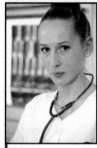

Edw/Shutterstock.com

Billy, a 5-year-old with leukemia, was admitted to the hospital for fever and neutropenia (low white blood cell count). Since his chemotherapy treatment started, he has eaten very little due to nausea. He has lost weight and has had little energy. He seemed very sad when Lisa, his nurse, came in to draw his blood work. The first vein became hard to target on the first attempt, and then the second attempt to get blood failed. The third time, Lisa was successful.

Billy started crying and said he wanted a Popsicle. He asked when his mother was coming. Lisa put the paperwork in with the tube of blood and hurried to get the Popsicle. She planned to spend some time calming Billy down. An hour later, the laboratory called and said they had received an unlabeled blood sample for a complete blood count CBC, and because they could not verify the patient, they would have to redraw from all patients who were not identified. Lisa's heart sank. Because she was distracted by Billy's crying, she forgot to put the name label on the tube. Now the whole ordeal had to start again!

CORE COMPETENCY

Describe risks to quality care and safety in nursing.

LEARNING OUTCOMES

1. Define safety and quality in nursing care.
2. Analyze the U.S. health system and the safety risks within the system.
3. Describe efforts to improve the safety and quality of health care, both within and outside of organizations, through foundations and credentialing bodies.
4. Integrate components that would be included in an ideal nursing practice environment.

Nurses are the heart and soul of healthcare delivery. With over 3 million nurses in the United States, they should command a strong voice in healthcare policy at the local and national levels (ANA.org, 2012). However, the U.S. healthcare system is complex, and decisions affecting nurses are rarely made by the nurses who are giving care at the bedside. This book proposes strategies to encourage nurses to be active participants in decision making and describes best nursing practice models used to ensure the many facets of safety and quality health care.

The State of Health Care in the United States

The U.S. healthcare system exists in a paradox of excellent high-technology care delivery paired with poor patient outcomes due to adverse events or preventable errors in care. The most current technologically advanced treatments are available to a select few, which contrasts with high morbidity and mortality rates in vulnerable low-income patients. Most patients assume that when they receive care at a hospital, their care will be provided to a high standard. The reality is that although healthcare providers want to relieve suffering and contribute to the health of their patients, there are barriers to doing so. The Committee on the Robert Wood Johnson Foundation Initiative on the Future of Nursing, at the Institute of Medicine (2011, p. 30) stated that "To ensure the delivery of safe, patient-centered care across settings, the nursing education system must be improved … nurses need to attain requisite competencies to deliver high-quality care." To attain this level of practice, the committee urges nurses to achieve higher levels of education and training, gain better collaborative partnerships with physicians and other healthcare professionals, and develop mastery of workforce planning and policymaking, data collection, and information infrastructure.

The 3 million nurses comprise the largest group of health professionals in the care delivery system. Nurses are the heart of the care delivery in the United States, and nursing remains among the most trusted occupations by U.S. citizens. Nurses enter the most private and vulnerable spaces in people's lives. They have the ability to heal, calm, educate, and provide reassurance to patients and their families. (See Figure 1-1.) When nurses practice in environments with good communication, adequate resources, and realistic patient responsibilities, the art and science of nursing is exhibited. In contrast, when there are too few nurses, poor communication, unrealistically long shifts, no breaks, and too many patients to care for, the care can be compromised, resulting in harm, infection, or death.

The Institute of Medicine Report on the State of Health Care

In 2000 the Institute of Medicine (IOM) report *To Err Is Human* estimated that as many as 98,000 people die in any given year from medical errors or adverse events in hospitals (IOM, 2000). That is more than die from motor vehicle crashes, breast cancer, or AIDS—three causes that

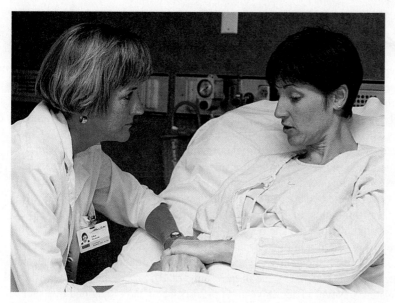

Figure 1-1 Good patient–provider communication increases the quality of care.

receive far more public attention. The number of deaths from hospital-caused errors is equivalent to more than 10 jumbo jet airliners crashing each week (Denham & Bugg, 2010).

To ensure safe healthcare systems, the IOM (2000) recommends adopting five critical principles:

- Provide leadership.

- Recognize human limits in process design.

- Promote effective team functioning.

- Anticipate the unexpected.

- Create a learning environment.

Although the IOM critical principles seem logical and intuitive, they are not common elements in all healthcare settings. The principles apply to both leaders of hospitals and staff nurses. All levels of leadership must be strong. The chief nursing officer needs to promote effective team functioning just as much as the night charge nurse and the on call medical resident. All team members should be flexible and understanding in their work processes. Finally, as is emphasized in Magnet recognition accreditation, the learning environment must be positive and supportive. When bad outcomes occur, the focus should be on examining the process to prevent future occurrences, not focusing on blame. The team spirit should be focused on the best interests of the patient and the best outcomes.

CASE STUDY: *Cindy*

Cindy, a veteran neonatal intensive care unit (NICU) nurse, was at the end of her 12-hour shift when she was called to her sickest patient's bedside and proceeded to attend to increasing ventilator settings on Maggie, who had been in the NICU for 5 weeks. Maggie had a sudden onset of desaturations (low oxygen in the blood) and bradycardia (low heart rate) and needed more oxygen and increased ventilation rates. Cindy called Agnes, the float nurse from the labor and delivery unit, and asked that Cindy give a quick heparin lock to Cindy's other patient, Justin, the 36-week-old premature infant who was scheduled for removal of his central venous line in the morning. Justin's parents were hoping to take him home by the end of the week. The line needed to be flushed every 4 hours with heparin solution (10 units/mL). Agnes found no heparin at the bedside, so she called down to the pharmacy and had a vial rushed up to the unit. In less than 10 minutes, the heparin was at the desk, and Agnes drew up 0.5 mL and administered it to Justin. About an hour after the heparin was given to Justin, Cindy arrived at the bedside and saw the vial of heparin used to administer the flush. She knew immediately that an error had occurred. Now what should be done? She gently questioned Agnes and found out that the heparin was 10,000 units/mL. Justin received 5,000 units instead of the 5 units of 10 unit/mL heparin. One thousand times the dose was administered. Never in her 28 years of practice had Cindy imagined that such a mistake could have happened.

Tracking the Root Cause of Errors

When an error is made, the most important action, after responding to any emergency or health concern is tracing back to the events that led to the error. This process is called root cause analysis and should be done with each error in a nonpunitive way. In cases of medication error, the responses of all those involved determine what the long-term effects of the error will be. If the mistake is viewed in a punitive context, nurses may not report future events or take actions to rescue a patient. Hiding mistakes or punishing staff members for unintentional errors helps no one. The response should be a logical, consistent, focused review of the events leading up to the error. Finally, the participants should develop the root cause analysis summary and develop a plan to prevent future errors. This chapter provides an overview of select approaches aimed at increasing the level of safety in hospital settings.

In Cindy's case study, several issues should be considered. First, inadequate staffing appeared to be an issue since the nurse from labor and delivery was floating (i.e., pulled to another unit where she had little expertise). In the IOM context, leadership may not have been strong. Second, the absence of heparin at the bedside should have prompted Agnes to ask Cindy where she could find the appropriate vial. In the IOM context, the human limitation was Agnes, the nurse who was not familiar with the unit's supplies. Last, the pharmacy should not have sent up heparin without an appropriate order including the dose, concentration, patient's name, and medication schedule. The team of nurse, physician, pharmacist, and ancillary messenger or secretary may have been able to prevent the error. Bar coding could have prevented the mistake if the order had been properly written. There are multiple factors in a situation that can predispose the nurse to adverse events. But the most important lesson is the focus on not placing blame. One must use situations with poor outcomes as learning opportunities to ensure future mistakes do not occur. In Chapter 2, the issues of medication reconciliation and nonpunitive reporting of medication errors are discussed. Luckily, most times the error is caught before it is delivered.

The Institute for Safe Medication Practices analyzed a cluster of heparin overdose incidents and placed blame on the learning culture in the hospital. The organization's report stated: "Workers must possess the willingness and competence to draw responsible conclusions from robust internal and external safety information systems and make substantial changes when necessary. Absent shared learning, the same heparin error will likely occur in other hospitals." (ISMP, 2007, para 8).

Heparin dosing errors were a concern in the years leading up to 2008. After the similarity in the bottles of heparin was identified as a primary factor in several errors throughout the United States, the manufacturer, Baxter, recalled the bottles and redesigned the product so that the difference between the two doses was more noticeable.

Evidence for Best Practices: Medication Administration

Recent studies have confirmed that fewer mistakes occur and more catches of near misses happen with bar code scanning of patient identification bracelets and medication bar codes linked with the patient's pharmacy data, allergies, and medications (Paoletti et al., 2007). In addition to bar coding, safety measures used in the airline industry have been adopted by nurses during medication administration. Using signals such as wearing a brightly colored vest and standing in a designated quiet zone while preparing medications, nurses have fewer distractions and provide safer medication administration (Pape, 2010). When combined, these documented improvements in safety, one based on technology and one focused on behavior, provide an excellent practice for the safest medication administration.

A replication study was conducted at St. James's Hospital (Dublin, Ireland) on a 59-bed medical–surgical unit in which nurses wore red aprons, followed a specific medication administration checklist, and posted "Do Not Disturb" signs when administering medications. There was a significant association between the overall interruption and distraction rate and the interventions. The rate of interruptions per hour postintervention was less than half the rate before the interventions were implemented. For observations, the institution used the Medication Administration Distraction Observation Sheet instrument developed by Dr. Pape.

Researchers and hospital quality department personnel contact Dr. Pape almost monthly about the medication administration checklist, and they ask for advice on using it in their own facilities. Some of the facilities working on implementation include: Texas Health Presbyterian Hospital–Denton in Denton, Texas; Texas Health Presbyterian Hospital–Plano in Plano, Texas; Midland Memorial Hospital in Midland, Texas; Princeton Healthcare System in Princeton, New Jersey; Children's Hospital of Philadelphia in Philadelphia, Pennsylvania; and New York–Presbyterian Hospital in New York, New York. The Joanna Briggs Institute in Queensland, Australia, has been using the "Do Not Disturb" signs with great success for some time. Changi General Hospital in the Republic of Singapore uses a vest based on a 2001 MedSafe study (AHRQ, 2011).

Root cause analysis—the backtracking of events surrounding the medication error—is useful in establishing policy in the NICU, pharmacy, and whole hospital system. McDonald and Levhane (2005) described the method of root cause analysis to identify the coexisting factors that lead to mistakes. When the factors are identified, the proper responses can be deployed to decrease risk and increase quality. Retrospective analysis of the causes for medication errors can range from noncompliance with policies or procedures to physician's illegible writing, wrong transcription of drug administration times, failure to check for the right patient, wrong identification of similarly packaged and labeled drugs, or distractions. Nurses in practice may regard the standard practice of the "golden rule" of three checks and five rights (right patient, right dose, right drug, right route, and right time) for drug administration as impractical because of time constraints, staffing shortages, and too many patients. In 2005, the IOM recommended a common safety report format that should be followed in all settings. The safety report includes discovery; the event; narrative, including contributing factors; ancillary information; causal analyses; and lessons learned (McDonald & Levhane, 2005).

Sentinel Event Tracking

In April 2008, the Joint Commission issued a sentinel event alert (SEA), or warning, to focus on the strategies needed to address the causes of serious medication errors within pediatric institutions. The SEA, called "Preventing Pediatric Medication Errors," was the first Joint Commission focus specifically on infants and children. This focus was triggered in part by the cluster of cases involving neonatal heparin overdoses. The incidents of heparin overdose followed a pattern: Vials of 10,000 unit/mL heparin were used in place of 10 unit/mL heparin flush solution. The SEA has resulted in a new approach for all children's hospitals to re-evaluate their systems for preparing, administering, and monitoring medication preparation and administration (Buck, Hofer, & McCarthy, 2008).

The process of sentinel event tracking focuses on the nonpunitive investigation of errors or near-miss errors. The purpose is to identify trends in potential errors and then intervene to prevent additional errors. The sentinel events must be significant enough to catch the attention of the healthcare institution's administration and critical units, such as the pharmacy, nursing units, and any other units that could possibly be involved in the risk.

Responses to the 2000 Institute of Medicine Report

Multiple responses have emerged to the IOM report *To Err Is Human*. Organizations such as the Robert Wood Johnson Foundation (RWJF), the Joint Commission, the American Hospital Association, the American Organization of Nurse Executives, and the American Nurses Association have established new efforts or collaborated on solutions to end the high level of adverse events. However, the multiple efforts must work collaboratively and form a coordinated effort to develop a standard, evidence-based approach to improving safety. Uniformity is required to address preventing threats to patients' health and well-being. Consistent methods and outcome measures are necessary to accurately track progress made toward diminishing adverse events.

Transforming Care at the Bedside Project

A model collaboration that will be referred to throughout this book is the Transforming Care at the Bedside (TCAB) project, a five-year project funded by the RWJF and the Institute for Healthcare Improvement (IHI). (See Box 1-1.) The TCAB project focused on medical–surgical units because the incidence of adverse events are highest in that area. Threats to quality and safe care that were addressed in TCAB included harm from falls, high turnover rates for hospital staff, high levels of nonnursing activity, ineffective communication between nurses and multidisciplinary teams, adverse events related to medication administration, and codes with poor outcomes. Over its lifespan, TCAB worked to develop a comprehensive model to address these risks. Using a multidisciplinary approach, the model included a rapid cycle, focused change process in which nurses providing direct patient care identified problems and proposed easy solutions that were tested over a few weeks, then either adopted or dropped. The common aims were to create early detection and response teams, such as rapid response teams (RRTs), prevent adverse drug events and falls, and build an environment that lessens the risk of adverse events. Figure 1-2 depicts the general safety and quality goals set by the TCAB project, which is discussed more fully in Chapter 8.

The TCAB project proved that simple structural changes such as interprofessional rounds and collaboration can dramatically decrease adverse events. However, one of the most challenging obstacles is getting cooperation from physicians. Their concerns are focused primarily on diagnosing and treating illness, and they tend to recoil when administrative programs are required. Even when patient safety is at the core of quality and safety efforts, physician buy-in remains elusive. The Patient Protection and Affordable Care Act signed into law by President Barack Obama in 2010

BOX 1-1	BUILDING A SAFER HEALTHCARE SYSTEM

An estimated 35% to 40% of unexpected deaths in hospitals occur in high-risk nursing units (mainly medical–surgical adult units) where nurses work long hours and have high turnover (RWJF). Finkleman and Kenner (2009) identified strategies to decrease the estimated 1.5 million adverse drug events (ADE) and unexpected deaths that occur every year in the United States. Their recommendations have been integrated into the TCAB model established by RWJF and the Institute for Health Care Improvement (IHI). The RWJF and IHI joined forces with multiple clinical sites throughout the country in the first two phases of TCAB and added schools of nursing as partners in the third phase. TCAB supports nurse-driven solutions designed to develop quality nursing care that includes efficient use of time, evidence-based practice, and multiple strategies to improve processes in health care.

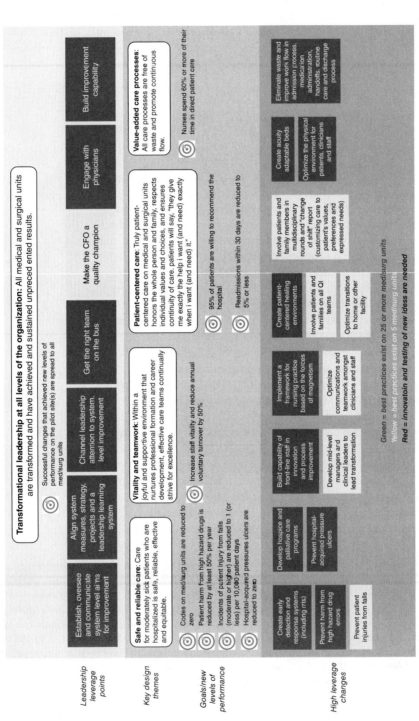

Figure 1-2 Transforming Care at the Bedside focused on safe and reliable care, vitality and teamwork, patient-centered care, and value-added care to promote safety in nursing environments.

Source: From Lee B, Shannon D, Rutherford P, Peck C. *Transforming Care at the Bedside How-to Guide: Optimizing Communication and Teamwork.* Cambridge, MA: Institute for Healthcare Improvement; 2008.

implemented pay for performance programs for select Medicare diagnoses. As a result, physicians and healthcare organizations would no longer be paid for patients' care if adverse events occurred, providing incentive to hospitals and other institutions to take measures to ensure safe care.

Paradoxical Health Care in the United States

Our health system can do marvelous work on the most premature infants, effectively treat cardiovascular disease with less-invasive technology, and diminish rates of death from cancer. But the day-to-day setbacks of hospital-acquired infection, the wrong dose of medication or the wrong drug, and failure to report a patient's slow demise can erase the allure and promise of high-technology care. The cost of medication errors is estimated to be $3.5 billion per year (IOM, 2011). That money could be used in much more productive ways.

Despite having excellent state-of-the-art technology and the best-trained physicians, our nation has the worst outcomes for those who live in extreme poverty. Those with access to excellent health care and good health insurance can expect to enjoy the best health care. In contrast, the poor and uninsured are coming to hospitals sicker than ever before, with multiple layers of health and social problems. However, even for those with excellent healthcare access, health promotion behaviors and compliance with medication regimens remain poor.

The most consistent predictor of long-term health and longevity remains a healthy weight. Despite this knowledge, the rate of obesity in the United States remains very high. The obesity epidemic has triggered predictions of children dying before their parents due to comorbidities of diabetes, heart disease, and kidney disease. The paradox of high-technology care paired with the reality of the obesity epidemic are difficult to reconcile. There is a limit to technological health care and cure-ability. The best healthcare intervention is the individual's own self-care and responsible health promotion activities. Nurses must be knowledgeable about such paradoxes in health care and able to provide health promotion teaching at each encounter with patients, inside or outside of the hospital setting.

Healthcare providers must be aware of the gravity of this situation. Health promotion focused solutions are best created by nurses with a mechanism for standard interventions and a consistent measure of outcomes, such as smoking cessation, indicating success (Blouin, 2010). For example, the Joint Commission (see Box 1-2) has a hand hygiene initiative that includes an acronym of HANDS for habit, active feedback, no one excused, data, and standards. Included in the initiative is a data driven framework that creates an easy flow toward compliance. Reviewing adverse events can help identify factors that contribute to the high number of patient deaths due to preventable occurrences such as medication errors, infections caused by hospital exposure to pathogens, and negligent safety practices that cause falls. A clear delineation of strategies that identify and minimize risks of adverse events must occur. These strategies are outlined in this book.

BOX 1-2   THE JOINT COMMISSION

Ann Blouin, RN, PhD, is executive vice president in the division of accreditation and certification operations at the Joint Commission. She is the first nurse to hold the position. The Joint Commission visits and reviews, then accredits, more than 15,000 healthcare organizations nationwide. To get reimbursement from insurance companies, healthcare organizations must have Joint Commission accreditation. Leadership is key to making sure that accreditation is ongoing and that mistakes do not occur. Blouin (2010) contends that workers do not commit errors on purpose. Systems and processes, combined with worker stress or lack of experience, can lead to mistakes. Nurses need to take leadership roles as Blouin has done and become proactive in the campaign for safety in health care.

Pulling It All Together

Mistakes happen, and the way people respond to mistakes shapes the outcomes and the risk of future poor outcomes. The healthcare environment must provide a culture of understanding and transparency related to adverse events. If workers are not willing to admit to errors, the pattern of increasing adverse events and poor quality care will continue. When there is a structure in place to review the events related to errors and develop solutions so that the same events will not happen in the future, workers feel valued and motivated to improve care. This should decrease the risk of adverse events.

Environment

The environment the nurse works in has a significant impact on nurse satisfaction and the outcomes of the patients. Many studies have confirmed the relationship between acuity of patients (how sick they are), the number of patients the nurse is caring for during the shift, and patient outcomes. Staffing formulas, which are complex and vary from hospital to hospital, determine how many and what acuity level of patients a single nurse cares for during the 8- or 12-hour shift. Beyond the staffing ratios, the general support and collegial climate on a unit significantly affect the nurse and patient care. Even though such concepts seem intuitive, they are important considerations when thinking about the safest care environment for both nurses and patients. (See Box 1-3.)

Safe Numbers

A simple solution to ensure safety is lower patient-to-nurse ratios. As Suzanne Gordon (2008) asserts in *Safety in Numbers*, dramatically improved outcomes go hand in hand with safe patient assignments. When an over-stressed nurse with too many patients administers medication, especially to an unfamiliar patient, the risk of a poor outcome increases. Even though safe patient-to-nurse ratios are an obvious and intuitive solution, hospital administrators hesitate to increase budgets to accommodate nursing salaries. The California Nurses Association lobbied for safe ratios of patients to nurses and won a pivotal victory in 2004. California is now the only state with mandatory maximum patient assignments.

BOX 1-3	THE IDEAL WORK ENVIRONMENT

Creating an ideal work environment provides a model to begin learning about best practices in nursing that are aimed at decreasing risks to safety and improving quality patient care.

With the ideal work environment, administrators ensure that safe care is practiced and that nurses are working under minimal stress. The following components of an ideal work environment can be used in nursing education and in real-life work environments to critique clinical systems.

- Full staffing based on national standards with safe nurse-to-patient ratios

- Nursing work hours and breaks that ensure off-unit time to rest, eat, and get away from the stress of caregiving

- Acuity-adaptable rooms and units

- Consistent nursing care, such as is discussed in the primary nursing model, where a nurse has the same patient consistently to ensure that care is optimal for the same patients every day and from admission to discharge

- Minimal floating to units that are outside the nurse's area of expertise

- Bar coding medication delivery to dramatically reduce medication errors

- Excellent communication with families and across all disciplines, including physicians, social workers, physical therapists, administrators, and nurses

- Pay that rewards excellence and benefits that encourage health promotion and self-care

- No mandatory overtime and limited length of shift, maximum 12-hour shifts

- Access to the best information systems for documentation of care, resources for learning, and tracking patient compliance

- Charge nurses and administrators that advocate for nursing practice

Stress, Long Hours, and No Breaks

The risk of adverse events caused by neglecting to discuss medications with patients and their families is greatest in scenarios where patient-to-nurse ratios are high and nurses work long hours without breaks. In high-stress, understaffed environments or environments in which shifts are longer than 8 hours, workers may be less careful when checking the accuracy of a drug, a dose, or a route. As recently as 2007, Nevada passed a nurse safety act banning mandatory overtime for nurses. Presently in Nevada nurses are not allowed to work over 12 hours in a 24-hour period and no more than 80 hours in a 2-week period. In the past, nurses were required to stay on shift for many hours past their 12-hour shift.

If successful companies like Target and Walmart make sure their cashiers and workers take frequent breaks, why do nursing units fail to provide the same? Much more is at stake in the healthcare environment than in a discount store. Most nurses refuse to take the time allotted for breaks if their patients are not doing well or if the other nurses are not taking breaks. It is up to the manager of the unit to make sure that nurses go on frequent breaks and that during breaks, patients are looked after by another staff member.

Risks and threats to safety in the nursing environment can include factors such as similar names—for example, Juan Gomez and Juan Gonzalez, Sue Miller and Sam Millard—medication errors, and neglecting patient needs, to more complex issues such as high nurse turnover high stress caused 12-hour shifts and mandatory overtime, and poor transdisciplinary communication and collaboration. The risks need to be highlighted for all healthcare professionals so that a unified effort to reduce harm is launched before another life is affected.

Concept Analysis of Safety and Quality

The words "safety" and "quality" have been used frequently in the past decade in discussions related to health care as Table 1-1 illustrates. Safe and quality health care, including the care nurses provide, is assumed to be the goal of all healthcare providers. The word "safety" is more clearly defined and less abstract quality. Safety is little or no risk for harm. Quality is much more elusive to define. The concept can be understood to mean the general standard or grade of something or the highest or finest standard. In health care, quality can have different meanings to patients and providers.

New standards for quality, as delineated in the National Hospital Quality Measures (NHQM) established in 2002, require nurses to be proficient in analysis of comparative quality data and able to design new patient care approaches to safe care so that hospitals will maintain their accreditation and continue to be reimbursed for services (Matthes et al., 2010). Without such competencies, nurses will find themselves in dangerous settings with little or no support.

In *Teaching IOM: Implications of the Institute of Medicine Reports for Nursing Education*, Finkelman and Kenner (2009), who are both nurses, explore the notion of quality care. As they discuss, the IOM has published multiple reports focused on quality care. In the IOM reports, safety and quality emerge as key components of healthcare administration. In 2000, *To Err Is Human* targeted the patient safety issue and proposed a comprehensive plan to address safety. At the time, safe care meant increasing the likelihood of better quality health care, and the primary focus was on process improvement to reduce errors instead of focusing on the individual patient. IOM publications evolved to focus more on organizational safety and quality care than on individual provider and patient safety actions. Ultimately, the IOM moved toward developing broader frameworks focused on the need for a national effort for data collection on quality health care.

Emerging Trends in Safety and Quality

Several responses have emerged in response to the IOM publications, including:

- American Association of the Colleges of Nursing (AACN)–accredited baccalaureate and masters education programs now

TABLE 1-1 ■ Definitions of Quality and Safe Care

Source	Quality Care	Safe Care	Setting or Context
To Err Is Human, IOM (2000)	Safety is the minimum standard required for quality care but does not comprise all aspects of it. Safe care does not signify that the care qualifies as quality care but increases the likelihood of it.	There are five critical principles related to designing safe healthcare systems: 1. Leadership is key. 2. Human nature can limit consistency in process design. 3. Team functioning is essential. 4. Anticipating the unexpected must be a continual state of mind. 5. Creating a learning environment that is nonpunitive improves safety.	Systems need to be the focus. Individual providers are not the only ones who make mistakes.
Crossing the Quality Chasm, IOM (2001)	Quality is a goal of healthcare systems that includes the six properties of care: 1. Safe care 2. Effective care 3. Patient-centered care 4. Timely care 5. Efficient care 6. Equitable care	Safety is the first component of quality.	All healthcare providers and stakeholders should be dedicated to raising the level of quality care.
Envisioning the National Health Care Quality Report, IOM (2001)	Quality is "the degree to which health services for individuals and populations increase the likelihood of desired health outcomes and are consistent with current professional knowledge" (p. 41). Structure, process, and outcome are the focus.	This source does not discuss the definition of safety. The focus is on an individual's health.	The report provides a framework for data collection on quality health care and served as the impetus for the creation of the Foundation for Agency for Healthcare Research and Quality (AHRQ).
Patient Safety: Achieving a New Standard of Care IOM (2004)	Quality will improve with better awareness of safety issues.	Safety is "freedom from accidental injury" (p. 53). To improve patient safety, changes must be made in safety and quality of care.	This report pertains to inpatient settings.
Preventing Medication Errors, IOM (2006)	The focus on patient–provider relationship is an integral part of quality care. Fewer errors result when strong patient—provider communication exists.	Patients taking a more active role in their own health can advance safety.	Inpatient and outpatient settings.
Patient Protection and Affordable Care Improvement Act (HR 3590 Health Care Quality Improvement)	Accessibility of comprehensive quality healthcare is the necessary origin of quality care.	Improved accessibility of comprehensive primary healthcare promotes compliance with yearly exams and avoidance of late-stage medical interventions.	"Quality measure means a standard for measuring the performance and improvement of population health or of health plans, providers of services, and other clinicians in the delivery of health care" (p. 692).

Amer 2012 (adapted from multiple references on quality and safety) require curriculum threads that focus on core competency in safe and quality nursing. The organization has responded to the need for more quality and safety education in nursing schools by developing the Quality and Safety Education in Nursing (QSEN) group to provide support for nursing educators to integrate safety and quality competencies into all nursing programs (see Chapter 3). QSEN has an extensive Web site full of resources for all levels of nurse educators.

- Quality-focused changes in the healthcare environment that include adopting standard checklists for procedures such as central line insertion or protocols for screening all admitted patients for antibiotic-resistant infections. Most hospitals have implemented some level of quality improvement plan.

- Transforming Care at the Bedside (TCAB) and the empowerment of clinical nurses to design and implement change. TCAB was a funded project that assisted nurses in designing solutions to safety issues on specific units. The innovations were tested for a short time and evaluated, then either adopted or dropped.

Patient care can be improved when front line nurses identify problems and implement incremental system solutions focused on safety. Nurses need the knowledge and tools to begin to affect change in their environments. Such changes can increase the efficiency of nursing care, help nurses spend more time with patients, and create safer environments.

CHAPTER HIGHLIGHTS

- Nurses are most able to identify risks and threats to safe nursing care.
- Transforming Care at the Bedside (TCAB) empowers nurses to address threats to quality and safe care by using rapid cycle change to improve care in medical–surgical units.
- There is a strong relationship between the structure of the U.S. healthcare system and the quality of healthcare delivery.
- The ideal work environment in nursing includes adequate staffing, collaborative practice, and a culture that values safety and quality.

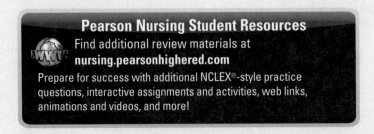

Pearson Nursing Student Resources
Find additional review materials at
nursing.pearsonhighered.com
Prepare for success with additional NCLEX®-style practice questions, interactive assignments and activities, web links, animations and videos, and more!

REFERENCES

Agency for Healthcare Research and Quality (AHRQ). (2011). Retrieved from. http://innovations.ahrq.gov/content.aspx?=1799

American Nurses Association (ANA). (2012). Retrieved from http://www.nursingworld.org/FunctionalMenuCategories/AboutANA

Blouin, A. (2010). Helping to solve healthcare's most critical safety and quality problems. *Journal of Nursing Care Quality, 25*(2), 95–99.

Buck, M.L., Hofer, K.N., & McCarthy, M.W. (2008). Improving pediatric medication safety part 1: Research on medication errors and recommendations from the Joint Commission. *Pediatric Pharmacotherapy, 14*(11), 1.

Denham, C. (Producer) & Bugg, S., (Director). (2010). *Chasing Zero: Winning the War on Healthcare Harm*. USA: Discovery Channel. Retrieved from. http://discoveryhealthcme.discovery.com/zero/zero.html.

Finkleman, A. & Kenner, C. (2009). *Teaching IOM: Implications of the Institute of Medicine Reports for Nursing Education* (2nd ed.). Silver Springs, MD: American Nurses Association Press.

Gordon, S., Buchanan, J., & Bretherton, T. (2008). *Safety in numbers: Nurse-to-patient ratios and the future of health care*. Ithaca, NY: ILR Press.

Institute of Medicine (IOM). (2000). *To err is human: Building a safer health system*. Washington DC: National Academy Press.

Institute of Medicine (IOM). (2001). *Crossing the quality chasm: A new health system for the 21st century*. Washington DC: National Academy Press.

Institute of Medicine (IOM). (2001). *Envisioning the National Health Care Report*. Washington DC: National Academy Press.

Institute of Medicine (IOM). (2004). *Patient safety: Achieving a new standard of care*. Washington DC: The National Academies Press.

Institute of Medicine (IOM). (2010). *The future of nursing: Leading change, advancing health*. Washington DC: National Academies Press.

Institute for Safe Medication Practices (ISMP). (2007). Another heparin error: Learning from mistakes so we don't repeat them. November 29, 2007 issue. Retrieved from http://www.ismp.org/newsletters/acutecare/articles/20071129.asp

Matthes, N., Cheng, J., Ogunbo, S., Reilly, C., Wilbon, A., & Wood, N. (2010). National hospital quality measures data supporting nurses' key roles in organizational performance improvement. *Journal of Nursing Care Quality, 25*(2), 127–136.

McDonald, A., & Levhane, T. (2005). Drill down with root cause analysis. *Nursing Management, 36*(10), 26–31.

Paoletti, R. D., Suess, T. M., Lesko, M. G., Feroli, A. A., Kennel, J. A., Mahler, J. M., & Sauders, T. (2007). Using barcode technology and medication observation methodology for safer medication administration. *American Journal of Health System Pharmacy, 64*(5), 536–543.

Pape T.M. (2003). Applying airline safety practices to medication administration. *Medsurg Nursing,12*(2), 77–93.

Pape T.M., & Richards, B. (2010). Stop knowledge creep. *Nursing Management, 41*(2), 8–11.

QUALITY AND SAFETY MODELS

Kim Siarkowski Amer

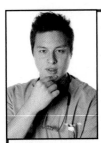

ZanyZeus/
Shutterstock.com

Ms. Turkel was recovering from gall bladder surgery and had abnormal electrolytes due to vomiting prior to surgery. Louis knew his patient's potassium was slightly low on admission two days ago at 3.2 mEq/L. The doctor ordered two vials of potassium to be injected intravenously. The pharmacy sent up two vials of 40 mEq each.

Louis was using his computer on wheels medication administration system and did not have potassium injections in the system. So he bypassed the computer, did not scan the drug, and injected two 20-mL vials of 40 mEq of potassium chloride intravenously. Two hours later, the patient had several episodes of ventricular fibrillations.

When Louis thought about the potassium and checked the dose, he realized the pharmacy had sent up the wrong vial. Ms. Turkel was supposed to get only 8 mEq of potassium chloride, not 80mEq.

CORE COMPETENCY

Apply safety and quality models to improving nursing practice.

LEARNING OUTCOMES

1. Describe efforts to increase safe nursing care, including safe medication administration and fall prevention.
2. Apply multiple models of safe quality nursing to a specific safety risk.

3. Integrate a change process into a high-risk clinical nursing situation.
4. Examine the best practices for quality improvement in nursing.

Nurses must be in charge of their practice, as Florence Nightingale proclaimed in *Notes on Nursing* (1860):

> *How few men, or even women, understand,*
> *Either in great or in little things,*
> *What it is the being "in charge."*
> *From the most colossal calamities,*
> *Down to the most trifling accidents,*
> *Results are often traced to*
> *such want of some one*
> *"in charge."*

Poor leadership, or the "want of some one in charge," can influence safe care and patient safety outcomes. Nurses must be educated and socialized to be competent in direct, safe, quality patient care, and knowledgeable leaders must be ready to evaluate and challenge the structure of the healthcare system. Nurses need supportive conditions and systems that support their practice. Conversely, when conditions are not ideal, nurses should be politically and socially aware of model systems that can be followed to decrease the risk to both the patient and the nurse.

Safety First

Safety is the most critical issue in nursing care. Too many lives are lost due to human error, adverse events, or acts of omission. Creating a safe nursing practice environment can be complicated and must include many levels of discipline and effective communication, collaboration, and attention to problem solving. But it can be done, especially when it is familiar and a priority for nurses and is included in the nursing curriculum. More nursing schools are beginning to integrate safety awareness into their curricula. According to a study by Chenot and Daniel (2010), all students in the nursing schools surveyed reported being taught at least three of six of the Quality and Safety Education for Nurses (QSEN) competencies, which are described later in this chapter. Although implementing change is complicated, often simple approaches to solve safety issues can have remarkably positive outcomes.

A simple but important example of transforming care developed in conjunction with the Transforming Care at the Bedside (TCAB) project is hand hygiene compliance by nurses and physicians. It has been shown that nurses' hand hygiene practices improve when they have a shelf on which to place supplies. Whether the shelf is above the sink outside of the room or next to the sink inside the room, having an easy place for temporary storage helps free hands for thorough hand hygiene. This is not a complex idea, but inadequate hand hygiene remains a major threat to patient and nurse safety. Infections acquired in hospitals remain a major cause of morbidity and mortality. The Centers for Disease Control

---

Evidence for Best Practices: Hand Hygiene

Why is hand hygiene compliance so difficult? Hand hygiene compliance ranges from 40% to 60% in hospitals. The Joint Commission developed a participant group of eight healthcare organizations and did a project to improve hand hygiene using the Robust Process Improvement system, which was developed by the Joint Commission for generating fact-based systematic data-driven methods. The first step of the project, as reported by Scott Blouin (2010), described barriers to proper hand hygience, including poor placement of dispensers and sinks, poor hand hygiene compliance data collected, lack of accountability, lack of a safety culture that encourages hand hygiene, ineffective education about when and how to perform hand hygiene, perception that hand hygiene is not needed if wearing gloves, and distractions, delays, and forgetting. All of these barriers must be overcome to increase compliance with hand hygiene.

and Prevention (CDC) estimate that 1 out of every 20 patients who are hospitalized will contract a hospital-acquired infection, and the associated costs range from $28.4 billion to $33.8 billion per year after adjusting for the consumer price index in 2007 (Scott, 2009). Even though it may seem simple and intuitive, hand hygiene is key to providing safer and less expensive care.

The Ideal Work Environment

A simple change such as increased adherence to hand hygiene can influence patient and staff outcomes and affect morbidity and mortality. But the structure of encouraging hand hygiene (as illustrated previously) is only one piece of a complex puzzle. An optimal work environment can integrate multiple factors that increase quality and safety. Nursing safety and quality care can be best understood when an ideal nursing practice environment is envisioned. A few components of optimal conditions include adequate staffing, a positive collaborative environment or supportive nursing culture, and resources that encourage ongoing learning. In contrast, staffing shortages, poor communication among healthcare teams, and long hours of practice consistently lead to adverse events (Gordon, Buchanon, & Bretherton, 2008). Poor communication between nurses and physicians doubles the risk of bad outcomes (Leonard, Graham, & Bonacum, 2004). Communication failures, which are usually unintentional, can be related to the complexity of multidisciplinary teams working with very sick patients. Such errors can occur in any setting. Since many levels and types of practitioners are involved in patient care, the ideal environment includes collaborative decision making by the whole team through regular communication. In the old model of physician-centered decision making, with no input from team members, communication was often fragmented, and care was compromised.

Quality and Safety Education in Nursing (QSEN)

A first step in ensuring that safety and quality concepts are learned universally is integrating them into all nursing programs. The Quality and Safety Education in Nursing (QSEN) project, which is supported by the American Association of Colleges of Nursing (AACN) and the Robert Wood Johnson Foundation (RWJF), has developed specific competencies and associated educational activities focused on ensuring positive communication and collaboration among all healthcare workers. Hundreds of nurse educators have participated in intensive two-day conferences that culminate in a QSEN certificate. This intensive updating of nursing faculty has increased the awareness of the importance of quality and safety in nursing curricula. The QSEN competencies are now integrated in both baccalaureate and master's education essentials for nursing education. The competencies include (1) patient-centered care, (2) teamwork and collaboration, (3) evidence-based practice, (4) quality improvement, and (5) safety and informatics (Finkelman & Kenner, 2009). Each competency is an area necessary for safe nursing care. Presently, practicing nurses do not consistently demonstrate mastery of the competencies. Thus, teaching these practice essentials is critical for nursing education so that in future years all practicing nurses will be knowledgeable about all aspects of safety. (QSEN will be discussed more extensively in Chapter 5.)

Patient-centered care, discussed in Chapter 10, can revolutionize nursing care by developing shared decision making between healthcare providers and patients. Even though patient-centered care may seem intuitive, in the past, patient care focused on telling patients what to do without getting their input. Improved collaborative teamwork could potentially prevent more than 50% of errors (Baker, Day, & Sales, 2006). Strategies such as consistent formats for handoffs—reporting from nurse to nurse—and the use of objective communication tools such as SBAR (situation, background, assessment, and recommendation) for nurse-to-physician communication provide simple solutions to improve patient safety. Nursing students who are nervous about contacting a provider in the clinical setting can organize their thoughts with the SBAR tool. First, a student describes a patient situation, for example, increased respirations in a person with asthma. Next, the student gives a brief history of the illness and any pertinent contextual information. For the third step, the student provides an objective assessment, for example, increased wheezing and more rapid respirations compared to previous assessment. Finally, the student provides a recommendation, for example, starting oxygen therapy or giving a nebulizer treatment.

Evidence-based practice and quality improvement go hand in hand. Both the evidence for providing interventions and the continual focus on monitoring quality are essential for nursing care at all levels. In the next decade, daily nursing care will continue to improve and nurses will be even more motivated to integrate best practices based on evidence and monitoring quality care. Both evidence from research and quality improvement monitoring will become easily accessible with new information systems in healthcare environments. Such standards of care will be essential for Joint Commission accreditation and Magnet status.

Magnet Recognition

The American Nursing Credentialing Center (ANCC) awards Magnet status to an elite few healthcare organizations that provide two years of evidence indicating educational and research support for nurses and support from colleagues, administrators, and physicians. Magnet status is important because nurses in institutions awarded that label are recognized as care coordinators and can provide a unique focus on contributing to quality outcomes.

Few hospitals achieve and maintain this level of nursing excellence. For those that are not at Magnet level, the criteria can be used to focus on improving patient care and nursing satisfaction within the organization. Nurses need to shed their complacency and become advocates for better nursing conditions to optimize patient-focused care and enhance their careers.

Nursing Exemplars That Support Quality Health Care

There are many quality monitoring models in health care. The common elements of most models include viewing safety and quality as a nonlinear process, having benchmarks for progress, using best practices based on the best evidence that is focused on safe quality care, incorporating a team of all levels of nurses, and involving all pertinent healthcare team members. Such models demonstrate excellent communication, collaboration, and coordination of care.

If an institution is not committed to having strong nursing leadership or has little support from its administration, it can focus on one or two of the Magnet areas to begin a journey toward improved safe quality care. There is wide variation in the level of safety and quality in hospitals across the United States. The work needed to improve patient safety remains significant. The first step to improvement is raising the awareness of safety education among nursing students and practicing nurses. Their piqued awareness will lead to greater interest in learning how to improve safety and ultimately to competent and excellent nursing care.

COPA Model for Nursing Practice

One conceptual model to help to raise awareness about outcomes-focused education is Lenburg's Competency Outcomes and Performance Assessment Model (COPA Model). (Lenburg, Klein, Abdur-Rahman, Spencer, & Boyer, 2009; Lenburg, Abdur-Rahman, Spencer, Boyer, & Klein, 2011). The framework of this model includes eight core practice competencies that are critical to contemporary practice (see Box 2-1).

The competencies focus on active learning. When mastered, the competencies in the COPA model should promote safe care that leads to better quality nursing. One principle of COPA is to replace typically passive

BOX 2-1 THE COMPETENCY OUTCOMES AND PERFORMANCE ASSESSMENT (COPA) MODEL

1. **Assessment and Intervention Skills**

   a. Safety and protection
   b. Assessment and monitoring
   c. Therapeutic treatments and procedures

2. **Communication Skills**

   a. Oral skills

      1 Talking, listening; with individuals
      2 Interviewing; history taking
      3 Group discussion, interacting
      4 Telling, showing, reporting

   b. Writing skills

      1 Clinical reports, care plans, charting
      2 Agency reports, forms, memos
      3 Articles, manuals

   c. Computing skills (information processing; using computers)

      1 Related to clients, agencies, other authorities
      2 Related to information search and inquiry
      3 Related to professional responsibilities

3. **Critical Thinking Skills**

   a. Evaluation; integrating pertinent data from multiple sources
   b. Problem solving; diagnostic reasoning; creating alternatives
   c. Decision making; prioritizing
   d. Scientific inquiry; research process

4. **Human Caring and Relationship Skills**

   a. Morality, ethics, legality
   b. Cultural respect; cooperative interpersonal relationships
   c. Client advocacy

5. **Management Skills**

   a. Administration, organization, coordination
   b. Planning, delegation, supervision of others
   c. Human and material resource utilization
   d. Accountability and responsibility; performance appraisals and QI

6. **Leadership Skills**

   a. Collaboration; assertiveness, risk taking
   b. Creativity, vision to formulate alternatives
   c. Planning, anticipating, supporting with evidence
   d. Professional accountability, role behaviors, appearance

(continued)

| BOX 2-1 | THE COMPETENCY OUTCOMES AND PERFORMANCE ASSESSMENT (COPA) MODEL (*continued*) |

7. **Teaching Skills**
   a. Individuals and groups; clients, coworkers, others
   b. Health promotion; health restoration

8. **Knowledge Integration Skills**
   a. Nursing, healthcare, and related disciplines
   b. Liberal arts, natural and social sciences, and related disciplines

learning objectives with learning outcomes that include the eight core competencies, all of which are essential to safe, quality patient care. This approach to learning can be applied universally in education and practice environments. Each competency category can incorporate a flexible array of related skills that can be adapted to a specific practice level or specialty area. All the competencies are listed in Box 2-1. However, because we are currently focusing on safety, only the first four of the eight competencies will be described here.

The first of the eight core practice competencies is assessment and intervention skills with safety and protection as the first priority. Instead of simply passively recording a patient assessment, the nurse could also engage in a discussion about health promotion goals with the patient and family. The focus on safety is enhanced by engaging the patient in a discussion that is integrated with the assessment, monitoring, and treatment.

The next two COPA Model competencies—communication and critical thinking skills—focus on actively talking, listening, and demonstrating care practices, and adapting nursing practice to patient and family needs. Such skills are critical to develop and evaluate in the first year of practice and continue to be important for veteran nurses. The fourth competency—human caring relationship skills, incorporates advocacy and respect for others, and sensitivity regarding differences in culture, age, and gender. When nurses implement the COPA competencies they promote patient safety and quality care that also embraces essential knowledge as discussed throughout this book.

Adequate Staffing for Nurses

In practice nurses can reluctantly accept unreasonable assignments due to a feeling of duty and service. Nurses may not know that they have a right to refuse an unsafe assignment with too many patients. To refuse an assignment, the nurse must know the chain of command and must feel confident enough to speak up to a charge nurse.

CASE STUDY: *Betty*

Betty, a novice nurse working night shift on a bone marrow transplant unit was shocked to find her patient assignment of four very sick patients on her second night shift. Each patient on a bone marrow unit is very high acuity and needs extensive care, including a strict isolation environment, to prevent infections. The acuity is similar to that found in intensive care units (ICUs). The usual assignment is two patients per nurse unless one nurse is covering for a nurse on break for 20 to 30 minutes, in which case one nurse takes on four patients. On this night, Betty was one of two staff nurses on the unit for eight patients, and when her colleague went on break, the ratio became eight patients to one nurse.

While Betty covered the eight patients during her colleague's 30-minute break, two patients had irregular cardiac rhythm patterns on the cardiac monitor, and their emergency alarms went off and kept ringing. One of the two patients had to be transferred to the cardiac intensive care unit (CICU). Another patient, who had received chemotherapy two days previously, was vomiting blood. Two patients needed to get up to go to the bathroom with assistance. The remaining three of the eight patients slept without any problems.

When her colleague returned, Betty was tired, agitated, and frustrated. Her colleague said, "Why didn't you page me? I would have come back from the cafeteria." The two nurses did not talk the rest of the shift, and Betty did not take a break.

The unreasonable expectations for nurses, as illustrated in Betty's case study, create situations that benefit no one. Nurses cannot possibly care for complex patients and meet all their needs when there are inadequate resources, including time. When one patient becomes sicker and near death, the nurse will focus attention on that patient to the neglect of others. This can lead to disaster. Who is to blame for this state of overwhelming responsibilities? All levels of nurses and administrators are responsible. Nurses must become adept at articulating the language of acuity and staffing numbers (patients assigned per nurse) and the resulting poor outcomes in the wake of overwhelming assignments.

Nurses in intensive care settings increasingly need standards or mandates for patient safety and nurse staffing ratios. The acuity status of intensive care patients is much higher than in past years (Gordon et al., 2008). Previously, patients stayed in the ICU for a week after they had a heart attack. Now, patients who become stable may be transferred in one day to a general floor, where there may be six to eight patients being cared for by one nurse. This situation becomes problematic for both nurses in the ICU and on the floor. ICU nurses are caring for high acuity patients for shorter periods of time with high patient turnover, while the non-ICU acute care units may have to care for more patients who are sicker with higher acuity.

Numbers Can Be Deceiving

Even staffing that appears reasonable can be deceiving. For example, a nurse may have three patients, which seems manageable. But consider what happens when two of those patients are discharged to home, a process that requires extensive preparation and paperwork. Two new patients are then admitted to the unit, and the nurse needs to do extensive assessments on the two new patients, including a health history, and orient the patients and their families to the unit. Even though at any one time throughout the shift, the nurse appeared to have three patients to care for, she ended up providing care for five separate patients (two discharged and two admitted), four of whom required extensive care. There is a significant difference between caring for three patients for 12 hours and five different patients throughout the shift. New patients who are admitted require a labor-intensive admission process and thorough assessment. Some newly admitted patients may take more than an hour of nurse time to get settled in their new environment. The nurse is also the primary communicator between the family, patient, medical team, and the other nurses. A "simple" assignment of three patients per nurse can become a very different assignment if admissions and discharges are involved.

If an adverse event or a poor outcome such as death results from an unsafe staffing situation, and the patient or patient's family files a lawsuit, the primary focus would be on whether the nurse's conduct was in line with the current standard of nursing care. The court would be looking at the case in the context of whether the defendant (nurse) gave the plaintiff (patient) care equal to that given by a reasonably well-qualified and prudent nurse in the same or similar circumstances. The hospital's responsibility to adequately staff the unit would not be in question.

Taking Action

Recently, neonatal intensive care units (NICUs) have come under more scrutiny for nurse staffing. Nurses who care for babies on ventilators need to make frequent adjustments on the ventilators, do frequent blood draws, and manage fluids. Such intensive care is provided in a safe manner when nurses have only one or two patients. What happens when a nurse comes to work and gets an assignment of three to four patients in the NICU? Many nurses think that they have no choice but to take the assignment and do the best they can. But a variety of steps can be taken if an assignment seems overwhelming.

First, a nurse can contact the direct supervisor. If there is no change in assignment, then the nurse may move up the administrative ladder and continue to object to the assignment. There is no need to practice in a situation that is not safe. The chain of command should be well known to all nurses in practice.

Legislating Safe Care Ratios

The most critical need related to providing safe patient care is for consistent standards for each practice area to be implemented and required by law. A NICU staffing ratio of one-to-one, or at most one nurse to two NICU patients, is required under current California legislation. According to reports from All Children's Hospital in California, before this legislation was implemented, one-to-one ratios were rare for a department that handles some of the sickest newborns in the state. Regulators monitored the NICU's staffing levels during three site visits from 2003 to 2007, with monthly reviews from 2005 to 2007. During that time, state mandated staffing ratios went from 77% to to 92% (www.calnurses.org 2/2/2012). This suggests that monitoring compliance with staffing ratios can positively impact hospital practices. Some argue that ratios are only one piece of the complex puzzle. Acuity and other factors need to be added to the policies and procedures used to determine safe care.

The Evidence Is In

Research clearly shows that care is safer when nurse-to-patient ratios are reasonable. Nurses who frequently feel stressed and that they are providing unsafe care often make the decision to leave bedside nursing altogether. More patients with higher acuity and rapid turnaround with discharges and admissions make nursing practice more stressful than ever. The corporate model for replacing older and more seasoned workers, who are paid more, with less experienced nurses to save money does not work in life-and-death situations. Nurses need the support of administrators and colleagues, reasonable assignments, regular breaks for rest and meals, and most important, a voice within the unit and institution regarding their practice environment.

Frith (2010) reported decreased length of stay and fewer reported infections in patients when nurse staffing adhered to staffing standards. Aiken and colleagues (2010) have also reported consistent patterns of improved outcomes related to safe staffing ratios in California over the first several years following implementation of staffing legislation (2005 to 2009). This evidence should result in an immediate response to ensure safe staff ratios. However, the reality is that change, and policy change in particular, takes considerable time and effort.

Higher nurse staffing has also been documented to improve outcomes such as functional status, lower mortality rates, fewer pressure sores, less use of restraints and long-term catheters in long-term care settings, and less antibiotic use (Lippincott, Williams, & Wilkins, 2008). Staffing also affects adverse drug events (ADEs). ADEs can be injuries related to medication without any error by the practitioner, or they can be related to professional practice or procedural issues. Most medication errors do not cause harm. Some may cause a temporary reversible reaction without long-term effects. It is prudent to keep in mind, however, that whenever a wrong dosage or wrong drug is given, results can range from minimal to dire. (Dlugacz, 2006).

Quality and Safety Competencies in Nursing Education

Quality education in nursing is key to improving nursing care. Nursing education innovations are included in QSEN, which has focused nursing educators on the emergent need to prepare nursing students as leaders who will ensure safety in clinical nursing settings and become competent in assessing quality nursing care. As Ironside and Sitterding (2009, p. 659) assert, "Nursing work environments are considered high hazard settings with little margin for human error, and nursing work is cognitively demanding." Nursing students have limited opportunities to experience the real-life demands of clinical nursing, such as having a full patient assignment, handling difficult family members, and reporting concerns to doctors. Current and future nurses will need to become competent in these organizational skills.

Patient simulation may facilitate building such competencies. Simulation labs present scenarios with high-fidelity "dummies," or simulated patients. Nursing students can practice communicating with the patient, role-play with the doctor, and monitor real-time demise of a patient through the computer-simulated program. This type of education builds on classroom knowledge, and debriefing after such a simulation helps build confidence. Feedback from peers and instructors can help identify both strengths and weaknesses in communication. Another advantage is having a clinical instructor in a lab observing six to eight students at one time instead of moving from student to student in a clinical setting.

Sears, Goldsworthy, and Goodman (2010) explored the relationship between human patient simulation in nursing education and medication safety. They studied the effect of simulation scenarios in an experimental group versus a control group (no simulation). The authors reported compelling evidence that students in clinical placement generated fewer medication errors and near misses if they had prior exposure to a related simulation-based experience than students who did not. The numbers were 24 errors in the control group sample of 30 students versus seven errors in the treatment (simulation experience) group sample of 24 students.

Nursing and Lifelong Learning

Quality and safety education needs to begin in nursing school and continue throughout nurses' career progression. Nurses should be encouraged to become lifelong learners. Continuous educational support is one of the criteria of Magnet status, and the focus on continuous learning must be nurtured in all nursing settings. This requires a scholarly approach to nursing by administrators and fellow nursing colleagues.

A unique model that supports such lifelong learning is the nursing profession's sabbatical program in New Zealand (www.nzno.org, 2/12/12). Staff nurses are eligible for a leave of one month once per length of employment, with pay, to explore a new area of knowledge. This program enhances nurses' loyalty to hospitals since they are supported in their need for a respite period, enriches the energy of the staff, and provides all staff with new resources and new perspectives. Veteran nurse Jane Hinds notes that understaffed nurses who lack adequate support services may become burned out, which can lead to cynicism, a lack of emotional connection to their work, and resentment of patients. In addition to pay that still does not seem commensurate with the work, Hinds suggests that stress and exhaustion are major problems for nurses. However, with support for ongoing education, the workplace becomes a more supportive and positive environment.

Many different changes can be learned and implemented to improve nursing care. Analysis of each proposed change should be based on evidence and the uniqueness of each setting. Changes that aim to improve safety in nursing care can range from implementing daily huddles—brief meetings with nurses at change of shift along with residents, physicians, dietitians and other healthcare providers—to system-wide changes such as implementation of bar coding for medication administration. Even though the length of time needed to implement simple versus complex changes varies, basic principles of change apply in both situations. Acquiring knowledge about evidence and integrating it with the unique characteristics of the healthcare setting need to be priorities in all nursing situations.

Rapid-Cycle Change and Continuous Quality Improvement

Rapid-cycle change, in which nurses who provide direct care decide what safety concerns exist and then propose a solution, is based on other models, including continuous quality improvement (CQI). CQI is one of the many models focused on transforming healthcare settings. CQI advocates a circular pattern that includes intervention, evaluation, and reassessment of the intervention or change. The change is dynamic and is never viewed as an endpoint. The process is nonpunitive and involves all levels of personnel.

Consider the following example of the use of CQI to address the issue of accurate and consistent patient identification and medication reconciliation. When patients have the same or similar last names, it is more likely that a medication error will occur. The potential for error is high when, for example, two Mr. Smiths are on the same unit, in rooms 588 and 586. The potential for error needs to be recognized, and nurses need to design a "red flag," or alert, that cues nurses and doctors to the similarity in names and the added risk for error. Moving patients to a distinct room far from the patient with the similar name, assigning a different nurse to each patient, and flagging the charts help to decrease the likelihood of error. CQI can include an assessment of the risk of same names, a plan for distinguishing between the two patients, and a continual evaluation of whether the methods to decrease adverse events indeed worked. The nonpunitive nature of CQI is vital so that the team freely reports errors and process improvements are authentic.

CASE STUDY: *Elda*

Elda is a new graduate nurse who is working in the surgical ICU at a trauma center. After a six-week orientation, she is caring for two to three ICU patients on her 12-hour night shifts. She enjoys the challenges of the unit and the new clinical knowledge she is acquiring.

This evening, she is caring for a patient with bowel cancer who was admitted for resection of the bowel earlier in the week and is now unstable with multiple drips of pressors, dopamine, fetanyl, and total parenteral nutrition. The pressor drips are titrated every hour.

Near the end of the night shift, Elda is feeling very tired. She does her hourly intake and output, assesses the large abdominal dressing, does pain assessment and neurological assessment, and monitors the drips and intravenous (IV) pumps.

Near the end of her shift, around 6:30 a.m., the attending physician approaches Elda and brings her into the patient's room. "How long has this hyperalimentation been running at 167 milliliters per hour? The rate was ordered to be at 67 milliliters per hour."

Elda thinks for a bit and says, "All shift. Why are you asking me?"

The physician yells at Elda and immediately calls Sherry, the nurse manager at home. The physician also fills out an incident report and calls Toni, the night supervisor for the whole hospital. Elda is devastated. She reviews the IV rate in her head over and over. Did she set that rate? Was that the rate before her shift? Why did she not check the machine every hour? The hyperalimentation was on a separate pump. The other eight drips were all on IV monitors on the opposite side of the patient.

The physician brings in a copy of the incident report for Elda to sign and states, "We are meeting with you on this unit at 12 p.m. tomorrow. Be prepared to explain this grievous mistake."

Elda thinks about resigning before the meeting, but instead she goes, only to be shamed and demeaned. The physician tells her she lacks integrity and honor, and that she may have killed the patient. Sherri, the nurse manager also uses strong language, calling her "incompetent, lazy, and dangerous." The incident lingers in her mind.

After a month of self-doubt and feeling depressed, Elda decides to change careers and enrolls in cosmetology school. After four years of intensive study in nursing school and the promise of a long career, a much-needed, caring novice nurse is lost to the profession.

1. Was the response to an IV rate mistake appropriate?

2. Was the incident reported properly?

3. How should the nurse be treated?

4. Are new graduates not safe on night shift without proper mentorship, preceptors, or leadership?

Had this been a nonpunitive institution, the administrators would have backed up and reviewed all the events that led up to the incorrect rate. *What was the patient assignment like that night? Was there a support person for the nurse? What did the day nurse recall about the rate? How did the error affect the patient's status and ultimate outcome? What can be learned from this mistake?*

When a nonpunitive approach is used, learning occurs on all levels. The unit can develop checks and balances to ensure that such a mistake does not happen again. Instead of helping the nurse learn through the mistake, she was demoralized and quit her nursing career.

Strategies and Tools to Enhance Performance and Patient Safety (STEPPS)

What is missing in the case study about Elda? Many components that could have improved the situation are included in the Strategies and Tools to Enhance Performance and Patient Safety (STEPPS) program used at the Franciscan Sisters of Saint Mary (SSM) Health Care System based in St. Louis (Kosseff, 2008). This program is another model for addressing the critical safety and quality problems in health care. For safe care to be provided, the multiple providers of healthcare teams must act in a coordinated manner. Dr. Andy Kosseff, the Medical Director of System Clinical Improvement at SSM, implemented STEPPS throughout the SSM hospitals as a method for producing more effective medical and healthcare teams and achieving optimal patient outcomes. The need for STEPPS, he explained, is greater than ever because of four factors: disorganized or fragmented care, multiple initiatives for the same patient, implementation of electronic health records, and that care-giving providers are at the heart of a safe work culture. The success of the program is measured by the number of sentinel events, nurse turnover rate, provider satisfaction, and scores on the safety culture and global trigger tool surveys. The program's focus is on communication between nurses and physicians as well as ensuring that all team members focus on providing quality care. The tools used in this program include electronic medication delivery, continuous safety and quality monitoring, and feedback to all team members.

Multiple strategies are used for all team members, and an ongoing structure is implemented for continuity and ongoing program sustainability. The integration of human patient simulation, trainer development, and multidisciplinary approaches makes this program an ideal model for improved safety and quality health care.

Theoretical Perspectives in Safety and Quality

Safe care is the first and foremost step in providing quality health care. However, safety alone does not ensure high quality nursing care. Quality care is provided by superb nurses who are able to integrate "all at once" as described in Jean Watson's book *Postmodern Nursing and Beyond* (1999). The "all at once" is the ability to assess in a prioritized manner the patient's physiological status along with his or her social, psychological, environmental, and spiritual awareness. Such a whole view of patients and families requires an artful practice. To provide such artful care, the nurse must understand the coping and adjustment the patient and family need to draw upon, identify resources from within and outside of the hospital setting, and know how to communicate with the patient, family, and support staff.

The hierarchy of goal setting is critical for the nurse to master. Needs go from the most basic needs of air, water, and food to the highest level of self-actualization. The ability to determine appropriate goals for patients is critical. When clear understanding of the patient and family is mastered by the nurse, future goals and plans are easily elucidated.

What is the link between nursing theory and safe quality nursing care? Defining safety is easy, as is discussed in Chapter 1. Quality nursing care, however, is a much more difficult concept to quantify. Safe care may be described as no falls, no medication errors, and no rehospitalizations. Quality care goes far beyond a lack of errors, falls, and returns to the hospital after surgery. It is superb nursing care that integrates the whole patient, the family, scientific and intuitive knowledge, and the ability to gain a sense of the patient's experience in life and in the healthcare setting. Quality nursing care is the integration of spiritual, cultural, psychological, family, community, and situational factors into patient care. Quality care incorporates all aspects of the science of nursing including pathophysiology, psychology, alternative and complementary treatments, and social and ecological influences on health, just to name a few, into nursing practice. Quality care should be defined by the patient, family, and nurses. Family, caregiver, and patient views of quality care should shape those of the nurse and hospital administration. Even though each perspective may have a different focus, the spirit of quality should be similar.

Table 2-1 presents possible perspectives, definitions of safe and quality care, and potential outcome measures. The table is not intended to be all inclusive. The examples are provided to illustrate possible perspectives and definitions from hospital administrators, patients, nurses, physicians, and health insurance companies.

TABLE 2-1 ■ Quality Measures from Various Perspectives

Persons Measuring Quality Care	Definition of Quality Care	Definition of Safe Care	Outcome Measures
Hospital administrators	Patient satisfaction surveys	• No patient falls • No medication errors	• Low staff turnover • Cost containment with safe care
Patients	• Good bedside manner by providers • Good food • Caring nurses	Nurses or nurses aids answering the call light	Good experience at the hospital and an improved health status
Nurses	Providing the best care possible and meeting all goals made with patients	Environmental as well as physical and physiological risks minimized	Comprehensive care provision (not rushed) and patient improvement in health status; no readmissions
Physicians	Treating the underlying illness and the patient	No mistakes	Patients go home satisfied with experience
Health insurance companies	Good health care in short stay with minimized cost	No readmissions or hospital-acquired infections	Home as soon as possible

CASE STUDY: *Rosa*

Rosa works on the adult oncology unit and has many primary patients. Primary nursing is a care model that encourages nurses to be the main nurse for patients with chronic health issues that cause them to have frequent hospitalizations. Rosa enjoys primary nursing because it helps to foster a strong bond between patient and nurse along with a high level of familiarity.

Rosa was working the night shift when her primary patient, Marilyn, a 68-year-old patient who had been in remission from breast cancer and had recently relapsed was admitted for fever and neutropenia. When Rosa weighed Marilyn, she noticed how bony and frail she looked. Over the past three weeks, Marilyn had lost 15 pounds, had developed mouth ulcers, and was fatigued from her new intensive chemotherapy regimen. Rosa completed her assessment and paged the doctor on call, Dr. Minks, a new fellow in oncology.

Dr. Minks came to the unit to see Marilyn for the first time and explained to Rosa that all her symptoms were normal for a person undergoing intensive chemotherapy. Rosa nodded and calmly explained that she had known Marilyn for eight years. Rosa told Dr. Minks about the decreasing weight trend, the mouth ulcers, and the appearance of fatigue and possible depression. She told Dr. Minks how Marilyn did very well a few years ago with a few days of total parenteral nutrition (TPN). She had the previous TPN order in hand from years ago with the dextrose, protein, fat, and electrolyte composition. Marilyn had tolerated TPN well, Rosa explained, with no hyperglycemia or electrolyte abnormalities.

Dr. Minks immediately ordered TPN, triamcinolone (Nystatin) for the mouth sores, and a soft diet. He then discussed with Rosa the possibility of starting an antidepressant for Marilyn. Rosa agreed to discuss the possibility at the next team meeting and then discuss it with Marilyn.

1. This case includes components of collaborative care, supportive resources for nursing, and a positive work environment. Provide an example of each.

2. What can Rosa implement independently as a nurse without exceeding the boundaries of scope of practice?

The range of perspectives and definitions regarding quality and safety should not be viewed as a negative or disconnected perspective. As long as all perspectives are known and respected, all parties can work together to try to meet multiple goals. When communication, mutual respect, regular multidisciplinary meetings, and continuous assessment of outcomes exist, patient safety improves. Conversely, in situations where one person or one discipline has all the power and decision-making authority, the ability to provide safe care becomes impaired. Power that is held by only one discipline leads to the nurse being ordered to perform a task or give a treatment or medicine without being allowed to question the possessor of that power, whether a physician or an administrator. No input from the nurse is requested by the physician, and the nurse is not allowed to question physician orders. Such a limiting practice environment stifles independent thinking and curiosity that encourages continuous lifelong learning, and it deflates pride in autonomous nursing care. (For more on empowerment in nursing, see Chapter 5.)

Methods of Change

Ensuring safe quality care requires changes in the present care delivery system. Change is not appealing to most people. Even when there is clear need for change, people resist it. The primary reason change is not appealing is fear of the unknown. It is easier for a person to imagine staying in a situation that is not ideal than to create a different and potentially better situation. The familiar is so much more comfortable than even a dreamy future because it is an unknown entity. People tend to stay in positions for many years even if advancement is not on the horizon. It takes a leap of faith to buy into a new situation, and the change means taking risks to get to a better place. Whether beginning a new relationship, a new educational degree, or simply taking a new route to work, most people need time, support, and courage to explore a new path.

Nurses tend to resist change more than other professionals. Even though evidence-based practice is a hallmark of modern nursing, the reality of day-to-day nursing care is one of "we always do it this way." An example of the resistance to change in nursing practice is exemplified by the decade-old research that explored the likelihood of IV catheters clotting when flushed with heparin versus a normal saline flush every two hours. The normal saline was equally effective in simple peripheral IV flushes. This was good news because risks related to normal saline are low. However, most units in hospitals have their own protocol that may or may not include heparin flushes for peripheral IVs. This resistance to change is a major barrier for the progress of safe nursing care.

Since nurses have access to a multitude of online resources, there should be no excuses for not implementing evidence-based practice, that is, best practices in nursing based on research. When a veteran staff nurse states, "We always use heparin for flushes," a new staff nurse can simply pull up an article from the ANA or a research journal such as *Nursing Research* to substantiate the claim that normal saline is better to use. Not using research and applying it to nursing practice is a weakness of the nursing profession. Nurses need to ensure that their status within their healthcare setting allows them to engage in a spirit of inquiry, so that they can allow their curiosity to guide them in getting answers to clinical questions. If no answers are available, the nursing staff can work as a team to develop its own solutions. Nursing and evidence-based practice will be at the forefront of future priorities for safe provision of care.

Safe care depends on having excellent nurses deliver comprehensive care that empowers patients and families. The nurse in Box 2-2 was able to evaluate multiple safety threats by appreciating the risks associated with toddler development, reviewing the physiological effects of chemotherapy and how to keep the child safe from infection, decreasing the stress on the parents and thus decreasing the risk of their health being compromised, identifying potential supports for the parents, and simply being available to answer questions and alleviate unsubstantiated fears. If the nurse had not been able to take the time to do the comprehensive

BOX 2-2 INTEGRATING ASSESSMENT DATA

Great nurses are able to integrate multiple assessment data simultaneously and immediately respond in a therapeutic manner. For example, a family with a child newly diagnosed with leukemia may be in the child's room when an assessment is due. The nurse comes into the room and interacts with the toddler in an age and developmentally appropriate manner, explaining all the tasks that will be done. The fear, anxiety, sadness, and uncertainty in the parents, who are at the bedside, are clearly palpable. The nurse engages the parents by allowing them to help with the assessment, asks them about the toddler's food preferences, and encourages them to take turns being at the hospital so that one of them gets some sleep. There is also discussion about other family members. The nurse asks questions about who lives at home, pets, siblings, and availability of extended family support. The work demands of both parents are then assessed based on the time needed for hospitalization and outpatient treatments. The nurse introduces the parents to resources in the hospital for parents of children with cancer and then follows up with an open, honest discussion about what to expect during the next few hours and days, helping to ease the parents' anxiety and giving them information that can help guide them through their new journey. Chemotherapeutic agents and side effects are briefly discussed, including neutropenia and risk of infection. The mother asks whether the toddler will become deaf from the chemotherapy because her grandmother became deaf after she had cancer of the throat. The nurse provides information about the risks of chemotherapy and describes a low risk for deafness.

During the 10 to 15 minute assessment, the nurse was able to integrate the following:

- Physical status of child

- Risk for falls or safety issues

- Developmental theory applied to assessment and explanations to child

- Psychological coping of parents

- Encouraging parents to care for self

- Including parents' input regarding the plan of care to ease anxiety and decrease feelings of loss of control

- Support systems in extended family

- Potential work stressors of family

- Need for social work, pastoral care, support groups for parents

- Parents' perceptions of the plan of care

- Parents' views of the impact of the illness on the family

---

assessment, multiple stressors could have festered and become larger issues. When parents and families are listened to and valued, the safety and quality of care is improved.

Models for Change

In popular books such as *Who Moved My Cheese* and *Soft Power,* people have been writing about theories and models for change for decades. The basic concepts remain similar throughout the various methods or theories. First, top-down dictums for change do not work. Workers need to take part in designing change and ideally produce ideas for change on their own. Second, change is difficult and frightening, and there will be resistance. Last and most important, if implemented well, the stakeholders will adapt, especially if there is a transition that is respectful of the workers and support throughout the change period.

An example of ideal change was observed on a cardiac telemetry floor at a children's hospital. New documentation systems were being implemented, and many nurses were frantic. All nurses went through a series of workshops over a period of months. The pace of implementation was scheduled with input from the nurses, and the workshops were interactive. The workshops were led by support people who were on the units during the transition. This provided an added level of comfort for the nurses. The combination of slow-paced workshops, familiar instructors who were also nurses, and the presence of support staff on the units instead of being at a "help line" all provided for an excellent transition.

Several models of change have been discussed in this chapter, including TCAB, the STEPPS program, and implementing safe-staffing models. Elements common to all of these models are that all critical persons are equally involved, the pace of the program is appropriate, and a process for planning, implementing, and evaluating is used, starting again with new goals.

The case studies included in this chapter provide examples that are not dramatic medication errors or overwhelming infection from safety breaches. They involve errors in potassium administration, too much hyperalimentation, and culturally sensitive comprehensive care. Patients and families can have serious problems if safety protocols are not followed. Nurses need to be aware of the need for comprehensive care for patients and families, and the goal should be to improve each encounter of care delivery. Change can be difficult, but it is well worth it when people suffer less, or when lives are saved.

Change Theories

A variety of change theories have been generated to explain the process needed to implement change. The classic theory is that of Lewin's force-field analysis (1951). It remains useful for nursing practice and other facets of the nursing profession.

Lewin's force-field analysis is most commonly used to provide a framework for problem solving and planned change. The theory discusses forces that are opposing, like a tug of war, that are status quo when both sides are equal but change when one side is stronger than the other. As Lewin describes, driving forces equal to restraining forces produce equilibrium (1951). Persons are most comfortable with equilibrium. Opposing forces that are strong may produce unplanned and negative change, whereas driving forces that are built on consensus create a positive change environment. The Lewin model frames change in relation to the culture in which one is working. It includes the resistance to change from workers and administrators, the willingness to be open to change, and the assessed need for change. The vision of what the new situation should look like is also included. When one needs to change a cube of ice to a cone of ice, the initial cube needs to be melted, just as the culture needs to be opened up and transformed for the new culture or situation to become a reality.

The classic Lewin model of unfreezing, moving, and then refreezing provides a mental picture of a change process that produces a different product or environment. Change that is acceptable can be exemplified by a Popsicle that has been left out of the freezer but is still in its wrapper, intact. The Popsicle has the wooden stick and the essential syrup, and the wrapper is keeping the contents intact. But when the Popsicle is refrozen, the shape and substance are different, and the resulting shape and taste may be difficult to adjust to initially. When a person discovers that the taste is good, even though the shape is different, the person eats the Popsicle with pleasure. Various people with different personality types will react in different ways to the new Popsicle. Some may toss the thawed Popsicle and forget about anything that is not how it is supposed to be. Some people may be willing to try to refreeze the Popsicle but may be opposed to the new product and then throw the Popsicle out. Last, those people who are open-minded and willing to try new adventures will try the new shape and enjoy it. The important thing to recognize is that all of these people may react in a different manner if they are encouraged or discouraged by peers or other colleagues.

If a supervisor insists that all staff eat the oddly shaped Popsicles, they may do it but resent the command. If a friend is eating the newly shaped Popsicle and likes it, staff may be willing to try it and like it. If the majority of staff say that the Popsicles are bad and should not be eaten, most others will go along with the crowd.

Other models play upon Lewin's force-field model, modifying its application. Havelock (1973) describes a modified Lewin phase series of change that includes these steps:

1. Building a relationship

2. Diagnosing a problem

3. Acquiring the relevant resources

4. Choosing the solution

5. Gaining acceptance

6. Stabilizing and undergoing self-renewal.

   Smith (2002) developed seven levels of change:

1. Being effective: Doing the right things

2. Being efficient: Doing things right

3. Improving: Doing the right things better

4. Cutting: Doing away with things

5. Copying: Doing things other people are doing

6. Being different: Doing things no one else is doing

7. Doing the impossible: Doing things that cannot be done

An example of how Havelock's and Smith's models for change can be used together involves Connie and Jose, both day shift nurses. They are finding it difficult to get all care done, medications administered, care plans updated, crash cart checked, and supply room stocked. At the brief lunch they have in the break room, they talk about feeling overwhelmed. In their conversation, they pair Havelock's building a relationship and diagnosing a problem with Smith's being effective and being efficient. They do not want to complain to the night shift, so they develop a plan for the night charge nurse to delegate the crash cart checks and supply room stocking to the night shift staff. They involve all staff in their proposal and decide to implement Havelock's steps of acquiring the relevant resources, choosing the solution, and gaining acceptance along with Smith's levels of being efficient (doing things right), improving (doing the right things better), cutting (doing away with things), and copying (doing things other people are doing). In developing a proposal and getting input, they are engaging the staff without alienating them. Staff members can speak up and suggest alternatives or provide supportive comments.

After the proposal is approved, the staff members implement the changes and then evaluate how well they worked. When the day shift nurses have the added time to provide care to patients, they are much more content, and the night shift nurses receive recognition for being open to new ideas and helpful. There may be a rocky road with such a change process, but the approach and the resulting reception of the proposal can be pivotal in how well the unit ultimately runs and becomes more effective, efficient, and safe.

When the concept of Lewin's opposing versus accommodating forces is applied to other theories, a practical progression of change implementation can be constructed. To use and adapt these models, nurses need to have the support of all levels of management, including their willingness to change practice. When front line nursing staff engages in identifying strengths and weaknesses in the staff, system, and care processes, a better process of change can be developed.

The Amer Hybrid Model of Change described in Table 2-2 uses a scoring system to evaluate the likelihood that a nursing unit will be willing to implement a change in care delivery. The five elements include communication, culture, collaboration, common goals, and ability to appreciate one another's perspective. The levels of each element can range from zero to two. Total scores in the eight to ten range indicate being most likely and ready for change. Scoring in the six to seven range indicates a

BOX 2-3 WHERE PATIENT SAFETY REALLY COUNTS—AT THE BEDSIDE

A Conversation with Pam A. Thompson

By Pat Muccigrosso

March 18, 2010—Patient safety is not a new topic. It has been making headlines and driving practice reviews and changes for nurses for years. It has also been the object of intense research and study by organizations like the Agency for Healthcare Research and Quality (AHRQ).

Pam A. Thompson, MS, RN CENL, FAAN, chief executive officer of AONE, believes patient safety starts with nurses.

Every year since 2003, AHRQ has released a report on healthcare quality which tracks several measures, including patient safety. Although progress has been made overall, findings released in their most recent report revealed that, "... reporting of hospital quality is leading improvement but *patient safety is lagging*."

Other organizations like the National Patient Safety Foundation (NPSF) have mounted a concerted effort to raise awareness of safety initiatives and provide resources for hospitals and healthcare providers to use, such as Patient Safety Awareness Week, March 7-13, 2010. But for Pam A. Thompson, the focus of a lot of these efforts is on nurses—the women and men doing battle on the front lines at hospitals across the country.

Thompson, MS, RN CENL, FAAN, is chief executive officer of the American Organization of Nurse Executives (AONE), a national professional organization which has been providing leadership, advocacy and research to advance nursing practice and patient care since 1967. She believes patient safety starts with nurses.

Q: There are a lot of health care workers involved in caring for a patient. Why are nurses considered so pivotal to improving patient safety?

A: Nurses are at the intersection of where all the work takes place and managing that intersection is the key role that nurses do in their practice. When you sit at the intersection, as nurses do, then it is incumbent upon you to be able to manage all those people coming and going at the patient's bedside.

Other roles come and touch the patient, move the patient, interact with the patient, but there is really no role in the hospital that is with the patient as the nurse is. They manage that environment in which the patient is living while they are in the hospital. They are the one professional there 24 and 7. It is their responsibility for being the advocate for the patient around patient safety.

Q: What is the nurse's primary role relative to patient safety?

A: The nurse is the one that provides that direct care. They are direct participants in the delivery of therapeutic care to patients so they are the users of the systems that we design. They provide the medications. They do many of the treatments that are provided. They support nutrition. So, a priority of the nurse is the provision of the therapy that the patient is to receive or the care of the patient after surgery or major therapeutic intervention. They are at the place where they can influence the ability to assure that what reaches the patient is safe.

Q: Why is patient safety so important that organizations like NPSF and AONE are involved?

A: The ability to provide safe care in these complex environments has become a challenge. As the environment has become more complex and the diseases that people are presenting with have become more complex, the importance of safety as a part of the culture has become more necessary and that's why you are seeing a significant amount of focus on it.

I think it has finally become more of a combined responsibility with attention to the importance of it in multiple areas across health care. That's why you are seeing so many different focuses on patient safety in a multitude of arenas.

(continued)

BOX 2-3	WHERE PATIENT SAFETY REALLY COUNTS—AT THE BEDSIDE (*continued*)

Q: The theme for this year's National Patient Safety Awareness week is "Let's Talk!"—why "Let's Talk?"

A: Good communication is one of the key foundations for any patient safety discussion. Research has told us that is an area where sometimes we have problems with patients' safety—not being clear in our communications, making sure that what we are communicating is understood and the multiple levels of communication that happen. And there has to be really good, clear communication between them [the levels]—physician to physician, physician to nurse, nurse to nurse—all of the people that are involved in the care of the patient.

Q: These are economically tough times for health care. How can hospitals reduce costs and still improve patient safety?

A: Costing less doesn't mean there is a direct correlation to the quality of the care. One of the key ways we can lower costs and improve quality at the same time is to take waste out of the system. Providing the right care at the right time to the right patient and in the right manner is really where you can control costs and make sure that all your costs are going to the provision of safe care.

I think that one of the key ways we can do that is really looking at the processes of care and the way in which we deliver the care—the flow of the care and making sure that is as efficient as possible. Make sure that every effort put forward is at the essential place it needs to be and we don't have a lot of unnecessary work taking place or complicated processes.

Q: If nurses are looking at the process for efficiency, are they looking at the process for its effectiveness as well? Can that reveal some issues that could affect patient safety?

A: That kind of vigilance is used at every place in the system. One of the key criteria is asking: Is the care safe if we use this process or can we improve the safety if we change the process? Safety becomes the guiding principle in the work that we do in designing our systems, modifying them and continuing to work on them.

TABLE 2-2 ■ Amer Hybrid Model of Change

Constantly Shifting Factors	Excellent (2 points)	Good (1 point)	Poor (0 points)	Not Applicable
Communication patterns and relationships between disciplines				
Culture in the workplace includes openness to learning and being listened to				
Collaborative problem solving				
Common goals				
Ability to appreciate another's perspective				

middle level readiness for change, and a score of two to five indicates fair to little readiness for change. Zero to one indicates very poor change potential.

In conclusion, multiple factors need to be present to change nursing practice and to increase safe delivery of care. The models of safety and quality need to begin with clear definitions that can be used by all team members. Once the definitions are agreed upon, the priorities of safety and then quality need to be conceptualized in a standard model of quality improvement.

The necessary components of a standard model include the practice environment of the nurse, support staff and administrative collaboration and communication, patient perspectives, and the openness of nurses to change (see Box 2-3). In a high-technology, rapidly changing world, all nurses need to adjust to provide the best care possible. Whether it is bar coding for safe medication administration or simply encouraging staff innovation, the process and method will help guide nurses into the next age of safer and better quality care. The best model to use will be that which is the most simple and palatable to all involved in health care.

CHAPTER HIGHLIGHTS

- The concepts of safety and quality are identified and applied to environments that support or detract from the safest health care.

- Efforts to help nursing students and practicing nurses learn about quality and safety, such as QSEN and Magnet recognition, support nursing and the goal to make nursing care safer.

- National programs aimed at changing the culture of healthcare environments are used to develop models for care, such as the Competency Outcomes and Performance Assessment Model (COPA), that can be adopted by all nurses.

- Change theory can be applied to nursing, resulting in dramatic benefits that include less severe illness and prevention of death.

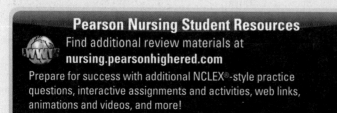

REFERENCES

Aiken, L. H., Sloan, D. M., Cimiotti, J. P., Clark, S. P., Flynn, L., Seajo, J. A., & Smith, H. L. (2010). Implications of the California nurse staffing mandate for other states. *Health Research and Education Trust.* doi 10.1111f. 1475-1773

Baker, D. P., Day, R., & Sales, E. (2006). Teamwork as an essential component of high-reliability organizations. *Health service Research, 41*(4), 1576–1578.

Blouin, Scott A. (2010). Helping to solve healthcare's most critical safety and quality problems. *Journal of Nursing Care Quality, 25*(2), 95–99. www.calnurses.org 2/2/2012

Chenot, T. M. & Daniel, L. G. (2010). Frameworks for patient safety in the nursing curriculum. *Journal of Nursing Education, 49*(10), 559–568.

Dlugacz, Y. D. (2006). *Measuring health care: Using quality data for operational, financial, and clinical improvement.* Jossey-Bass. Hoboken, NJ.

Finkelman, A. & Kenner, C. (2009). *Teaching the IOM: Implications of the IOM reports for nursing education.* (2nd Ed.) Washington, DC: American Nurses Association Publishing.

Frith, K.H. (2010). Effects of nurse staffing on hospital-acquired conditions and length of stay in community hospitals. *Quality Management in Health Care, 19*(2), 147.

Gordon, S., Buchanan, J., & Bretherton, T. (2008). *Safety in numbers: Nurse-to-patient ratios and the future of health care (the culture and politics of health care work).* Ithaca: ILR Press/Cornell University Press.

Havelock, R. G. (1973). *The change agent's guide to innovation in education.* Englewood Cliffs, NJ: Educational Technology Publications.

Ironside, P. M., & Sitterding, M. (2009). Embedding quality and safety competencies in nursing education. *Journal of Nursing Education, 48*(12), 659–660.

Kosseff, A. (2008, September). *STEPPS: Producing effective medical teams to achieve optimal patient outcomes.* Retrieved from www.ahqr.gov.

Lenburg, C.B., Klein, C., Abdur-Rahman, V., Spencer, T., & Boyer, S. (2009). The COPA Model: A comprehensive framework designed to promote quality care and competence for patient safety. *Nursing Education Perspectives, 30,* 312–317.

Lenburg, C.B., Abdur-Rahman, V., Spencer, T., Boyer, S., & Klein, C. (2011). Implementation of the COPA Model in nursing education and practice settings: Promoting competence, quality care and patient safety. *Nursing Education Perspectives, 32,* 290–296.

Leonard, M., Graham, S., & Bonacum, D. (2004). The human factor: The critical importance of effective teamwork and communication in providing safe care, *Quality and Safety in Health Care, 13*(1) 85–90. doi 10.1136/qshc2004.010033

Lewin, K. (1951). *Field theory in social sciences.* New York: Harper and Row.

Lippincott, Williams, & Wilkins. (2008). *Evidence-based nursing guide to legal and professional issues.* Philadelphia: Lippincott, Williams, & Wilkins.

Nightingale, F. (1860). *Notes on nursing: What it is, and what it is not.* New York: D. Appleton and Company.

Scott, R. D. (2009). *The direct cost of healthcare-associated infections in US hospitals and the benefits of prevention.* Retrieved from http://www.cdc.gov/HAI/pdfs/hai/Scott_CostPaper.pdf.

Sears, K., Goldsworthy, S., & Goodman, W. M. (2010). The relationship between simulation in nursing education and medication safety. *Journal of Nursing Education, 49*(1), 52–55.

Smith, R. (2002). *The 7 levels of change: Different thinking for different results.* Austin, TX: Tapestry Press.

Watson, J. (1999). *Postmodern nursing and beyond.* Toronto, Canada: Livingstone.

CHAPTER 3

TRANSITION TO PRACTICE: AN ESSENTIAL ELEMENT OF QUALITY AND SAFETY

Nancy Spector

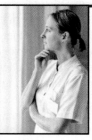

Yuri Arcurs/
Shutterstock.com

Debbie is a new graduate registered nurse (RN) who is in charge of the oncology unit during the night shift two months after starting her position as a nurse. She is managing admissions from the emergency department (ED) and has five patients with cancer. One of them, Brenda, who is 64 years old, has breast cancer in remission but has a fever and pneumonia. In the middle of the night, Brenda puts on her call light.

When Debbie gets to Brenda's room, she finds Brenda cyanotic and gasping for air because her oxygen mask is off. Debbie sits her up and replaces her mask. She tells Brenda to relax and that she will be back in a few minutes.

Meanwhile, Debbie's other patients are restless and need pain medications. There are three admissions from the ED, and one of the night nurses has gone home sick with the stomach flu. Debbie considers calling the night supervisor but keeps running around trying to keep everyone stable.

Two hours later, Debbie checks in on Brenda and finds her pulseless and not breathing. Debbie calls a "code blue," but it is too late. This is a fail to rescue situation, and help should have been called much sooner. Debbie is a novice nurse with very little clinical experience. She will carry this experience with her for the rest of her career.

CORE COMPETENCY

Articulate the value of transition to practice models and the safety implications for both novice and expert nurses.

LEARNING OUTCOMES

1. Analyze evidence for and against use of transition to practice models in all healthcare settings.

2. Identify times during the first year of practice that a new nurse graduate may face potential challenges.

3. Compare and contrast the U.S. transition to practice guidelines to those of other developed countries.

4. Discuss legal and ethical implications and nursing practice ramifications of neglecting transition to practice recommendations.

This chapter presents a compelling argument for adopting a standardized, regulatory model for transitioning all new nursing graduates to practice, with an emphasis on quality and safety. The National Council of State Boards of Nursing (NCSBN) has developed such a model, which will be discussed later in this chapter

In the healthcare workforce, nurses are considered the patient's last line of defense (Benner, Sutphen, Leonard, & Day, 2010). It only makes sense that their transition from education to practice should be carefully orchestrated. Other health professionals, such as physicians, pharmacists, and those in pastoral care, have standardized residency programs that are funded by the Centers for Medicare and Medicaid (CMS). Further, according to the American Association of State Colleges and Universities (2006), 30 or more states have a mandatory standardized teacher induction program for novice teachers, and 17 states fund this mentoring. Yet the research shows that transition programs in nursing are variable, depending on the setting and level of education of the graduate, and sometimes they are completely nonexistent (NCSBN, 2003; NCSBN, 2006b; NCSBN, 2006c; Scott, Engelke & Swanson, 2008). It is the responsibility of nurse leaders in regulation, education, and practice to work together to provide all new graduates with support during their critical transition period.

Safety and Quality Are Prompting This Movement

Health care is becoming increasingly complex, and there is a need to look beyond the patient at larger systems that affect patients. Such systems include families, communities, healthcare organizations, and insurance coverage. Nurses need to broaden their thinking beyond the hospitalized patient. Today's patient population is more diverse, sicker, and older than in the past, and patients are presenting with multiple conditions. Technology is growing exponentially, and nurses are working at a "staccato" pace (Wiggins, 2006). Patients are discharged so soon that they go home with complex medical, social, and economic issues. This complex and increasingly seriously ill patient exists in a healthcare system with challenging nursing care issues as well. Concomitantly, there is a nursing shortage looming in the future, and a faculty shortage that is predicted to continue for many years to come (Clarke & Cheung, 2008), though Auerbach, Buerhaus, and Staiger (2011) found that the nursing workforce is getting younger and therefore the shortage might not be quite as dire as has been predicted.

Furthermore, as discussed earlier in this book, medical errors are a pervasive problem in all of health care today. Since 1999, the Institute of Medicine (IOM) has released reports on patient safety issues in health care, making recommendations on how to improve the system. Yet a recent report (IOM, 2012) asserts that not much progress has been made since the 1999 IOM report *To Err Is Human* (Kohn, Corrigan, & Donaldson, 1999) estimated that 44,000 to 98,000 lives are lost in the United States each year due to medical errors. One study found adverse events continue to occur in as many as one-third of hospitalized patients (Classen et al., 2011). Another study suggests that more than 27% of Medicare patients will experience adverse events during their hospitalizations, and one-half of those will be severe adverse events (HHS, 2010). Additionally, another IOM report estimates that 1.5 million preventable adverse drug events occur annually (IOM, 2006).

Medical errors do not just take place in hospitals; they also occur in ambulatory care settings, physician's offices, long-term care facilities, pharmacies, urgent care centers, and home care. While there is not much data on the extent of the problem outside of hospitals, it is likely medical errors in these settings are common. For example, a recent review of malpractice claims concluded that 52% of all paid malpractice claims for all physician services involved ambulatory services, and almost two-thirds of these claims involved a major injury or death (Bishop, Ryan, & Casalino, 2011).

Related to patient safety and healthcare outcomes, we may soon be experiencing the "perfect storm" in nursing if we do not take action soon (Orsolini-Hain & Malone, 2007). The "expertise gap" that we are facing will most likely continue into the future. First, increasing numbers of experienced nurses will retire, which will lead to an increased ratio of newly graduated nurses to seasoned nurses. From numbers of nurses reporting they will retire between 2011 and 2020, Dracup and Morris (2007) predict there will be a 50% turnover in the nursing profession in a little more than a decade. Berkow, Virkstis, Stewart, and Conway (2008) report that currently 10% of a typical hospital is staffed by new graduates. This is significant because 89.2% of newly licensed RNs and 23.5% of newly licensed practical nurses (LPNs) work in hospitals (NCSBN, 2009a). Concurrently, there is a shortage of experienced nurse educators and insufficient research to determine best practices in nursing education.

Health policy and patient safety implications are serious with shortages of seasoned nurses because novice and inexperienced nurses are caring for more complex patients, under trying circumstances, as described previously. Multiple studies have confirmed that fewer nurses in areas such as intensive care units (ICUs) increase the risk of patient morbidity and mortality (Aiken, Clarke, Sloane, Lake, & Cheney, 2008). Statistics show that if new nurses fail to recognize changes in patient status, those patients can deteriorate quickly. When CPR is needed, for example, only 27% of pediatric patients and 18% of adult patients survive in-hospital resuscitation efforts (Nadkarni et al., 2006). Therefore, our current situation presents serious implications for the future of health care.

One Solution: A Standardized Transition to Practice Program

A standard six-month transition to practice residency with a preceptor is one solution toward improving patient safety and healthcare outcomes during these challenging times. Such a residency provides all nurses, across all levels of education, and throughout all settings with a standardized postgraduation transition to practice program. Many healthcare organizations in the United States and other countries have some level of transition to practice program in place.

Status of International Transition Programs

The international community is interested in transition to practice, as is evidenced by the following programs. Portugal has developed a regulatory model referred to as a professional development program. While not in place yet, it is being considered by the government. The new graduate is given a provisional license and participates in a nine-month supervised practice. At the end of the nine months, the new nurse writes a reflective report, and the supervisor writes a report. Both reports are reviewed by a body separate from the board of nursing, which makes a recommendation to the board for permanent licensure. If the recommendation is not made for permanent licensure, the new nurse is given a second chance for three more months. This separate body certifies all supervisors and accredits each facility placement. It should be noted that the government would fund this model, and the whole country has only 59,000 nurses.

Scotland is currently evaluating a voluntary online model (http://www.flyingstart.scot.nhs.uk) called Flying Start, which incorporates an online mentorship. The elements of this model include communication, teamwork, clinical skills, safe practice, research for practice, equality and diversity, policy, reflective practice, professional development, and career pathways (Roxburgh et al., 2010).

Australia, which implemented national licensure in July 2010 (http://tinyurl.com/y99mqf3), has incorporated a yearlong graduate transition program into their system, though it is voluntary. Canada has done good work with preceptorships and mentorships (http://www.cna-nurses.ca/CNA/default_e.aspx) for new graduates, and the Canadian Nurses Association sent a representative to the NCSBN Transition to Practice Committee meetings to learn about practices in the United States. Ireland has taken a different approach. In this country, a transition program that is part of students' last year of school includes a 36-week internship period (http://www.nursingboard.ie/en/education.aspx). Employers pay students during this internship period. Although the time period provided for various transition to practice programs is variable, the essence of the programs is similar. Whether the program is included at the end of the nursing program, used as part of the licensure process, or included in the first year of orientation for new practitioners, the primary focus is on building a strong foundation for developing expert practitioners that are satisfied in their positions.

Status of U.S. Transition Programs

In the United States, supporting new graduates in their transition to practice is not new. It was first discussed in the 1930s, when Townsend (1931) wrote about the need to integrate theory into the nurse's curriculum. However, that took a toll on practice, she wrote, and there was a resultant "... gap between the doctor's lecture and the actual nursing problem in the condition he lectured about" (p. 1183). Yet it was not until the 1970s that transition to practice was studied in depth. In 1974, Marlene Kramer, in her renowned book *Reality Shock: Why Nurses Leave Nursing*, crystallized the concept. Kramer described the difficulties new graduates face when they begin to work, and she called this reality shock. Kramer describes reality shock as "...shock-like reactions of new workers when they find themselves in a work situation for which they have spent several years preparing and for which they thought they were going to be prepared, and then suddenly find that they are not" (pp. vii–viii). A major reason nurses have difficulty moving into the workforce, Kramer says, is because of their perception of the role. While they are taught about maintaining professional standards, this is in stark contrast to the hospital's bureaucratic role where there is more emphasis on technical and administrative skills. She then proposes and assesses strategies to ameliorate reality shock, develop interpersonal competency, and define lines of action for constructive conflict resolution. Similarly, in 1978, Patricia Benner began an august line of study of the nurse's transition from novice (first year of education), to an advanced beginner (new graduate), to the competent stage (one to two years in practice), and then to proficiency and expertise (Benner, 2004).

More recently, there has been significant work on developing national transition to practice programs, and the Commission on Collegiate Nursing Education (CCNE) has developed a national accreditation process for residency programs (Beecroft, Kunzman, & Krozek, 2001; Williams, Goode, Krsek, Bednash, & Lynn 2007; www.aacn.nche.edu). Additionally, the Joint Commission, the Carnegie Study of Nursing Education report, the American Association of Colleges of Nursing partnering with the University HealthSystem Consortium (AACN/UHC), and the IOM Future of Nursing report (IOM, 2010) have made calls for a national standardized transition program for newly licensed nurses. The recommendation from the Carnegie study suggests lower entry-level salaries as a way to fund this residency program, while the recommendation from the IOM Future of Nursing report suggested that CMS stop funding nursing diploma programs and funnel that money into residency programs for nurses. The IOM report also recommended a yearlong nurse residency program to be funded by CMS (Joint Commission, 2002; Benner et al., 2010; Goode, Lynn, Krsek, & Bednash, 2009).

Transition experiences vary across the United States, across all levels of education, and across settings. NCSBN (2006c) investigated transition experiences in a geographically representative sample of 628 newly licensed registered nurse graduates and 519 newly licensed practical nurse graduates. They found that while a majority of the graduates reported having some sort of orientation or transition program, RNs spent an average of only 11.4 weeks in transition programs, while LPNs and licensed vocational nurses (LVNs) spent 4.72 weeks. This difference was statistically significant. More RNs reported participating in comprehensive transition programs (39.7%) than LPNs and LVNs (15.3%). Most RNs practice in hospitals after graduation, and only 40.9% participated in comprehensive transition programs that included an orientation to the hospital and unit, as well as an internship, preceptorship, or mentorship. Similarly, most LPNs and LVNs work in long-term care facilities following graduation, and only 12.7% of them participated in comprehensive transition programs. Surprisingly, 3% of the RN sample and 7.4% of the LPN and LVN sample reported not receiving any type of transition program, including orientation (NCSBN, 2006c). Of the RNs reporting having no type of transition program, all graduated from associate degree nursing (ADN) programs. Other studies had similar findings (NCSBN, 2003; NCSBN, 2006b; Scott et al., 2008) related to the variability of transition programs in the United States.

Is it time for nursing to take a giant step forward and design and implement a national standardized transition program? Obviously this initiative would have to be implemented collaboratively with nursing practice, regulation, and education. Regulators have authority over new nurses and could take the step of requiring a transition program for license renewal. However, nursing regulation does not have authority over nursing employers. Therefore, practice and education leaders would have to stand by the regulators and convince huge hospital systems, small rural community hospitals, nursing homes, legislators and other policymakers, and consumers that this action must be taken to improve the quality and safety of health care. Can nursing mount such an enormous effort? The nursing profession would have to come together with one voice, like never before, and articulate the necessity of this major change in how nurses are educated and regulated.

It is imperative to stress that this movement toward developing a national standardized transition program is not occurring because the education programs are failing to adequately prepare our nurses for practice. Our nurse educators are working harder, and smarter, than ever before to educate sufficient and qualified nurses during this intense faculty shortage. Nor is the need for this regulatory transition model because practice settings are failing and are expecting new nurses to hit the ground running. Many practice settings have developed their own individual programs because they are concerned about transitioning new graduates. Yet research has shown that the caliber of these programs varies (NCSBN, 2006b; Scott et al., 2008). This need for a national standardized transition program has arisen because of the tremendous changes in health care in the past 20 years. Healthcare agencies need to commit to adopting transition to practice models even though there is a perceived high expense. Even though orientation for new nurses may seem expensive, the benefit of safer care and retention of quality nurses far outweighs the initial expense.

Identifying the Evidence

Research on transition to practice programs remains in the formative stage. Requiring substantial evidence before implementing new models can be a barrier to innovation. The following review includes a variety of the evidence that is currently available, such as expert opinions and consensus statements, unpublished reports, results from interviews with those who have implemented successful programs, and published research papers, all of which add depth to the inquiry.

The guide to reviewing the evidence for transition to practice (Spector & Echternacht, 2010) was Sackett's widely accepted definition for evidence-based practice. Sackett and colleagues describe evidence-based practice as the integration of the best research evidence with clinical expertise and patient values (Sackett et al., 2000). The available evidence was identified by searching the literature systematically, as well as by contacting those who have developed transition programs. The following levels of research were considered, and they are consistent with other NCSBN work (NCSBN, 2006a).

- Level I: A properly conducted randomized controlled trial, systematic/integrative review, or meta-analysis

- Level II: Other studies, such as quasi-experimental, correlation, descriptive, survey, evaluation, and qualitative

- Level III: Expert opinions or consensus statements

Of the available evidence, there were several Level II and Level III studies or projects, but none were Level I. One study, by Hofler (2008), synthesized national reports on transition to practice, but the methodology was not rigorous enough to consider it a systematic or integrative review. It is common in health care, health policy, and nursing research not to find randomized controlled trials because they are not always feasible or ethically possible. Expert opinions and consensus statements (such as standards by a professional organization) can be important supportive data, especially in an area as complex as transition to practice.

Safety and New Nurses

When nurses' mistakes are analyzed, reasons for errors are most often linked to lack of knowledge of hospital procedure and unfamiliarity with patients. Unfamiliarity with patients and units as well as first-time experiences were cited by the Massachusetts Board of Nursing (Board of Registration in Nursing, 2007) and Ebright, Urden, Patterson, & Chalko (2004) as reasons for near misses or errors. This is significant because novice nurses who do not take part in transition programs notoriously have a high turnover rate, which will be discussed later in this chapter. Research reports link new nurses to patient safety issues such as near misses, adverse events, and practice errors (Berens, 2000; Bjørk & Kirkevold, 1999; Board of Registration in Nursing, 2007; Del Bueno, 2005; Ebright et al., 2004; Johnstone & Kanitsaki, 2006; Johnstone & Kanitsaki, 2008; NCSBN,

BOX 3-1	FINDINGS FROM THREE MILLION STATE AND FEDERAL COMPUTER RECORDS ON NURSING ERRORS

Michael Berens (2000), a *Chicago Tribune* staff writer, compiled findings from three million state and federal computer records to report the following:

- From 1995 to 2000, the following occurred from the action or inaction of RNs across the country:

  - 1,720 hospital patients were killed.

  - 9,584 hospital patients were injured.

- Some specific errors that occurred nationwide between 1995 and 2000 included:

  - At least 418 patients were killed and 1,356 were injured by RNs misusing infusion pumps.

  - At least 216 patients were killed and 429 were injured because RNs failed to hear alarms on lifesaving equipment.

  - At least 119 patients were killed and 564 were injured by unlicensed nurse aides.

- Some specific cases include:

  - In Chicago, a 2-year-old child received a deadly overdose of sedatives from a newly graduated nurse who was left alone to perform a delicate medical procedure without training.

  - In Denver, a 78-year-old patient was killed when a nurse, overwhelmed with the care of 15 patients, inadvertently delivered a fatal dose of drugs into an intravenous line.

  - In Wichita, Kansas, a 38-year-old patient bled to death after a hysterectomy. She complained for hours of pain but attempted to endure the ordeal after the nurses said she was fine by whispering to herself, "I am not a wimp. I can take this."

  - In Chicago, a pediatric nurse worked as an agency nurse on a geriatric unit of a hospital, where she received no orientation. She was charged by the board of nursing with neglect after not monitoring a 67-year-old woman who had complained of chest pain. The patient's condition deteriorated, and she died of a heart attack.

2007a; NCSBN, 2007b; Orsolini-Hain & Malone, 2007). Berens (2000) reviewed three million state and federal computer records related to safe nursing practice, citing several statistics related to patient deaths due to the actions or inaction of all nurses (Box 3-1), not just novice nurses. However, specifically related to novice nurses, Berens (2000), after reviewing Illinois state disciplinary data, reported that temporary nurses (those filling in when novice nurses leave) were increasingly the focus of investigations. Therefore, when these nurses leave, they are often replaced by temporary nurses who tend to make more errors.

Others report newly licensed nurses have significant job stresses (Elfering, Semmer, & Grebner, 2006; Fink, Krugman, Casey, & Goode, 2008; NCSBN, 2007a; Williams et al., 2007), and this stress has been linked to patient errors (NCSBN, 2007a; Elfering et al., 2006). Investigators in Sweden studied 23 novice nurses from 19 hospitals for two weeks and found job stressors and low job control to be risk factors for patient safety. The most frequent safety issues, related to job stressors, were incorrect documentation, medication errors/near misses, delays in patient care delivery, and violence among patients or toward nurses. In another study, newly licensed nurses who reported higher stress also reported making significantly more errors than new nurses who reported lower stress levels (NCSBN, 2007a). Interestingly, in the NCSBN national study (2007a) of newly licensed nurses, the stress levels of new nurses were highest at the three- to six-month period of practice. This is often the period when new nurses are no longer in any kind of transition or orientation program. In the study of the AACN/UHC yearlong residency program, stress gradually decreased over the year (Williams et al., 2007). These results indicate that a comprehensive yearlong transition program may decrease stress, which in turn is related to safe patient care.

Disciplinary procedures tend to be less severe for novice nurses (those who have been working from zero to 12 months) versus those in practice for 10 or more years because it is expected that the latter group is more knowledgeable, but that they also have a longer time frame or opportunity to make errors. New nurses are often treated more leniently when being reported for errors. Further, there is a difference in the severity of discipline prescribed for minor errors or near misses; the latter is more often seen with new nurses, both RNs (Ebright et al., 2004) and LPNs (Board of Registration in Nursing, 2007). The NCSBN Nursys data on discipline in the boards of nursing (NCSBN, 2007a) found that 4.1% of discipline was for novice nurses. For all nurses, there was a trend of increased discipline from 1996 to 2006, which supports Institute of Medicine (IOM) reports of increased practice errors in health care. The Massachusetts findings on discipline data from 77 nursing homes (Board of Registration in Nursing, 2007) had no novice RNs in the analysis. However, of 44 LPNs disciplined, seven were novices. In the Massachusetts study, the researchers concluded that errors made by new nurses were linked to inexperience, lack of familiarity, and lack of consistent preceptors. They recommended more supervision and support for new nurses.

A study conducted in Australia (Johnstone & Kanitsaki, 2008) found that incident reporting increased during the novice nurse's first year in a supportive transition program because they were taught about the importance of reporting errors and near misses for root cause analyses. These nurses were able to integrate patient safety into the system within three to four months of this 12-month program. Supporting findings from Ebright and colleagues (2004) and the Board of Registration in Nursing (2007) discussed previously, the key indicators Johnstone and Kanitsaki used to validate this integration included new graduates' familiarity with the following:

- Hospital layout
- Hospital policies regarding risk assessment tools

- Processes of evidence-based practice

- Incident reporting

New nurses often engage in concrete thinking and focus on technology (Benner, 2004; Orsolini-Hain & Malone, 2007), thereby missing the bigger picture. They may miss subtle indicators of patient decline or serious health concerns. This can be devastating during these complex times in health care (Benner et al., 2010; del Bueno, 2005; Ebright et al., 2004). With the increased ratio of novice nurses to seasoned nurses, as discussed earlier in this chapter, it is possible that novices are assisting each other, thus putting them in situations where errors in judgment are not corrected by more experienced colleagues (Ebright et al., 2004; Orsolin-Hain & Malone, 2007). Indeed, in a well-designed prospective study, Bjørk and Kirkevold (1999) found how patient safety can be compromised when effective transition programs are not in place. They conducted a longitudinal study in Norway, videotaping nurses as they practiced and conducting interviews with nurses and patients. Four nurses were followed for eight to 14 months as they performed dressing changes and ambulated new surgical patients. The nurses had only a short orientation to their units. While the nurses reported they had become efficient and rated themselves as better nurses over time, the analysis of their practice revealed that they made the same practice errors (such as contaminating wounds and unsafely removing wound drains) at the end of the study as they made at the beginning. According to the researchers, the nurses considered themselves practiced nurses and assumed they knew what they were doing. There were no opportunities for feedback from expert nurses or opportunities to reflect on their practice, thus preventing them from learning from their mistakes. Another study (Ebright et al., 2004) found that of 12 recruited new nurse participants, seven reported at least one near-miss event, while one nurse described two events. Some of the identified themes related to near-misses or adverse event cases include the following:

- Minimal ability for clinically focused critical thinking

- Lack of seeking assistance from experienced nurses

- Lack of knowledge of unit and workflow patterns

- First-time experiences

- Time constraints

- Handoffs

- Influence of peer pressure and social norms

- Losing the big picture

- Novices assisting novices

Inexperienced nurses who are not supported can also impact patient safety because of missed nursing care. Kalisch (2006), in a qualitative study, investigated missed nursing care, identifying a main issue of lack of patient surveillance. Using focus groups, Kalisch (2006) also identified many reasons for missed care, including poor use of existing staff resources and ineffective delegation. The focus group members reported there were too many inexperienced nurses with inadequate orientations. They also reported inconsistent assignments, meaning that novice nurses did not have the opportunity to get to know their patients well enough to recognize changes. When nursing care is omitted, patient outcomes can be adversely affected, thus promoting falls, failure to rescue, and pressure ulcers.

Similarly, Benner and colleagues (2010) recommended a yearlong transition program for new nurses in part because in educational programs, students do not have the opportunity to follow up with their patients. Therefore, novice nurses are often weak in detecting subtle changes in patient conditions, and when nurses fail to recognize changes in patient status, those patients can deteriorate quickly. For example, Ashcraft (2004), in presenting three cases, discusses how crucial pattern recognition is when patients are in prearrest states. Novice nurses take longer to "put the pieces together" and would benefit from consulting with an experienced nurse in these critical situations. A supportive transition program would assist new nurses to identify subtle changes and avoid practice errors.

As reported in a NCSBN national study, when transition programs in hospitals addressed specialty care, new nurses reported making significantly fewer practice errors. Similarly, when nurses perceived they were more competent, they reported making significantly fewer practice errors, and this was especially true when they reported more competence in clinical reasoning abilities, communication, and interpersonal relationships (NCSBN, 2007a).

When involving new nurses in clinical risk management systems in Australia, outcomes improved as reported by Johnstone and Kanitsaki (2006) and Johnstone and Kanitsaki (2008). The authors stress the importance of not teaching new graduates deficit education; that is, do not assume the transition program needs to re-educate new nurses. Instead, nurses need to learn, by experiential means and with the support of qualified nurses, how to manage risks in practice. These researchers found that when the new graduates were introduced to clinical risk management, none of them were involved in a preventable adverse event that resulted in patient harm. Unfortunately, the researchers did not compare these findings to new nurses who were not introduced to clinical risk management.

Competence and New Nurses

Nursing education cannot prepare new graduates for acculturating into their workplace and for using their recently acquired new language (Keller, Meekins, & Summers, 2006). Keller asserts that new graduates are expected to become skilled in a wide range of absolutely necessary skills, and gain a sense of the wider world of their organization and health care. She describes some of these necessary skills as being self-aware and learning about team dynamics, leading teams, coordinating care, managing conflict, understanding the psychological effects of change and transition, communication, evidence-based practice, systems thinking, and financial pressures. Neophyte nurses become overwhelmed and stressed with all of these expectations (NCSBN, 2007b; Williams et al., 2007), and, as stated previously, stress in the first year of practice is significantly related to practice errors (NCSBN, 2007b).

There is excellent empirical data about what can happen when new nurses do not have supportive transition programs. Employers report new graduates are not ready to practice. NCSBN studies found that fewer than 50% of employers reported "yes, definitely" when asked if new graduates are ready to provide safe and effective care (NCSBN, 2002; NCSBN, 2004). Similarly, Berkow and colleagues (2008), from the Nursing Executive Center, conducted a survey of more than 5,700 front line nurse leaders, asking about employer perceptions of new graduates on 36 competencies. Improvement was needed across both levels of education, ADN and bachelors of science in nursing (BSN). For example, 53% of employers were satisfied with the top-rated competency (utilization of information technologies), while only 10% were satisfied with the last-rated competency (delegation of tasks). The researchers noted that the bottom-rated competencies would be better taught in an experiential environment, such as a transition to practice program. (See Table 3-1.)

There is evidence, however, linking competence to the need for effective transition programs (Benner et al., 2010; Beyea, von Reyn & Slattery, 2007; Bjørk & Kirkevold, 1999; del Bueno, 2005; NCSBN, 2009a; NCSBN, 2007a; Orsolini-Hain & Malone, 2007; Williams et al., 2007). NCSBN (2007a) reported that new graduates were significantly more likely to self-report practice errors when they also reported decreased competence and increased stress. In this study, three to six months after hire was the vulnerable period when nurses reported more stress and less competence, and therefore were at risk for practice breakdown. Other research has demonstrated this V-shaped pattern, showing declines in novice nurse variables at mid-program, with subsequent gains (Halfer, Graf, & Sullivan, 2008; Williams et al., 2007), though in these studies the decline began at the six-month level. This evidence supports the vulnerable period of new graduates as being three to nine months after employment.

TABLE 3-1 ■ New Nurse Graduate Competencies Employers Find Lacking

Competency	Percentage of Employers Satisfied with BSNs	Percentage of Employers Satisfied with ADNs
Understanding of quality improvement	20	15
Completion of tasks within expected timeframe	20	16
Ability to track multiple responsibilities	14	11
Conflict resolution	14	11
Ability to prioritize	15	9
Ability to anticipate risk	13	10
Ability to delegate tasks	11	9

Source: Berkow, S., Virkstis, K., Stewart, J. and Conway, L. (2008). *Journal of Nursing Administration* (JONA).

In the Bjørk and Kirkevold (1999) study, as described previously, there were limited opportunities for feedback or reflective practice in the nursing settings studied, which likely would have improved the competence of these nurses. In the Dartmouth-Hitchcock transition program (Beyea, Slattery, & von Reyn, 2010), investigators measured confidence, competence, and readiness to practice, all of which significantly increased after nurses completed the transition program. This program uses simulation vignettes that highlight high-risk and low-frequency events, as well as commonly occurring clinical situations. According to the study, this is a highly effective way of developing competency and confidence in new graduates.

Mississippi's Office of Nursing Workforce (MONW, 2010) implemented a six-month transition program in some hospitals, using an interesting outcome measure that is indirectly related to patient safety and competence; they measured patient satisfaction and found a 10% increase after nurses completed a formal six-month transition program.

One-Year Turnover

Job retention is used by some as a measure of patient safety because while nurses may leave one job during the first year, they generally move to another position. However, the workplace that loses the nurse may already be affected because satisfaction is a predictor of anticipated turnover, which is also linked to healthcare outcomes (Beecroft, Dorey, & Wenten, 2008), though studies on outcomes when hospitals use temporary nurses have been conflicting. Aiken (2007) did not find temporary nurses affected quality and safety. Bae, Mark, and Fried (2010) found that there were significantly more falls on units with high levels of temporary nurses, but there were significantly fewer medication errors on those units, compared to those without temporary nurses. More research is needed to better understand the relationship between turnover and safety and quality outcomes.

Do these new graduates leave nursing altogether? Orsolini-Hain and Malone (2007) report that the 2004 National Sample Survey shows a trend of nurses leaving nursing altogether. In the late 1980s, only 4.5% of nurses were employed outside of nursing, whereas in 2004, 16.8% were employed elsewhere (Orsolini-Hain & Malone, 2007). However, this trend may not affect new nurses; evidence shows that 98% of nurses who pass the NCLEX exam are working two years later (Kovner & Djukic, 2009).

The literature reports moderate to high turnover rates during new graduates' first year of practice. Turnover rates have been reported as high as between 35% to 60% for one year in practice, depending on the report (Advisory Board Company, 2006; Beecroft et al., 2001; Halfer et al., 2008; Pine & Tart, 2007; Williams et al., 2007). Turnover rates are not reported the same across studies, and Kovner and Djukic (2009) discuss some of the problems with turnover rate statistics for newly licensed nurses. For example, some studies include turnover within the institution, while others report rates after institutions have developed comprehensive transition programs. Using unpublished raw data from the RN Work Project, Kovner and Djukic (2009) report a 26% turnover rate in two years, though they do not report what part of that percentage belongs to year one.

It is clear, however, that comprehensive transition programs are associated with significantly decreased turnover rates (Beecroft et al., 2001; Halfer et al., 2008; Pine & Tart, 2007; Williams et al., 2007). Some turnover is expected in the first year of practice because of normal life situations; from reviewing the literature, anything over 7% to 10% is most likely related to the job situation.

Turnover of newly licensed nurses is more often analyzed in acute care settings than in long-term care settings. The third American Health Care Association (2008) study of vacancy and turnover in long-term care settings, while not looking specifically at novice nurse turnover rates, reported high rates of turnover generally: 41% for staff RNs and 49.9% for LPNs. This certainly indicates the likeliness of high turnover rates for new graduates. Similar to NCSBN's beliefs about the transition to practice model, these authors conclude that high-quality care depends on a stable, well-trained workforce and that promoting sound fiscal policies designed to strengthen the workforce should be a top national priority.

As was stated earlier, data indicate that temporary nurses, who are often hired when a new nurse resigns, have an increased number of disciplinary complaints filed at boards of nursing (Berens, 2000) compared to nurses hired on a permanent basis. Similarly, errors made by novice LPNs in nursing homes (Board of Registration in Nursing, 2007) and near misses reported by RNs (Ebright et al., 2004) are linked to unfamiliarity with the workplace setting. Further, every study examined found that increased retention resulted from a formal transition program (Beecroft et al., 2001; Halfer, 2007; Keller et al., 2006; NCSBN, 2007b; Pine & Tart, 2007; VNIP, 2010; Williams et al., 2007), and that turnover rates, for the first year in practice, varied from 6% to 19%.

Promising Practices in Programs Transitioning New Graduates to Practice

There is no doubt the literature and research on long-term settings, and licensed and vocational nurses are not as strong as with acute care settings and registered nurses. One NCSBN report (NCSBN, 2006c) found that practical nurse transition programs averaged 4.72 weeks in length, which is so short that they most likely would not provide any insight as to what the effect of transition on practical nurses would be. Another study focused on discipline in nursing homes and concluded there is a need for improved transitioning of licensed practical nurses (LPNs) (Board of Registration in Nursing, 2007). A national survey on the nursing home workforce (My Inner View, 2008) calculated priority ratings on areas for needed improvement: (1) lower job stress, (2) management that listens,

(3) management that cares, and (4) training to deal with difficult residents. The study on issues in LPN practice points to the need for new nurses in long-term care, who in the future should receive more support through a standardized transition program. A transition program may lower job stress, as discussed previously. Further, with incorporation of specialty content, nurses would better learn how to care for difficult patients. The transition to practice model is of course only one factor in provision of quality nursing care. Many other factors complicate the equation of safety and quality in nursing care.

Transition Programs in Long-Term Care

While there are many descriptions in the literature of transition programs in acute care, exemplars of transition programs in long-term care are limited. Two voluntary statewide transition programs include long-term care sites (VNIP, 2010; WNRP, 2008), and these programs were discussed by personal communication with the project managers of each. Employers in long-term care and rural settings have responded positively to these programs. Similarly, reports from nurses involved with these programs have been positive, though there is no formal data on these outcomes. Practical nurses should also have transition to practice programs that focus on quality and safety in long-term care settings. Relying on the limited number of available studies on practical nurses and long-term care, and applying results from acute care settings and registered nurses, it is reasonable to include all settings and all levels of education in a transition model.

NCBSN's Transition to Practice Module

In response to evidence that changes must be made, the NCSBN developed a standardized regulatory model for transitioning all new nursing graduates to practice, with an emphasis on quality and safety. NCSBN's Transition to Practice (TTP) model was designed, in part, by the author to help with new graduate nurse adjustment to practice. It is also intended to help retain nurses in practice. (See Box 3-2.)

Recommended Elements

The five transition modules of the NCSBN's TTP model supported by the evidence (https://www.ncsbn.org/1603.htm) are based on the IOM competencies (Greiner & Knebel, 2003) and the Quality and Safety for Nursing Education initiative (Cronenwett et al., 2007):

- Patient-Centered Care

- Communication and Teamwork

- Evidence-Based Practice

- Quality Improvement

- Informatics

| BOX 3-2 | GOAL, GUIDING PRINCIPLES, AND DEFINITIONS FOR NCSBN's TRANSITION TO PRACTICE MODEL |

GOAL

To promote public safety by supporting newly licensed nurses during their critical entry period and progression into practice

GUIDING PRINCIPLES

- The mission of the boards of nursing is the protection of public health, safety, and welfare.

- Nursing regulators recognize the value of evidence-based models in their responsibility of public protection.

- Transitioning new nurses to practice is best accomplished when practice, education, and regulation collaborate.

- Transition to practice programs should occur across all settings and all education levels.

- Regulation criteria for transition programs should reflect minimum requirements and be the least burdensome criteria consistent with public protection.

- Transition program outcomes are consistent with the knowledge, skills, and attitudes required for safe and effective provision of nursing care.

DEFINITIONS

- **Competent:** Clinical competency encompasses the ability to observe and gather information, recognize deviations from expected patterns, prioritize data, make sense of data, maintain a professional demeanor, provide clear communication, execute effective interventions, perform nursing skills correctly, evaluate nursing interventions, and self-reflect for performance improvement within a culture of safety.

- **Deliberate practice:** Focused learning with an engaged learner that involves repetitive performance of psychomotor or cognitive skills, coupled with rigorous assessment, informative feedback, and the opportunity for reflection.

- **Orientation:** The process of introducing staff to the philosophy, goals, policies, procedures, role expectations, and other factors needed to function in a specific work setting. Orientation takes place both for new employees and when changes in nurses' roles, responsibilities, and practice settings occur. This is consistent with the American Nurses Association (ANA) Scope and Standards of Practice for Nursing Professional Development.

- **Preceptor:** A nurse who has had the preceptor training module and is assigned to work with a newly licensed nurse for the first six months of practice to provide expert feedback, to foster reflective practice, to role model safe and quality patient care, and to socialize the novice nurse into the role of a nurse. The preceptor can work on a one-to-one basis with the new graduate, or some institutions might utilize a team preceptorship model.

- **Preceptorship:** A formal relationship between a qualified preceptor and a newly licensed nurse that facilitates active learning and transition into practice.

- **Transition to practice:** A formal program of active learning, implemented across all settings, for all newly licensed nurses (registered nurses and licensed practical/vocational nurses) designed to support their progression from education to practice.

Source: National Council of State Boards of Nursing (https://www.ncsbn.org/TransitiontoPractice_goals_081911.pdf)

As Johnstone and Kanitsaki (2006) points out, these should not be taught as deficit education, meaning that they should not be presented under the assumption that students did not learn the content in the first place, or did not learn it well. Instead, these concepts should be incorporated into the new nurses' experiences so that they continue to learn, from preceptor role modeling, how to think like a nurse. While these could be presented separately as modules, they should be integrated throughout the transition program.

Patient-Centered Care

Among the aspects of patient-centered care that should be emphasized are specialty content as well as prioritizing and organizing care. The shift in focus is on the patient's perceptions, needs, and schedule preferences versus the nurse's need to provide or impose care on a rigid schedule. For example, patients who are stable may value being able to sleep until 10 a.m. instead of waking at 7 a.m. for vital signs and baths. (See Chapter 9 for more on patient-centered care.) Specialty content in a transition program has been linked significantly to self-reporting of lower practice errors (NCSBN, 2007a). Other research supports integrating specialty practice into transition programs (Beecroft et al., 2001; Benner et al., 2010; Beyea et al., 2007; Flying Start, 2010; Halfer, 2007; Joint Commission, 2002; Keller et al., 2006; Pine & Tart, 2007; VNIP 2010).

Prioritizing and organizing is a part of clinical practice that is often a weakness for novice nurses (Berkow et al., 2008; Halfer, 2007; NCSBN, 2004; NCSBN, 2006a; Williams et al., 2007), most likely because of lack of experience. Specifically, the AACN/UHC residency program measured ability to organize and prioritize before and after their program and found significant increases at the end of the program. Prioritizing and organizing are integrated throughout most of the transition programs that focused on specialty content.

Communication and Teamwork

Communication and teamwork are essential in any regulatory model. The 2003 IOM report Health Professions Education (Greiner & Knebel, 2003) stressed the importance of teaching healthcare students to collaborate across professions. McKay and Crippen (2008) report that in hospitals where collaboration occurs, there is a 41% lower mortality rate than would be predicted. In other hospitals, McKay and Crippen (2008) report, where collaborative communication does not take place, mortality rates were 58% higher than would be predicted. Similarly, enhanced communication in hospitals has been linked to nurse satisfaction, lower costs, and greater responsiveness of healthcare providers (McKay & Crippen, 2008). Along the same lines, one NCSBN (2007b) study found that new nurses perceived they made significantly fewer practice errors when they reported being more competent in communication and interpersonal relationships. Yet prelicensure nursing programs provide students with few opportunities for interprofessional communication (Benner et al., 2010). Most reports of transition programs that were reviewed recommended a purposeful integration of communication, including interprofessional relationships, into transition programs (Beecroft et al., 2001; Beyea et al., 2007; Flying Start, 2010; Halfer, 2007; Keller et al., 2006; Pine & Tart, 2007; Williams et al., 2007; WNRP, 2010).

The communication and teamwork module also includes role socialization, which is an important concept for regulation. New nurses must have a good understanding of their scope of practice, as well as that of others on the healthcare team. Role socialization has been studied by O'Rourke (2006) for a number of years, and she has developed a program and some metrics for measuring outcomes. Role socialization was an integral element of many of the transition programs reviewed by the NCSBN (Flying Start, 2010; Keller et al., 2006; Kentucky Board of Nursing, 2010; Pine & Tart, 2007; VNIP, 2010; Williams et al., 2007).

Closely related to role socialization is the need for new nurses to develop a better understanding of delegating and supervising. Since 2002, NCSBN studies of new nurses have consistently found that new nurses report a lack of understanding of delegation (NCSBN, 2004; 2006b; 2007a; 2009a), as do others (Berkow et al., 2008). NCSBN's position paper on delegation and supervising provides background for this module (NCSBN, 2005). Transition programs may be incorporating delegation and supervising into their curricula, though not many specifically indicate that. Of those the NCSBN reviewed, only the Wisconsin Nurse Residency Program (WNRP, 2010) and the UHC/AACN (Williams et al., 2007) model identified delegating and supervising as elements of their programs. NCSBN's regulatory model will require experiential learning of delegation principles and practice.

Evidence-Based Practice

Another essential experiential module is evidence-based practice because nurses are expected to base their practice on the evidence (Cronenwett et al., 2007; Greiner & Knebel, 2003). Yet research has shown that new nurses are weak in this area (NCSBN, 2006a; NCSBN, 2006b). In the Launch into Nursing program in Texas, new nurses participate in an evidence-based project and present the results to their hospital unit (Keller et al., 2006). The international and national programs previously cited support incorporating evidence-based practice into transition programs (Beecroft et al., 2001; Flying Start, 2010; Williams et al., 2007), as do individual programs (Pine & Tart, 2007; WNRP, 2010).

Quality Improvement

Quality improvement is another module incorporated into NCSBN's TTP. With healthcare institutions focusing on safety and improving their systems, novice nurses need experiential learning related to quality improvement processes, such as Six Sigma, a model improvement process based on corporate manufacturing and elimination of mistakes. Berkow and colleagues (2008) surveyed educators and practice leaders about the emphasis of 36 competencies taught in nursing programs, compared to how prepared new nurses were related to those competencies. They found that quality improvement (as well as priority setting and delegation) was not emphasized enough in nursing education and concluded it is best learned in a practice setting with experiential learning. Additionally, Barton, Armstrong, Preheim, Gelmon, & Andrus (2009) conducted a national research survey to determine the progression of quality and safety competencies. They identified the following knowledge and skills that should be introduced in the advanced phase of a nursing curriculum, which also would include transition to practice programs:

- Give examples of tension between professional autonomy and system functioning.

- Explain the importance of variation and measurement in assessing quality care.

- Describe approaches for changing processes of care.

- Participate in a root cause analysis of a sentinel event.

- Practice aligning the aims, measures, and changes involved in improving care.

- Evaluate the effect of change.

Informatics

In this module, newly licensed nurses learn how to identify the electronic information that is available at the point of care and learn how to access information that is not readily available but is needed. The Technology Informatics Guiding Educational Reform initiative (TIGER, 2010) is used as a resource. Confidentiality of information is stressed in this module.

Safety Threads Throughout the Curriculum

Teaching safety is an essential part of a transition to practice regulatory model, and is threaded throughout all the modules. Johnstone and colleagues (2006 & 2008) in Australia have reported on the importance of experientially teaching risk management to new nurses. Cronenwett and colleagues (2007), using the expertise of national healthcare leaders across disciplines, have described in detail a module on safety that could be used in transition programs. This consensus opinion document, Quality and Safety Education for Nurses (QSEN), can be considered excellent evidence for this transition model. The Massachusetts Board of Nursing (Board of Registration in Nursing, 2007) findings on nursing home errors called attention to addressing safety issues in transition programs, based on their review of discipline of new practical nurse graduates. Likewise, an NCSBN study (NCSBN, 2007b) found that, according to self-reports, practice errors made by new graduates were prevalent. Many of the successful transition programs focus on safety (Beecroft et al., 2001; Beyea et al., 2007; Flying Start, 2010; Halfer, 2007; Pine & Tart, 2007; Williams et al., 2007; WNRP, 2008). Funding for TTP programs must be provided with the same urgency as aviation safety infrastructure. Without adequate investment in TTP, the cycle of adverse events will continue.

Clinical Reasoning

Clinical reasoning, also sometimes referred to as critical thinking, is another essential part of a transition to practice regulatory model that is integrated throughout the modules. As the Carnegie study (Benner et al., 2010) points out, critical reasoning is where nurses learn to think like a nurse. The Dartmouth program (Beyea et al., 2007) is exemplary as it uses simulation to assist novice nurses in making decisions during common clinical events or events that are uncommon but life threatening. Some transition programs specifically report integration of clinical reasoning and critical thinking (Beecroft et al., 2001; Halfer, 2007; Keller et al., 2006; Mississippi Office of Nursing Workforce, 2010; Pine & Tart, 2007; VNIP, 2010; Williams et al., 2007; WNRP, 2010). However, interviews with project managers of transition programs indicated that all programs examined attempt to integrate clinical reasoning.

Feedback and Reflection

Feedback and reflection are important threads in the transition to practice model and are formally maintained during the six-month transition program, as well as during the six months that follow. Bjørk and Kirkevold's (1999) longitudinal study, discussed earlier, showed the importance of feedback and reflection. If new nurses do not receive feedback on their practice, along with an opportunity to reflect, their practice will not improve. As was seen in Bjørk and Kirkevold's study (1999), without those opportunities, new graduates are at risk of making the same mistakes time and time again. It is important for preceptors to be taught how to provide constructive feedback and how to foster reflective practice. Many of the transition programs included in the literature review for this chapter did provide opportunities for feedback and reflection (Beyea et al., 2007; Flying Start, 2010; Halfer, 2007; Keller et al., 2006; NCSBN, 2006a; Pine & Tart, 2007; Williams et al., 2007; WNRP, 2010). For fostering reflection, journaling and personal inventories were described as successful strategies.

Preceptor–Nurse Relationship

The evidence is overwhelming that transition to practice programs are most successful when they incorporate the use of preceptors. All programs detailed on the NCSBN's TTP model implementation document (https://www.ncsbn.org/1603.htm) used the preceptor model. In the Massachusetts study (Board of Registration in Nursing, 2007) of nursing errors, one practical nurse commented that during her orientation to the unit, she "worked with three different nurses on three different days," after which she worked alone and was encouraged to ask questions of other nurses as needed. This pattern will not allow for the consistent feedback that is so essential to this model. However, if well designed, team preceptorships have been proven successful (Beecroft et al., 2008), and therefore this would be an acceptable strategy in this model.

The evidence also supports that preceptors need to be skilled in the role. In many transition programs, orienting preceptors to the role is important; however, the Vermont Nurse Internship Program (2010) is an exemplary model of preceptor education. It has developed this model since the beginning of its initiative in 1999, and it now credentials all its preceptors. There are also other models available in the literature (Nicol & Young, 2007). Often, preceptors feel unprepared and unsupported for the preceptorship role. For example, in one study of 86 preceptors, researchers found preceptors reported they were unprepared to precept new graduates, and they needed more support and recognition (Yonge, Hagler, Cox, & Drefs, 2008). An online preceptor course, with credentialing, also has been successfully accomplished (Phillips, 2006). In areas where preceptors are not available (very small workplaces, remote geographic areas, or organizations with preceptor burnout), a national web site could be designed to connect preceptors, through a remote interface, to novice nurses. This innovative approach has been successfully implemented in Scotland's Flying Start program (2010) and could provide new nurses with opportunities for feedback, reflection, and support even when preceptors are not geographically available.

Once a national transition model is implemented and all nurses are precepted, it is expected that the culture of nursing will change. Nurses will see precepting as an important part of their role, and it is anticipated that facilities will no longer experience "preceptor burnout," or a shortage of available preceptors.

Length of the Transition to Practice Program

While the time period for the preceptorship will be six months, the preceptor, having been trained, will be able to evaluate how much support the new graduate needs during the preceptorship. Some novice nurses will need more support than others.

Evidence for Best Practices: How Long Do I Need for My Transition to Practice?

After all the research is reviewed and discussed, the question becomes how long should transition to practice programs be for new graduates? The answer needs to be discussed with regard to cost, research, existing structure for building preceptor relationships with mentees, and developing a professional identity (Kovner & Djukic, 2009). The likelihood of turnover, or having a nurse leave a position within the first two years, is lower in hospitals that have transition to practice programs (Beecroft et al., 2001; Halfer et al., 2008; Pine & Tart, 2007; Williams et al., 2007). So the best evidence shows that at least six months to one year is ideal. However, three months is better than no transition.

In an NCSBN study (2007a) of newly licensed nurses (with variable types of transition and/or orientation programs), researchers found that the three- to six-month period after hire was the most vulnerable time for new graduates because they perceived the most stress and the least competence, most likely because they were beginning to practice independently. In the UHC/AACN study of their yearlong residency program (Williams et al., 2007), investigators found that while stress decreased over the yearlong residency program, both control over practice and satisfaction measures started high, dipped at six months, and then increased. The authors believe this is because during the first six months in practice, many new nurses have specialty classes and might feel overwhelmed by the amount they must learn. This would be similar to the phenomenon of reality shock that Kramer (1974) described. Because of this evidence and because a regulatory program should reflect minimum requirements, it was decided that an effective transition program should last at least six months, with institutional support for one year. Interestingly, even in programs that are less than one year in length (Beecroft et al., 2001; VNIP 2010), project directors often indicate continued support after the program ended, and in some cases the preceptorships continued.

Formalized support systems should be built into the last six months of the new nurse's transition program, and the NCSBN has devised strategies for assisting employers to support newly licensed nurses during their second six months in practice. Johnstone, Kanitsaki, and Currie (2008), from Australia, have written extensively on providing support to new graduates. They define support as "a process that aids, encourages, and strengthens and thereby gives courage and confidence to a new graduate nurse or a group of new graduates to practice competently, safely, and effectively in the levels and areas they have been educationally prepared to work" (p. 53). Some of the components of support, according to Johnstone and colleagues (2008), include being available and approachable; being able to ask questions without being ridiculed; being prompted to engage in best practices; providing benevolent surveillance, which is keeping an eye on the new graduate; providing constructive feedback and reflection; and having backup when there are problems.

Putting It All Together

If there were consensus within the nursing community to implement a regulatory model for transitioning new graduates to practice, that model could incorporate the evidence-based best practices that were presented earlier in this chapter. The TTP model shown in Figure 3-1 was designed to be flexible, so there are many different ways of implementing it, depending on the organization, area of the country, type of setting, availability of preceptors, and other factors. For example, a large urban medical center might want to partner with a local nursing program to develop its transition program. In a small rural community hospital, new graduates might use a national web site for connecting to preceptors and delivery of the modules. Both institutions would meet the criteria

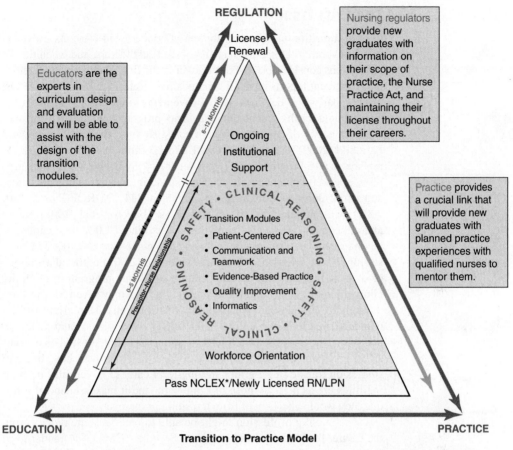

REGULATION

Nursing regulators provide new graduates with information on their scope of practice, the Nurse Practice Act, and maintaining their license throughout their careers.

Educators are the experts in curriculum design and evaluation and will be able to assist with the design of the transition modules.

License Renewal

Ongoing Institutional Support

CLINICAL REASONING • SAFETY

Transition Modules

- Patient-Centered Care
- Communication and Teamwork
- Evidence-Based Practice
- Quality Improvement
- Informatics

Practice provides a crucial link that will provide new graduates with planned practice experiences with qualified nurses to mentor them.

Workforce Orientation

Pass NCLEX*/Newly Licensed RN/LPN

EDUCATION

PRACTICE

Transition to Practice Model

Figure 3-1 Education, practice, and regulation are the three cornerstones of the NCSBN's Transition to Practice Model.

set forth in the model, but how they accomplished that would be very different. Similarly, the model has been designed to be robust; that is, it will include all levels of prelicensure education, from practical nurse education through baccalaureate education. All patients deserve a nurse who has been effectively transitioned to the nursing role.

A Collaboratively Designed Model

The TTP model was a collaboratively designed model whereby NCSBN committee members sought informal feedback from boards of nursing, as well as formal responses at NCSBN's midyear and annual meetings. Additionally NCSBN collaborated with more than 35 nursing organizations and stakeholders, with committee members presenting the model to the organizations and listening to their concerns and suggestions.

The Cost Issue

Cost of transition programs is an area of concern and warrants consideration. Several of the reports have addressed cost factors, and when the organizations consider the cost of turnover in the first year of practice, return on investment reports have all been positive. Return on investment (ROI) is a comparison of net financial improvements to the cost of the program. The formula for this calculation equals net program benefits (i.e., consider turnover costs) divided by program costs. Kovner, Brewer, Greene, and Fairchild (2009) report that it costs 1.2 to 1.3 times the one-year salary to replace an RN. Program costs (Keller et al., 2006) include staff, office supplies, speakers, photocopying, journal subscriptions, refreshments, texts, and so on. One study looking at ROI found an 884.75% ROI (Pine & Tart, 2007), while another found an ROI of 67.3% (Beecroft et al., 2001). Keller and colleagues (2006) estimated that it cost them $1,000 per resident in the internship program, while replacing one nurse cost $60,000. The Mississippi Nurse Residency Program (monw.org 2008) reported a savings of over $4 million with their six-month residency program through the elimination of agency and travel nurses. Further, they saved $1.1 million through decreased turnover. Similarly, the Children's Memorial Hospital (Chicago) yearlong residency (Halfer, 2007) saved that hospital $707,608 per year. The Transition to Practice Committee found no studies of transition programs that reported a negative ROI. While there have been no studies on transition programs in long-term care, turnover rates in these facilities are as high as those in acute care, and it makes financial sense that they would also benefit from transition programs.

The nursing profession might be able to receive some money from the Center for Medicare and Medicaid Services (CMS) if a standardized national program to transition new nurses to practice is designed that is inclusive of all new nursing graduates, or that the TTP model is adopted for all institutions. As mentioned earlier, other healthcare disciplines receive CMS funding for their standardized residency programs, so nursing should vie for this money as well. There may be other federal funding, at least for the beginning stages of designing and implementing this initiative. It is also important for the nursing profession to continue to analyze the costs of transition programs, and this is especially important in long-term care. Other options for paying for this program were suggested by business consultants and might include individual grants for start-up programs, charging each new nurse a fee, a healthcare service tax, providing continuing education credits to preceptors, or a hybrid of some of these ideas.

Next Steps

Because this is such a big step for nursing, NCSBN is studying the implementation of this model in three states: Illinois, North Carolina, and Ohio. The organization enlisted a national advisory panel of experts to plan and conduct a multisite, randomized study, and NCSBN is tracking outcome measures via an online data collection system. Further, NCSBN developed, with 15 experts in the field, five online, interactive modules for the new nurses and a training module for preceptors. There are separate modules for LPNs and RNs. NCSBN created an innovative web site where the new nurses and preceptors can take the modules and complete and submit their surveys. The new nurses can also have informal discussions with their preceptors or other new graduates. More information, including the timeline on this landmark study, can be found at www.ncsbn.org.

Implications for Educators

This chapter has presented the case for a postgraduate transition program for all newly licensed nurses. Educators, as has been emphasized throughout this chapter, should be an integral part of designing this program because if it is not collaboratively designed, it will not work.

But what can educators do to facilitate the transition to practice? Many already have designed excellent immersion courses, with preceptors, at the end of the program. This is highly recommended. Some worry about preceptor burnout if educational programs were to all have immersion programs at the same time that a standardized model was implemented. This would probably be the case for the first few years. However, as nurses become acclimated to being precepted in their first year of practice, they will see the importance of giving back and will themselves become preceptors. After a standardized preceptor model has been implemented for a few years, it is expected preceptors will be readily available.

Educators are strongly encouraged to develop practice partnerships where practitioners and educators can work together to design clinical and simulation experiences that foster a more seamless transition to practice. There is a movement now to transform clinical experiences from the oftentime randomness currently present to more focused learning experiences (Tanner, Gubrud-Howe, & Shores, 2008). Tanner and colleagues outline some new ways of delivering clinical education, including:

- Focused direct client care experience
- Concept-based experience
- Case-based experience
- Intervention skill-based experience
- Integrative experience

The Advisory Board Company (2008) has outlined some exemplars in clinical instruction where educators and practice partners have collaborated, and it has illustrated how partnerships have helped to design outstanding clinical experiences. The exemplars presented were in the following broad categories:

- Targeted clinical rotations
- Expert clinical instruction
- Exceptional student experiences

The Advisory Board Company, as previously noted, developed 36 mutually agreed upon competencies essential for safe and effective nursing practice (Berkow et al., 2008). To be included on the list, the competencies had to be specific, actionable, and reflective of current hospital demands. From this list, the competencies were identified by employers to be lacking in new graduates. While these particular competencies are best attained in an experiential program, such as a postgraduate transition program, educators certainly would want to introduce them into their curricula.

CHAPTER HIGHLIGHTS

- Safe, quality nursing care is promoted when a transition to practice (TTP) model is used.
- Data consistently documents the benefits of using TTP models.
- The NCSBN's TTP model can be applied and used in all healthcare settings.
- New nurse graduates face challenges during their first year of practice, especially at three to six months, when support may decline.
- Moral, legal, and ethical standards are important when using the transition to practice recommendations.

Pearson Nursing Student Resources

Find additional review materials at
nursing.pearsonhighered.com

Prepare for success with additional NCLEX®-style practice questions, interactive assignments and activities, web links, animations and videos, and more!

REFERENCES

Advisory Board Company. (2006). *Transitioning new graduates to hospital practice: Profiles of nurse residency program exemplars.* Washington, DC: Author.

Advisory Board Company. (2008). Bridging the preparation-practice gap: Volume II: Best practices for accelerating practice readiness of nursing students. Washington, DC: Author.

Aiken, L. H., Clarke, S. P., Sloane, D. M., Lake, E. T., & Cheney, T. (2008). Effects of hospital care environments on patient mortality and nurse outcomes. *Journal of Nursing Administration (JONA), 38*(5), 223–229.

Aiken, L. H. (2007). Study: Temporary nurses not a threat to quality. *Healthcare Benchmarks and Quality Improvement, 14*(11), 128–130.

American Association of State Colleges and Universities. (2006). Teacher induction programs: Trends and opportunities. *Policy Matters, 3*(10), 1–4. Retrieved from http://www.aascu.org/uploadedFiles/AASCU/Content/Root/PolicyAndAdvocacy/PolicyPublications/Teacher-Induction.pdf.

American Health Care Association. (2008). *Report of findings: 2007 AHCA survey nursing staff vacancy and turnover in nursing facilities.* Retrieved from http://www.ahcancal.org/research_data/staffing/Documents/Vacancy_Turnover_Survey2007.pdf

Ashcraft, A. S. (2004). Differentiating between pre-arrest and failure-to-rescue. *Medsurg Nursing, 13*(4), 211–216.

Auerbach, D. I., Buerhaus, P. I., & Staiger, D. O. (2011). Registered nurse supply grows faster than projected amid surge in new entrants ages 23–26. *Health Affairs, 30*(12), 2286–2292.

Bae, S., Mark, B. & Fried, B. (2010). Impact of nursing turnover on patient outcomes in hospitals. *Journal of Nursing Scholarship, 42*(1), 40–49.

Bae, S. H., Mark, B., & Fried, B. (2010). Use of temporary nurses and nurse and patient safety outcomes in acute hospital units. *Health Care Management Review, 35*(3), 333–344.

Barton, A. J., Armstrong, G., Preheim, G., Gelmon, S. B. & Andrus, L. C. (2009). A national Delphi to determine developmental progression of quality and safety competencies in nursing education. *Nursing Outlook, 57*, 313–322.

Beecroft, P. C., Dorey, F., & Wenten, M. (2008). Turnover intention in new graduate nurses: A multivariate analysis. *Journal of Advanced Nursing, 62*(1), 41–52.

Beecroft, P. C., Kunzman, L., & Krozek, C. (2001). RN internship: Outcomes of a one-year pilot program. *JONA, 31*(12), 575–582.

Benner, P. (2004). Using the Dreyfus model of skill acquisition to describe and interpret skill acquisition and clinical judgment in nursing practice and education. *Bulletin of Science, Technology & Society. 24*(3), 188–199.

Benner, P., Sutphen, M., Leonard, V., & Day, L. (2010). *Educating nurses: A call for radical transformation.* San Francisco: Jossey-Bass.

Berens, M. J. (2000). Dangerous care: Nurses' hidden role in medical error. September 10. P. 17 *Chicago Tribune.*

Berkow, S., Virkstis, K., Stewart, J., & Conway, L. (2008). Assessing new graduate nurse performance. *JONA, 38*(11), 468–474.

Beyea, S. C., Slattery, M. J., & von Reyn, L. (2010). Outcomes of a simulation-based residency program. *Clinical Simulation in Nursing, 6*(5), 169–175.

Beyea, S. C., von Reyn, L., & Slattery, M. J. (2007). A nurse residency program for competency development using patient simulation. *Journal for Nurses in Staff Development, 23*(2), 77–82.

Bishop, T. F., Ryan, A. K., & Casalino, L. P. (2011). Paid malpractice claims for adverse events in inpatient and outpatient settings. *Journal of the American Medical Association 305*(23), 2427–2431.

Bjørk, I. T., & Kirkevold, M. (1999). Issues in nurses' practical skill development in the clinical setting. *Journal of Nursing Quality Care, 14*(1), 72–84.

Board of Registration in Nursing, Division of Health Professions Licensure, Massachusetts Department of Public Health. (2007). *A study to identify evidence-based strategies for the prevention of nursing errors.* MA: Author.

Clarke, S. P., & Cheung, R. B. (2008). The nursing shortage: Where we stand and where we're going. *Nursing Management, 39*(3), 22–28.

Classen, D. C., Resar, R., Griffin, F., Federico, R., Frankel, T., Kimmel, N., et al. (2011). "Global trigger tool" shows that adverse events in hospitals may be ten times greater than previously measured. *Health Affairs, 30*(4), 581–589.

Cronenwett, L., Sherwood, G., Barnsteiner, J., Disch, J., Johnson, J., Mitchell, P., et al. (2007). Quality and safety education for nurses. *Nursing Outlook, 55*, 122, 131.

Del Bueno, D. (2005). A crisis in critical thinking. *Nursing Education Perspectives, 26*(5), 278–282.

Dracup, K., & Morris, P. E. (2007). Nursing residency programs: Preparing for the next shift. *American Journal of Critical Care, 16*(4), 328–330.

Ebright, P., Urden, L., Patterson, E. S., & Chalko, B. A. (2004). Themes surrounding novice nurse near-miss and adverse event situations. *Journal of Nursing Administration, 34*(11), 531–538.

Elfering, A., Semmer, N. K., & Grebner, S. (2006). Work stress and patient safety: observer-rated work stressors as predictors of characteristics of safety-related events reported by young nurses. *Ergonomics, 49*(5–6), 457–469.

Fink, R., Krugman, M., Casey, K., & Goode, C. (2008). The graduate nurse experience: Qualitative residency program outcomes. *JONA, 38*(7–8), 341–348.

Flying Start. (2010). Retrieved from http://www.flyingstart.scot.nhs.uk/.

Goode, C. J., Lynn, M. R., Krsek, C., & Bednash, G. D. (2009). Nurse residency programs: An essential requirement for nursing. *Nursing Economics, 27*(3), 142–147.

Greiner, A. C., & Knebel, E. (Eds.). (2003). *Health professions education: A bridge to quality.* Washington, DC: National Academies Press.

Halfer, D. (2007). A magnetic strategy for new graduate nurses. *Nursing Economics, 25*(1), 6–11.

Halfer, D., Graf, E., & Sullivan, C. (2008). The organizational impact of a new graduate pediatric mentoring program. *Nursing Economics, 26*(4), 243–249.

U.S. Department of Health and Human Services (HHS). (2010). *Adverse events in hospitals: National incidence among Medicare beneficiaries.* Washington, DC: Author.

Hofler, L. D. (2008). Nursing education and transition to the work environment: A synthesis of national reports. *Journal of Nursing Education, 47*(1), 5–12.

Institute of Medicine (IOM). (2006). *Preventing medication errors: Quality chasm series.* Washington, DC: National Academies Press.

Institute of Medicine (IOM). (2010). The future of nursing: Leading change, advancing health. Retrieved from http://www.iom.edu/Reports/2010/The-Future-of-Nursing-Leading-Change-Advancing-Health.aspx

Institute of Medicine (IOM). (2012). *Health IT and patient safety: Building safer systems for better care.* Washington, DC: National Academies Press.

Johnstone, M. J., & Kanitsaki, O. (2006). Processes influencing the development of graduate nurse capabilities in clinical risk management: An Australian study. *Quality Management in Health Care, 15*(4), 268–278.

Johnstone, M. J., Kanitsaki, O., & Currie, T. (2008). The nature and implications of support in graduate nurse transition programs: An Australian study. *Journal of Professional Nursing, 24*(1), 46–53.

Johnstone, M. J., & Kanitsaki, O. (2008). Patient safety and the integration of graduate nurses into effective organizational clinical risk management systems and processes: An Australian study. Quality Management in Health Care, 17(2), 162–173.

Joint Commission. (2002). White paper: Health care at the crossroads: Strategies for addressing the evolving nursing crisis. Retrieved from http://www.jointcommission.org/assets/1/18/health_care_at_the_crossroads.pdf.

Kalisch, B. J. (2006). Missed nursing care: A qualitative study. Journal of Nursing Care Quality, 21(4), 306–313.

Keller, J. L., Meekins, K., & Summers, B. L. (2006). Pearls and pitfalls of a new graduate academic residency program. *JONA, 36*(12), 589–598.

Kentucky Board of Nursing. (2010). Retrieved 2/12 from http://kbn.ky.gov/education/pon/entry/

Kohn, L., Corrigan, J., & Donaldson, M. (Eds.). (1999). *To err is human: Building a safer health system.* Washington DC: National Academies Press.

Kovner, C. T., Brewer, C. S., Greene, W., & Fairchild, S. (2009). Understanding new registered nurses' intent to stay at their jobs. *Nursing Economics, 27*(2), 81–98.

Kovner, C., & Djukic, M. (2009). The nursing career process through the first 2 years of employment. *Journal of Professional Nursing, 25*(4), 197–203.

Kramer, M. (1974). *Reality shock: Why nurses leave nursing.* Saint Louis: CV Mosby Company.

McKay, C. A., & Crippen, L. (2008). Collaboration through clinical integration. *Nursing Administration, 32*(2), 109–116.

Mississippi Office of Nursing Workforce (MONW). (2010). Retrieved from http://www.monw.org 2/12.

My Inner View. (2008). *2008 national survey of consumer and workforce satisfaction in nursing homes.* Retrieved from http://www.ahcancal.org/research_data/staffing/Documents/MIVConsumerWorkforceSatisfaction2008.pdf.

Nadkarni, V. M., Larkin, G. L., Peberdy, M. A., Carey, S. M., Kaye, W., Mancini, M. E., et al. (2006). First documented rhythm and clinical outcome from in-hospital cardiac arrest among children and adults. *JAMA, 295*(1), 50–57.

NCSBN. (2002). *Report of findings from the 2001 employers survey*. Chicago: Author.

NCSBN. (2003). *Report of findings from the practice and professional issues survey: Spring 2002*. Chicago: Author.

NCSBN. (2004). *Report of findings from the 2003 employers survey*. Chicago: Author.

NCSBN. (2005). Working with others: A position paper. Retrieved from https://www.ncsbn.org/Working_with_Others.pdf.

NCSBN. (2006a). Evidence-based nursing education for regulation (EBNER). Chicago: Author.

NCSBN. (2006b). *A national survey on elements of nursing education*. Chicago: Author.

NCSBN. (2006c). *Transition to practice: Newly licensed registered nurse (RN) and licensed/vocational nurse (LPN/VN) activities*. Chicago: Author.

NCSBN. (2007a). *The impact of transition experience on practice of newly licensed registered nurse*. Retrieved from https://www.ncsbn.org/1603.htm.

NCSBN. (2007b). *NCSBN's analysis of Nursys® disciplinary Ddata from 1996–2006*. Chicago: Author.

NCSBN. (2009a). *Post-entry competence study*. Retrieved from https://www.ncsbn.org/09_PostEntryCompetenceStudy_Vol38_WEB_final_081909.pdf.

NCSBN. (2009b). *2008 RN practice analysis: Linking the NCLEX®RN examination to practice*. Retrieved from https://www.ncsbn.org/08_Linking_the_NCLEX_to_Practice_Vol36.pdf.

Nicol, P., & Young, M. (2007). Sail training: An innovative approach to graduate nurse preceptor development. *Journal for Nurses in Staff Development, 23*(6), 298–302.

O'Rourke, M. W. (2006). Beyond rhetoric to role accountability: A practical and professional model of practice. *Nurse Leader*, June, 28–44.

Orsolini-Hain, L., & Malone, R. E. (2007). Examining the impending gap in clinical nursing expertise. *Policy, Politics, & Nursing Practice, 8*(3), 158–169.

Phillips, J. M. (2006). Preparing preceptors through online education. *Journal for Nurses in Staff Development, 22*(3), 150–156.

Pine, R., & Tart, K. (2007). Return on investment: Benefits and challenges of a baccalaureate nurse residency program. *Nursing Economics, 25*(1), 13–18.

Roxburgh, M., Lauder, W., Topping, K., Holland, K., Johnson, M., & Watson, R. (2010). Early findings from an evaluation of a post-registration staff development programme: The Flying Start NHS Initiative in Scotland, UK. *Nurse Education in Practice, 10*(2), 76 81.

Sackett, D. L., Straus, S., Richardson, S., Rosenberg, W., & Haynes, R. B. (2000). *Evidence based medicine: How to practice and teach EBM* (2nd ed.). London: Churchill Livingstone.

Scott, E. S., Engelke, M. K., & Swanson, M. (2008). New graduate transitioning: Necessary or nice? *Applied Nursing Research, 21*, 75–83.

Spector, N., & Echternacht, M. (2010). A regulatory model for transitioning newly licensed nurses to practice. *Journal of Nursing Regulation, 1*(2), 18–25.

Tanner, C. A., Gubrud-Howe, P., & Shores, L. (2008). The Oregon Consortium for Nursing Education: A response to the nursing shortage. *Policy, Politics and Nursing Practice, 9*(3), 203–209.

Technology Informatics Guiding Educational Reform (TIGER). (2010). *The TIGER Initiative*. Retrieved from http://www.tigersummit.com/Home_Page.php.

Townsend, L. B. (1931). Teaching the classes following the physician's lecture. *American Journal of Nursing, 31*(10), 1183–1186.

Vermont Nurse Internship Program (VNIP). (2010). Retrieved from http://www.vnip.org/. www.aacn.nche.edu

Wiggins, M. (2006). The partnership care delivery model. *JONA, 36*(7–8), 341–345.

Williams, C. A., Goode, C. J., Krsek, C., Bednash, G. D., & Lynn, M. R. (2007). Postbaccalaureate nurse residency 1-year outcomes. *Journal of Nursing Administration, 37*(7–8), 357–365.

Wisconsin Nurse Residency Program (WNRP). (2008). Retrieved from http://wnrp.org/.

Wisconsin Nurse Residency Program (WNRP). (2010). Retrieved from http://wnrp.org/.

Yonge, O., Hagler, P., Cox, C., & Drefs, S. (2008). Listening to preceptors. *Journal for Nurses in Staff Development, 24*(1), 21–26.

POWER, EMPOWERMENT, AND CHANGE

Paula N. Kagan

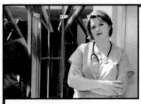

CHAPTER 4

Elena Elisseeva/Shutterstock.com

Kate, a staff nurse who has practiced for four years, has started work on a new medical–surgical unit on evening shift. She observes certain nurses giving limited report during the change of shift and assumes that they are in a rush to get home. Kate also notes that many 3 p.m. scheduled medications are not documented as administered. She has had to call nurses at home three or four times a week to make sure the medications were given. The nurses are often very irritated with her calls.

When Kate discusses the issue with her head nurse, he states that this has always been a problem and that Kate should remind the nurses to chart their medication administration before they leave. Kate has a few other ideas that may make it easier for the nurses to remember to chart medications and report off to the evening nurses with more thorough information. She presents a new flow chart reporting sheet based on SBAR, the communication tool using **S**ituation, **B**ackground, **A**ssessment, and **R**ecommendation, to the head nurse. The head nurse laughs and says, "Good luck with that!" Kate is frustrated and unsure how to progress.

CORE COMPETENCY

Analyze power structures in healthcare settings, society, and the healthcare system in the United States.

LEARNING OUTCOMES

1. Describe power in nursing and health care.
2. Determine how power dynamics form the basis of decision making affecting nursing and health outcomes.

3. Apply principles of change and emancipatory practice to specific safety issues.

Nurses' primary concern is for the well-being, safety, and care of patients. However, many nurses find a strong dissonance between what motivated them to enter the profession of nursing and what they encounter in the typical workplace, which for most nurses is the hospital. Future-focused nurses should consider more comprehensive care models focused on community and population health promotion.

Most care continues to be provided in hospitals despite research that indicates the public would enjoy better outcomes if the locus of health care moved away from biomedicine—where health care focuses on disease, cure, high-technology intervention, and the acute care setting—and into the community (Guidry, Vischi, Han, Raymond, & Passons, 2010). Still, most nurses find jobs in hospitals, and it is there that their values are challenged and safety and quality are at risk. Understanding how morbidity, mortality, nursing satisfaction (vitality, turnover, retention), and patient satisfaction and expectations influence patient safety and quality care is essential for understanding the relationship between power and safety in the context of nursing practice. (See Table 4-1 for definitions of power and other key concepts used in this chapter.)

Nurse educators have to begin teaching nurses in school and in the workforce that it is right to question established organizations for their motives and institutionalization of policy that interferes with safety and quality. While there are hospital practices, policies, and procedures that govern nursing care, they are neither derived nor evaluated from theoretically sophisticated and novel forms of nursing knowledge, in other words, from the experts on nursing care and patient safety, nurses. Methods for research and practice that employ emancipatory frameworks for care and analysis of power are required if substantial changes are to be made to reduce risk as well as enhance the safety and quality of health care for patients. To realize actual change, all interested parties must welcome such analysis. Nurses will be required to learn how to resist frameworks influencing practice that do not support the nursing agenda to enhance safety and quality of care and actively push for the changes informed by their expertise and knowledge from the discipline.

This chapter offers a path to developing a philosophical and theoretical foundation from which nursing students will be able to create practical plans and actions for improving safety and quality based on their values, expertise, and experience. The overarching learning goal is to provide a framework for analyzing power and understanding ways of self-empowerment to create and sustain change within the work setting for the betterment of nurses and their patients. Nurses can create change that enhances safety and quality of care in the hospital by looking at several philosophical and material perspectives to assist them in understanding the difficulty inherent

TABLE 4-1 ■ Definitions of Key Concepts

Power	A complex social process that constrains or enables human action; energy to accomplish tasks, objectives, to move forward through life; the ability to influence others and the environment
Power Dynamics	The social processes and results arising from power differences between people, communities, institutions, or nations based on relative levels and qualities of gender, class, race or ethnicity, and sexuality
Emancipation	Freedom and liberation, outside or beyond the often socially accepted dominance and power of others
Activism	Activity with the intention of creating and producing social change across all dimensions: personal, political, cultural, economic, social, environmental, and so on
Change	The process that creates different or new ways of social interaction, rituals, routines, beliefs, values, social status, and power dynamics
Empowerment	Advocating, educating, legislating, organizing, or otherwise enhancing the capability of persons and communities to choose and act on their behalf while lessening the power-over of others
Social Justice	The idea of equality and fairness in human endeavors; support and advocacy for universal basic human rights such as respect for diversity of gender, class, race or ethnicity, sexuality, multiculturalism, and access to food, shelter, sanitation, and health care
Diffusion of Innovation	How change and new ideas catch on and spread; how innovations are accepted
Praxis	The practice of social justice values and theory; professional practice that is explicitly guided and performed from social justice values and intentionally conducted for the good of persons and society
Resistance	Opposing or challenging the actions or ideas of others or institutions

Source: Contributor: Paula N. Kagan.

in moving large systems toward betterment for the health and well-being of patients. The theoretical foundations used to get to this end help to understand the key ingredient in making change happen: power.

Theoretical Foundations and Key Concepts

The theoretical basis for this chapter is derived from nursing paradigms that hold that humans are indivisible, ever-changing, unpredictable, and in mutual processes of health and quality of life with the environment and universe (Newman, Smith, Dexheimer-Pharris, & Jones, 2008; Parse, 1998; Rogers, 1970; Smith, 2002). Scholars in nursing who research and write on topics from emancipatory theoretical frameworks are significant because their work examines nursing practice and the commonly held notions of how health care is delivered, often suggesting possible routes to change. Critical social and critical feminist theories, postmodern and postcolonial discourses, and theories of change enhance the understanding of power and change as well as the relationship these concepts have to safety and quality.

Relevant literature from the nursing discipline specifically about power, empowerment, and change has emerged over the past two decades but is underutilized in the practice and education of most nurses. Examining this literature serves to strengthen awareness in the legitimacy of nursing values that support social justice, the enactment of nurses' professional autonomy and agency, and holistic care that enhances safety and quality, and to highlight what is needed to manifest those values in practice. Knowledge of power and change should be mandatory in nursing education and may increase the possibility that graduate nurses will understand and employ emancipatory approaches to the problems of safety and quality at the bedside, in research, and at policy and media levels.

Issues beyond the theoretical arise when considering power and empowerment for nurses and the potential for change in the workplace. Critical frameworks of thought encourage practice methods that can address and resolve "on-the-ground" nursing concerns about safety. However, in the hospital, nurses' autonomy and preferred practice methods are often obstructed, and hospitals may give various rationales for the subordinated way nurses are allowed to provide care and their expertise.

By obstructing empowerment and change, authorities outside of the discipline—or nurse managers who are unable to critically appraise nurses' workplace situations and therefore uphold the biomedical model of health care—impede nurses from practicing their ideological preference for holism and health promotion. A simple example is staffing and acuity models that override safety standards. If there is a budget concern, nurse positions may be cut and staffing levels raised to create a situation with unsafe, demanding care.

Safety should be at higher priority than budget. When nurses have too many patients to care for, each patient's care is less safe. Even though nurses know that they are not delivering the best and safest care, they hesitate to speak up or challenge administrators. Such impediments to nurses understanding and exerting power are fundamentally linked to safety and quality.

Other conditions that deter nurses from practicing according to their ideals are organizational constraints, lack of political activism, dominance of the medical business model, educational and social class differences within and outside of nursing, and assimilation by nurses of society's dominant discourses related to status, gender, and professional work (Falk-Rafael, 2005a). The quality of nurses' work environment, unfair management, and unwieldy organizational structure are just some of the issues that impact patient safety and quality of care.

Valuing Safety: Nurses' Professional Domain

Nurses have achieved many progressive accomplishments in health care. Nurses such as Nightingale, Wald, Dock, Sanger, and Ashley strove for emancipatory, political, and activist-driven change. Many contemporary nurses conduct research, build theory, and practice in activist and emancipatory ways that inspire and encourage other nurses toward empowerment and change. Today's nurses have a great capacity for innovation, change, and power to influence how health care is conducted and to strengthen safety and quality in all aspects of healthcare services.

Professional nurses value the healing, growth, and safety of individuals, families, and communities. They teach, comfort, advocate for, and provide emotional and physical monitoring and the intervention necessary to protect patients and promote health and healing. However, most nurses in the United States work in the industrial biomedical complex that is the healthcare system, which focuses on disease, intervention, cost containment, and often, the convenience of physician practice methods and administrators' supervisory concerns. Nurses are expected to execute the actual care and management of patients often without the decision-making power to implement strategies for care, particularly concerning safety and quality, according to their knowledge and expertise. To facilitate an examination of how nurses can function as agents of change, it is helpful to contrast the industrial biomedical complex that is the healthcare industry with the professional domain of the nurse, from which safety and quality naturally arise from the values that nurses hold.

While safety and quality of care is the domain of nursing, nurses sometimes face risks involved with speaking up and risks that stem from a silent nurse workforce. Cultural perceptions of nurses also contribute to the problem of lack of power and the difficulty nurses have in advocating for sustained change.

Relevance of Power, Empowerment, and Change to Safety and Quality

Since nurses' specific professional objective is the health, safety, and healing of individuals, families, and communities, it is therefore imperative that they be involved in the formation and oversight of safety and quality processes. Nursing's professional scope is not oriented to disease and cure, although those domains are part of nurses' purview. Nurses' specific expertise and knowledge base, while including medical and scientific knowledge, is always consistent with safety, quality, advocacy, and healing. As the model of business stands in most hospitals today, nurses do not have professional agency to freely enact their values, knowledge, and free will in the caring situations in which they find themselves every day. They live with and are complicit in compromised safety and quality as they adhere to external expectations, demands, and objectives that shape staffing ratios, decision making, documentation, and, most centrally, how nurses provide care.

The healthcare industry—more appropriately called an industrial complex because it concerns multiple business interests well beyond health care itself—has not adequately responded to research focused on improving safety. Health promotion and educating patients about taking charge of health are more beneficial approaches (Guidry et al., 2010; Kagan, Smith, Cowling, & Chinn, 2010). This point is important because it is precisely in the community and in homes that the core of nursing, the disciplinary art and science, can be implemented to the satisfaction of nurse professionals and the public. While the core of biomedicine is pathology and intervention is emphasized in acute care settings at the time of illness or crisis, the core of nursing holds the premise that each person or family is an integral whole, that is, a complex, dynamic ever-changing process of life to which respect and dignity are due. Personalized, nonroutinized care is an essential part of the core of nursing. Health promotion, education, and advocacy are key features to this core. Nurses have always been the most trusted of professionals, and this stems from the nurse's concern for not only what is *done* to patients but also *how* it is done and their acknowledgement that the quality of care and quality of life during and after medical intervention is of utmost importance.

This community-based health promotion model leaves room for nurses who enjoy acute care, critical care, and the hospital setting. The problem is that while the hospital remains the dominant healthcare setting, the art and science of nursing as well as the safety and quality of care available to patients is continually at risk and often compromised by system flaws or shortcomings and infrastructure that hospitals have created and strive to sustain (Aiken, Xue, Clarke, & Sloane, 2007).

"We're All Here for the Good of the Patient": What Is at Stake?

Kagan and Chinn (2010) discussed the public perception, and that of many health professionals, that hospitals are built for the good of the patient. However, some of the procedure and policy orientation of such settings is detrimental to continually enhanced safety and quality. Several examples that occur commonly are the inadequate ratio of registered professional nurses to patients, the inadequate screening for nosocomial infections, the growing cesarean birth rate in the United States—nearing 35% in 2008, which is up from 4% in 1965—and the distinct lack of nurses in high-ranking power positions who have the capacity to influence decision making and policy development. Hospitals have competing stakeholders with competing agendas, ranging from teaching medical students and residents and conducting biomedical research to providing income venues for physicians, administrators, suppliers, and myriad other businesses to … finally … providing patient care. Of the many hospital and regulatory organizations, both public and private, only a few represent safety and quality from nursing perspectives—that is, those perspectives that consider the whole

Evidence for Best Practices: Nurse-to-Patient Ratios

Does having one fewer patient per shift really influence nursing care? The California Nurses Association (CNA) has been a strong advocate for safe nurse-to-patient ratios. The CNA has pushed hard with lobbying and intense political activism, and in 2004 they were successful as the first state to mandate minimum nurse-to-patient staff requirements.

Aiken and colleagues reported in 2010 how nurse workloads, compared across states, affect patient and nurse outcomes. On average, California nurses cared for one fewer intensive care patient per shift than in other states and two fewer patients on medical and surgical units. The nurses' better evaluations of work environment were in California. In California, Pennsylvania, and New Jersey, nurses reported reasonable workloads. All of those states had workloads similar to California. Inpatient mortality over 30 days was lower, and the complaints from patients were lower in hospitals with lower patient ratios.

The progress toward safe ratios came out of much organizing and tireless work of nurses and their organizations. So to answer the question, yes, it appears that having even one fewer patient can have a dramatic effect on patient outcomes and nurses' satisfaction in their work and environment.

person and family and what is truly best for them, a holistic approach where the patient comes first before anyone else's agenda and goals.

While the Joint Commission and the American Hospital Association assess and provide policy and accreditation guidelines for safe delivery of health care in hospitals, nurses need to question the social-political investment and motivation within these organizations. Accreditation is for oversight of safety and quality, and as such hospitals are constantly playing catch-up as investigations bring to light the ever-present threat of adverse events as well as the actual events contributing to injury and death. Staffing ratio issues seem to be chronically underappreciated by administrators based on current standards criteria and common hospital practices despite research that suggests a correlation. (See Evidence for Best Practices: Nurse-to-Patient Ratios.) In other words, unsafe conditions are not addressed as urgent. In addition to inadequate professional nurse staffing, lack of detection of and intervention related to Methicillin-resistant *Staphylococcus aureus* (MRSA) and *Clostridium difficile* (C diff), diagnostic and interventional radiation errors, lack of facilities and staff for urgent care, and medical errors of all sorts are just some of the chronic issues leading patients to injury or death.

Among these myriad policy and procedural standards and the extant power structure present in the acute care setting, the professional nurse strives to use nursing agency to implement nursing knowledge and expertise to effect change in the health and quality of life for patients and families. This is exceptionally difficult given this context. Nurses are not entirely or even substantively in control of their professional decisions and actions. Hascup (2003), in a letter to the editor, reminded scholars of the harsh reality of working bedside nurses who speak up: They are often punished and stigmatized by nursing leadership and management. This is problematic in terms of patient safety and quality of care. Nurses who question high-risk conditions or suggest risk reduction that may be contrary to overall hospital business objectives may be put in their place and reminded that "We're *all* here for the good of the patient," implying that the nurses' concerns are petty, insignificant, and at worst selfish. Nurses who question such conditions repeatedly may be stereotyped, sidelined, passed over for promotion, or limited in their scope of influence or practice.

Hospitals Exist to Provide Nursing Care

Underlying all of this is the fact that hospitals exist predominately to provide nursing care in 24/7 fashion, yet the current infrastructure of hospitals supports the dominance of physicians, who provide the limited realm that is medical intervention, and of administrators, who are caretakers for the corporation. It is the physicians whose agency is freely enacted and the administrators' policies and procedures that not so much guide as direct nurses work. The very fact that nurses do not have "attending" status and still, in the twenty-first century, respond and adhere to "doctors' orders" reflects their second-tier status. This status continues unabated despite strides in gender equality and demonstration through research that it is nursing care, not medical intervention, that is foundational to persons getting better and healing (Aiken, Smith, & Lake, 1994).

Attending nurses have been suggested as a means of making visible the distinction between the discipline and professional purview of nursing and that of medicine. Attending status grants the legitimacy that recognizes the significant and essential contribution that nursing makes to the industrial biomedical complex. It means patients would be assigned or offered a choice of nurses as they are offered or assigned doctors. Nurses would manage all aspects of patient care, as they now do, but would have the recognition of this reality. Nurses would work on par as colleagues with doctors to determine the plan of care and intervention based on the holistic approaches favored by most nurses and patients rather than the biomedical approaches that have left both patients and nurses on the margins.

The surgeon may spend several hours on a difficult and highly technological procedure; however, it is nurses who prepare patients prior to surgery, monitor them in recovery, and care for them until they can be discharged. Nurses teach, comfort, advocate for patients, and provide emotional and physical monitoring and the intervention necessary to protect patients and promote health and healing. This is not to denigrate the importance of medical knowledge or skills, but it is time to stop the maintenance of a power structure that privileges one professional domain over another.

The stratification of professional domains and the dominance of nurses' time by tasks mandated by those with "power over" have an impact on more than social status. They influence experiences and outcomes for patients. They also influence whose voice is heard and who is at the table to provide input for policy on safety and quality as well as for infrastructure changes that are badly needed to improve safety and quality.

These ideas lead to a fundamental question: Why does nursing care in most hospitals *not* resemble the proposed care actions and outcomes acknowledged in research to enhance safety and quality? Consider how nursing activity might look if underpinned by nursing philosophy and theory and by the findings of studies that examine workplace conditions and resultant morbidity and mortality (Aiken, Clarke, Sloane, Sochalski, & Silber, 2002; Aiken, et al., 1994).

Another way to enhance the understanding of power and change along with the relationship these concepts have with safety and quality is to explore how employers, physicians, and the media perceive nurses. In media and society nurses are often misunderstood and objectified as representations of service or sexuality rather than expert professionals valued for their knowledge and skills. Repeatedly, in news stories and on television shows, doctors are given heroic status and credited for actions that are really performed by nurses (Kalisch, Kalisch, & Clinton, 1982; Kalisch & Kalisch, 1986). Additionally, the services provided by physicians are acknowledged as separate line items on a patient's bill, while nursing services are hidden, rolled into room charges, rendering their contribution invisible.

The power that nurses could have in supporting an enhanced agenda for safety and quality remains an illusive goal, discussed continually by nursing educators, administrators, and nurses but with little impact. One example is the decades-old discourse and lack of comprehensive implementation of the baccalaureate degree as the basic entry into professional nursing in the United States. Better educated nurses have been associated with lower morbidity and mortality rates in hospitals among other significant findings (Aiken, Clarke, Cheung, Sloane, & Silber, 2003). Better educated nurses are positioned to desire—and understand the meaning of—power and its association with safety, quality, and patient outcomes. Contributing to a disempowered nursing workforce is nurses' lack of understanding of power and change as well as the practical guidelines to implement change.

Support for the preceding ideas can be found in the contributions to the scholarly literature of two nurse researchers who have significantly and substantively focused on empowerment, workforce quality, and improving healthcare delivery as discussed in the next section.

Nursing Research on Empowerment, Safety, and Quality: Aiken and Laschinger

Nurse researchers have studied multiple factors to determine which indicators are predictive of the presence of an empowered work environment, good quality of care, and a high degree of safety. For almost two decades, two researchers have added much of what is known to nursing literature on workforce determinants of nursing and patient satisfaction as well as quality and safety.

In the United States, Linda Aiken (Heede, Clarke, Sermeus, Vleugels, & Aiken, 2007; Scott, Sochalski, & Aiken, 1999) has studied variables pertaining to workplace characteristics such as those of Magnet hospitals and other organizational structures, Medicare mortality rates relevant to the quality of nursing care, and patient satisfaction with how care is structured. In 2002 and 2003 respectively, Aiken and her team found that morbidity and mortality increased for each patient added to a nurse's care and that the educational preparation of nurses at the baccalaureate level was associated with lower rates of mortality in postsurgical patients.

In Canada, Heather Laschinger (Laschinger, Sabiston & Kutszcher,1997; Laschinger & Sabiston, 2000; Laschinger, Almost & Tuer-Hodes, 2003; Laschinger & Finegan, 2005) led a team of researchers at the University of Western Ontario, testing and contributing to what is known about Rosabeth Moss Kanter's (1977) structural empowerment theory. The theory posits that notions of informal versus formal information and domains of information, support, resources, and opportunity can be useful to analyze workplace conditions of power and empowerment.

Laschinger and colleagues, in light of cost-cutting measures, discuss strategies for empowering nurses to act according to their knowledge and expertise. Cost-cutting measures tend to implement strategies that minimize the importance of professional nursing, promoting low morale, decreased job satisfaction, and increased stress. The authors link Magnet hospital characteristics with those in the framework of Rosabeth Moss Kanter's (1977) structural empowerment theory. The goal of the study was to identify factors that make work conditions attractive to nurses, leading to retention, satisfaction, and quality of care. Empowering work conditions and the Magnet hospital characteristics of autonomy, control over practice environment, and positive nurse-doctor relationships were predictive of job satisfaction and supported the creation of empowering work environments.

Motivated by such literature and hundreds of medication errors and unintended patient deaths, the IOM recommended in 2003 (IOM, 2003) a common safety report format that should be followed in all settings. The safety report categories include discovery of the problem, description of the event, and a narrative including contributing factors, ancillary information, causal analyses, and lessons learned. This report can be adapted to document any risk or breach to potential safety before a serious error occurs and results in injury or tragedy. Reported incidents can range from too few nursing staff to too many floaters to not enough certified nurse assistants (CNAs) to assist the professional nurse. Nurses should be encouraged to conduct a power analysis and safety report as a routine nursing intervention on a continual basis. When safety or quality breaches do come to light, nonpunitive approaches, such as educational approaches, are encouraged to revise policy and procedures that would enhance safety and quality of care. This will require a cultural shift in many hospitals in general and nursing units in particular.

Becoming familiar with and understanding the research of Aiken and Laschinger is essential to increasing awareness of workforce and work environment issues as well as research findings. Barrett (1983, 2010) suggested that awareness is fundamental to participating in and creating change. Chinn's (2008) *Peace and Power* processes are good methods to use to start manifesting the freedom to choose to become an empowered nurse in action. At the same time, it is also essential to examine and understand the emancipatory and activist ideas that underpin the research and praxis as presented in this chapter.

It is important for nurses to be able to engage in several consciousness-raising activities. First, they should be able to cite the research on how an empowered nurse workforce changes morbidity and mortality. Second, nurses should understand and discuss the theoretical and philosophical ideas behind praxis actions to identify and articulate change opportunities in one's work life. Finally, nurses should work toward such change.

Nurses on Power, Emancipation, and Activism

The stories of several significant nurse activists may stimulate student nurses as they develop their own praxis. Lillian Wald, Jo Ann Ashley, Elizabeth A. M. Barrett, and Peggy Chinn share characteristics of a life of activism recognized by a focus on emancipation, equality, scholarship, and engagement across disciplines and professions. In addition to the work of research groups led by Aiken and Laschinger, these four extraordinary nurses are exemplars of the efforts toward empowerment as well as emancipatory research and practice that reveal a path to quality and safety.

Lillian Wald

Lillian Wald (1867–1940) was an American nurse who founded the Visiting Nurse Service and, in 1893, the Henry Street Settlement in New York City. She coined the term "public health nurse" and was instrumental, along with close friends Lavinia Dock, Adelaide Nutting, Florence Kelley, and Annie Goodrich, in her unrelenting pursuit of equality for women and for enhanced health services for the disenfranchised (Daniels, 1989). Wald was also a close associate of Jane Addams, reformer, American Pragmatist, and founder of Hull House in Chicago. Motivated by the Jewish values of her upbringing—such as *tzdekah*, giving to others, and *tikun olam*, repair of the world—and her lifelong commitment to women's equality, Wald was involved in numerous initiatives and organizations having to do with not only nursing but women's suffrage, labor organizing, education, national public policy formation, and the peace movement. Critical to truly appreciating Wald's exceptional contributions to nursing, public health, and society is the reading of her two books, *The House on Henry Street* (1915) and *Windows on Henry Street* (1934), as well as Daniels' critical and analytic biographical work, *Always a Sister* (1989). Wald's advocacy for radically inclusive healthcare policy was a major contribution to healthcare quality.

Jo Ann Ashley

Jo Ann Ashley (1939–1980) was an American nurse scholar, feminist, and historian with very different beginnings than Wald. Though Ashley was born to a farming family in rural Kentucky, she came to share many of the same domains that Wald focused on such as the education, power, and autonomy of nurses; the health of the public; women's equality; and the politics of health care. Like Wald, Ashley read widely from philosophy, feminism, politics, poetry, literature, and social criticism and published in both the lay and professional press. Unfortunately, her life was shortened by breast cancer, and she died at barely 40 years of age. However, Ashley was relentless in her pursuit of telling the truth about the establishment of medicine and hospitals in the United States and the power dynamics that situated physicians at the top of a hierarchy in which nurses had to struggle for autonomy and recognition of their science, expertise, and contribution to health care. Ashley not only wrote constantly but also was often on television and interviewed for news articles after her foundational study, *Hospitals, Paternalism, and the Role of the Nurse*, was published in 1976 (Ashley, 1976).

Ashley's book unveiled the gender and class bias that is purposive and inherent in an American healthcare system dominated by medicine and acute care in hospitals rather than collaborative practices of public health served in community settings. She was adamant that nurses recognize their own power and act politically and critically to change the system. Reading essential to understanding Ashley includes *Hospitals, Paternalism, and the Role of the Nurse* (Ashley, 1976); *Jo Ann Ashley: Selected Writings* (Wolf, 1997), and *Jo Ann Ashley Thirty Years Later: Legacy for Practice* (Kagan, 2006). Table 4-2 (Kagan, 2006), contains direct quotations from Ashley's many works constructed along the domains Barrett (1983) delineated in her Power Theory, including the concepts of awareness, freedom, choice, and action that are also thematic in Ashley's work. The domain of creativity, while implied in Barrett's work, was added because Ashley often emphasized the need for creative re-visioning of nursing and healthcare practices. Ashley's insistence on individual and systemic change was a major contribution to patient safety and quality of care.

Peggy L. Chinn

Peggy Chinn, also an American, is a nurse scholar, theoretician, educator, and feminist activist whose international recognition and reputation speak to her ability to make quality in nursing practice and in health systems a central theme throughout her life's work to impact heath care. The substantial social justice and empowerment messages seen in her vast body of work have influenced countless nurses around the world and run parallel with her emphasis that nursing practice be underpinned with explicit professional philosophies based on values that nurses embrace. Chinn was instrumental in the late 1970s and early 1980s for her efforts in creating the nursing group Cassandra Radical Nurses Network (Kagan,

TABLE 4-2 ■ Ashley on Power: In Her Own Words

Awareness	"A main goal of nursing's quest for power must be that of changing society's attitudes toward members of the profession. To do this nurses themselves will require social re–education along with political sophistication" as well as " knowledge related to the modes and methods of effective political activism" (Wolf, 1975/1997, pp. 47–48). "We must break away from outmoded conceptual views … if we are to develop meaningful theories and new knowledge to guide the expanding horizons of our practice and our persons" (Wolf, 1977/1997, p. 247).
Freedom	"Power and its companion, freedom, are never given to oppressed groups. Power and freedom must always be taken. Conformity, blind cooperation and the lack of the questioning of established policies are never avenues to progress or to the attainment of freedom" (Wolf, 1975/1997, p. 38). "Paradoxically enough, the medical profession, of all groups in the health field, has not for even a moment underestimated the power of nursing. Physicians have successfully harnessed the power of nurses and used it to advance their own cause" (Wolf, 1973/1997, p. 32). "It cannot be repeated often enough that the very structure of hospital and institutional staffing in nursing has traditionally been economically and not professionally determined. As a result, nurses have been limited, restricted, and confined to narrow spheres of technical functioning. Too few nurses have questioned the nature of the limitations placed upon them" (Wolf, 1975/1997, p. 38).
Choice	"Many contend that mass conformity is one of the most difficult dilemmas facing all humans" (Wolf, 1975/1997, p. 61). "The time is ripe for nurses to re-examine what is morally right and morally wrong in the health field. Lack of power and freedom on the part of nurses is a moral problem of major proportion and should be viewed as such" and "members of the profession are responsible to society for what they do or do not contribute through their practice. Yet their right to assume overt responsibility for practice is still not a reality in many settings" (Wolf, 1975/1997, pp. 40–41).
Action	"While working for changes in the law, nurses must consider taking the action of moving their practice out of the present economic structures in control of delivering nursing care. This will mean the creation of new institutions and new modes of practice within nursing" and "see nurses owning and controlling nursing homes, and establishing nursing centers in communities, centers designed solely for the production of nursing care for citizens who need and want it" (Wolf, 1976/1997, p. 134). "A systematic approach to the collection, evaluation, and exchange of information and ideas could lead to more creative and more productive means of delivering nursing care. This type of activity might prove to be far more meaningful to nurses than the development of 'new role' for them. 'Old' roles within hospitals and elsewhere need to be made more viable and stimulating. If this can be done staff turnover might lessen to a considerable degree. It is a burden for a profession constantly to be developing new roles for members when the potential in old ones has hardly been realized" (Wolf, 1975/1997, pp. 48–49). "We need to foster the creation of 'rebels' in our midst—rebels who have insightful knowledge, vision, and a cause, rebels with the inner courage to fight for it openly. We need nurses who will fearlessly and repeatedly raise questions about their 'place' in established institutions and in society" (Wolf, 1975/1997, p. 50). "We nurses need to begin making astute observations about what is wrong with our society. We need to set our sights on correcting some, if not all, of these wrongs. We need to begin shaping ourselves and our destiny. We need to begin the slow and tedious process of creating a different kind of society, a society fit for humans to live freely with a minimum of psychological, social, and physical distress. We cannot eliminate all distress, but we should at least prevent distress which can easily be prevented by professional nursing care" (Wolf, 1975/1997, p. 71).

TABLE 4-2 ■ *(Continued)*

Creativity	"Creativity has not traditionally been the major goal of nursing education, and it has certainly not been a goal in practice settings. It is time, however, for educational programs to make creativity their main objective in teaching, practice, and research" (Wolf, 1980/1997, p. 201).
	"Professional growth and development for nurses has not been congruent with the economic aims and goals of [hospital] institutions. Technical (manual) competence and efficiency have been valued. The creative productivity of [*nursing* sic] professionals has not been" and "staffing at the least expensive [level] devalue(s) and exploits(s) the potential of nurses who could constructively improve delivery systems" (Wolf, 1975/1997, p. 37).
	"In this age of evil, we live in a society that worships science and technology. We need to grow into a society that more fully appreciates the art of being human … it is time a number of nurses at all levels of practice become concerned about the artistic side of nursing practice. I say this because it will be the nurse as artist who will develop concepts most relevant to the subject of what it means to be human" (Wolf, 1975/1997, p. 78).
	"We need to turn away from an exclusive praise of science and dwell on the meaning of art … art, and art alone, teaches one not to suppress, repress, or kill the feeling side of life—the side of life that is most human. More than ever before, society needs the nurse as artist, whether the nurse applies knowledge from the arts or engages in artistic creation" (Wolf, 1975/1997, p. 78).

Reprinted and adapted with permission. Kagan, P. N. (2006) Jo Ann Ashley 30 years later: Legacy for practice. *Nursing Science Quarterly, 19*, pp. 317–327.

2009), whose news journal published quarterly between 1982 and 1989. For many nurses, this news journal was their only link to feminist and emancipatory ideas along with the colleagues who shared them. Today, that legacy continues online through a web-based initiative known as the Nurse Manifest Project (www.nursemanifest.com). A close friend and teaching colleague of Ashley, Chinn wrote the well-known book *Peace and Power: Creative Leadership for Building Community* (2012), now in its 8th edition, and together with Maeona Kramer, wrote the equally well-known *Integrated Theory and Knowledge Development in Nursing* (2010), a staple of many nursing theory courses. *Peace and Power* is an excellent best practice guideline to transformative and emancipatory group dynamics and should be required at all levels of nursing education and practice. *Peace and Power* considers how to engage in peaceful group dynamics. The book explores conflict resolution, building solidarity, praxis and integrity, rotating leadership, values-based decision making, critical reflection, conflict transformation, and communication. Chinn also identifies practical ways in which individuals and groups can use a peaceful power, not to control others or engage in greed but to encourage peace, diversity, and positive change. Chinn's dedication to the intersections of feminism, peace, and nursing is an invaluable contribution to quality and safety.

Elizabeth A. M. Barrett

A contemporary of Chinn and Ashley, Elizabeth A. M. Barrett is an internationally known nurse theorist who studied with Martha Rogers (1970), who developed the Science of Unitary Human Beings (SUHB). In 1983,

Barrett published her own theory (founded on the principles of SUHB) known as the Power Theory, which defines power as the capacity to knowingly participate in change. Barrett delineated four domains that underscore how humans create and live change in their lives. These domains are awareness, freedom, choice, and action. Barrett developed the Power to Knowingly Participate in Change Tool (PKPCT), an instrument that measures—through a series of questions representative of each domain—the level of power a person experiences and perceives in life. The tool is beneficial to use with people in health care contexts as a means of recognizing one's pattern of living awareness, freedom, choice, and action; in other words, living change. Barriers to creating desired change in life and health are illuminated during dialogue through the process of discussing a person's power score on the instrument. Change can then occur toward enhanced health and quality of life. In an update on her theory in 2010, Barrett contends that she wished to:

> derive a Rogerian theory of power that would be useful to nurses in understanding people and their worlds. This required embracing the acausal worldview, meaning a world that does not operate by the laws of cause and effect. I quickly learned that this meant I would need to be willing to buck the conventional system in healthcare, in nursing, and to some extent in all of life in the material world (p. 47).

Barrett's theorizing around power, as the capacity to knowingly participate in change, is a major contributor to quality and safety in nursing.

Other Nursing Scholars on the Topic of Power

Other nursing scholars have also contributed to this dialogue and have addressed the themes of privilege, discrimination, power, and change.

Falk-Rafael (2005a, 2005b) wrote in support of critical caring as an expansion of empowered caring. She argued that nurses practice at the intersection of public policy and personal lives, and she demonstrated the significance of links between social and economic inequalities and health inequities. Falk-Rafael identified four sources of positive power that nurses could utilize to "speak truth to power": credentials and credibility, association and alliances, research and knowledge development, and expertise and experience. Falk-Rafael also supported sociopolitical action as part of nursing history, a moral imperative, and a demonstration of caring.

Relevant to Falk-Rafael, Beagan and Ells (2009) conducted qualitative interviews to investigate nurses' moral experiences and also found that systemic challenges interfered with nurses' goals of enacting their values. Such challenges included professional hierarchies, organizational structures, infrastructure issues in the healthcare system, and power dynamics.

From 1990 to 2009, several other authors provided concept analyses on power, empowerment, and emancipation. Hawks (1991) provided an early examination of power that explicated definitions and meanings of the concepts "power over" and "power to." Underpinned by goal attainment theory, Hawks defined power as the ability to achieve goals within collaborative and mutual interpersonal relationships. Similarly, Koberg, Boss, Senjem, & Goodman (1999) considered the antecedents and outcomes of empowerment and used a variety of instruments (questionnaires) to examine which variables influence healthcare workers' perception of empowerment. Their study looked at personal characteristics, work group characteristics, and personal position in the workplace hierarchy. They concluded that persons feel empowered with increased tenure, an approachable leader, when their work group is valued by others and is effective, and when they hold a favorable position in the hierarchy of the organization. In addition, a concept analysis of emancipation in decision making (Wittmann-Price, 2004) was performed from critical social theory and feminist theory perspectives. The goal of this concept analysis was to apply the concept of emancipation to women making health decisions and to nurses' professional development. Findings from that concept analysis showed that antecedent to emancipation is oppression, and the defining attributes of emancipation emerged as empowerment, personal knowledge, social norms, reflection, and flexible environment. Finally, Du Plat-Jones (1999) conducted a literature review considering power and representation. Du Plat-Jones found consistency in the literature to support the idea that within the hierarchy of health care, empowerment and representation for both nurses and patients are obstructed. She suggests nurses use established codes of professional conduct to support the legitimacy of their professional knowledge and expertise in order to empower their advocacy and representation of patients and themselves.

Other nursing scholars have engaged in discussions of workplace and organizational power and empowerment issues. Kuokkanen and Leino-Kilpi (2000) and Kuokkanen and Katajisto (2003) used critical social theory, organization theory, and social psychological theory to explore how well the concept of empowerment could be used as a framework for nurses' professional development. They determined that given the myriad definitions and uses of the term, linkages to specific philosophical frameworks were necessary to enhance the value and utility of empowerment to frame nursing research and professional development. Zurmehly, Martin, and Fitzpatrick (2009) investigated the organizational characteristics that were conducive to nurses' empowerment. They found a correlation between empowered nurses and professional retention that is linked with high quality nursing care. They found that organizational characteristics such as availability of opportunity, support, information, resources, and nurses having formal as well as informal power were essential to an empowered nurse work force. Cornett and O'Rourke (2009) looked at organizational capacity and characteristics that enhance safety and quality in the workplace. The authors argue that utilization of professional models of practice helps identify purview and role of professionals such as nurses, provides support for their particular work, and ensures high quality care and safety.

Lastly, Knol and van Linge (2009), in their cross-sectional correlational study in the Netherlands, found a significant correlation between nurses' structural and psychological empowerment and their capacity for innovation. They suggest that workplaces establish and support conditions that empower nurses so that innovation that enhances healthcare delivery can occur.

Theory, Philosophy, and Safety: What Is the Link?

Although much is known and understood about power and change in nursing and across disciplines, such content is lacking in most nursing education. Nursing is not practiced atheoretically, meaning without any theoretical or philosophical foundation. The problem is that nurses often do not explicitly identify and articulate why they practice the way they do, from what standpoint.

To promote safer and higher quality care and care settings, nurses need to identify their values, the philosophical support for those values, and the consequences to patients of nurses being allowed to practice from those perspectives. That is how safety and quality will be achieved in hospitals. Table 4-3 presents theories that are consistent with empowerment and emancipation in nursing along with a short review of theories and philosophies that may help in understanding change and power from emancipatory perspectives that are relevant to nursing's goal of enhanced safety and quality. These theoretical propositions increase the understanding of power, knowledge, and change in the clinical setting. The table was developed by nurse scholars Kagan, Smith, Cowling, and Chinn (2010), who examined a web-based manifesto (www.nursemanifest .com) of nursing ideas that spoke to emancipatory nursing and activism. Table 4-3 summarizes the theoretical and philosophical foundations that emerged from their analysis of the manifesto, its core ideas, and relevant quotes from the manifesto itself that reflect values that embrace safety and quality of patient care as primary concerns of nursing practice, and more generally, health care.

To help bridge the connections between theory/philosophy and safety/quality, several concepts should be remembered about nursing. Nursing is a discipline that is a basic science, meaning scholars conduct research about the nature, conduct, and consequences of nurses' practice, and nursing has a practice application that can have a variety of philosophical underpinnings. For the purposes of emancipatory nursing practice, the premise is that safety and quality depend on nurses' ability to practice according to their values in holistic and humanistic ways. Practice based on such principles, as opposed to those of the biomedical model, takes into account the whole person, including the person's perspective on his or her own situation, and treats each person with respect and dignity, providing uniquely individualized and nonroutinized care to each person.

TABLE 4-3 ■ Ideas Influencing the Nursing Manifesto

Philosophies and Theories	Relevant Core Ideas, Values, and Worldviews	Illustrative Statements from Manifesto
Postmodern/Poststructural: Characterized by reacting to and transcending rigid thought forms, ideologies, and conventions that oppress creative emergence. Postmodernism may encompass reshaping traditional elements abandoned by the empirical, rationalist restrictions imposed in the modern era. Analysis of the social construction of institutions, values, rituals, and habitual ideas.	**Consciousness-raising:** Recognizing the limits of constructed practices and traditions, and reaching for new models and practices.	We call forth a repudiation of patterns that we create, or that are imposed upon us, that inhibit the full expression of our beings as nurses and persons. We call forth the passion of practicing nursing from [a] state of sovereignty and rightfully claim governance of our discipline.
Postcolonial: Analysis of power and domination of one group by another geographically, bodily, culturally, by language or political means. The critique of how power over designated "less-than" others is created, maintained, accommodated, resisted, and disrupted. The claiming of a distinctive identity that has been demeaned, subjugated, or co-opted by a more powerful group.	**Global-ecological:** Acknowledgement of the interconnectedness of persons from countries around the world and the interdependence of persons and our environment. **Diversity and inclusivity:** Values difference of all kinds (race, ethnicity, age, gender, class, physical ability, sexual identity) as important and enriching for any society.	We are opposed to colonization; that is, we do not wish to impose our views onto others. Our concern covers the world, and we seek to embrace a global perspective. We can no longer consider our values and actions out of the context of all beings. [Concerns about] persistent racism, sexism, classism, heterosexism, and hosts of other "isms" that prevail in nursing and health care, undermining our sensitivities to the fundamental humanness and value of all people everywhere.
Critical Theory/Feminist Theory: Recognizes knowledge as created within a social-political context and shaped by power dynamics. Values equality and subjugated (nondominant) ways of being and knowing. Support of [such] knowing is characterized by self-reflection, critique, emancipation, and the unity of knowing and doing. Consciousness raising, shared power/authority, and action are essential components of knowledge development. Feminist critique guarantees gender and experiences of women are included in content and methods.	**Participatory:** Recognizes that humans are cocreators of their lives. It unifies knower and known, and observer and observed. **Consciousness-raising and community building:** Approach to change through education, participation, and relationships.	The situation we find ourselves in has been created from an array of forces. While economic issues have helped create a situation in which nurses cannot practice nursing, we, as nurses, have participated by remaining silent. We are calling for nurses who share our concerns to join in collective consciousness-raising and action based on chosen values. We realize we can rely on each other as we seek conscience-based action to shape a new future for nursing and for health care.

(continued)

TABLE 4-3 ■ (Continued)

Philosophies and Theories	Relevant Core Ideas, Values, and Worldviews	Illustrative Statements from Manifesto
American pragmatism: Emphasizes the importance of experience, reflection, lifelong learning, and the relationship of theory to practice. The form that theoretical application takes to practice is intentionally acting to better society and the human condition, that is, praxis. Concern for democracy, education, nonhierarchical interpersonal and social structures. Challenges empiric-analytic positivist stances.	**Audacious optimism:** Belief in the goodness, creativity, and strength of human beings and our collective ability to solve problems and make a better world. Implement deliberate hope projects.	We believe that it is possible to find connection in the midst of alienation, to find inspiration in the midst of cynicism, to find nourishment and meaning in the midst of spiritual impoverishment, to find hope in the midst of despair, to find wholeness in the midst of fragmentation, to find peace in the midst of violence, to find enrichment in the midst of economic idolatry, and to find sovereignty in the midst of constraints.
Disciplinary foundations of nursing: Discourse that defines nursing as a distinct professional discipline, a field of study with the application/generation of knowledge in nursing practice.	**Caring:** Foundational knowledge and ethic for nursing that focuses loving, valuing, and nurturing self and others.	It is our firm conviction that there is a body of knowledge that is specific, if not unique, to nursing's concerns and interests. We think that this knowledge is grounded in appreciation of wholeness, concern for human well-being, and ways in which we accommodate healing through the art and science of nursing.
Unitary-Transformative Paradigm: A nursing paradigm that acknowledges the irreducible wholeness, connectedness of persons and environment, and the continuous and evolutionary process of health and healing.	**Holism:** Philosophy focusing on whole person wellness and the innate human potential for health and healing, consistent with Nightingale's perspective that nursing's role is to facilitate the natural emergence of healing. **Values and conscience-driven ethics based social justice:** Philosophy that deeply held convictions, discovered through self-reflection, guide actions toward the good for individuals and equality and justice for all.	We seek to recognize, appreciate, celebrate, and exploit this individual and universal wholeness in order to create health. The idol of the current healthcare system is symbolized by achieving measurable outcomes in an economically feasible manner in the shortest amount of time, at the expense and depletion of even more valuable resources such as caring, understanding, real human connections, and spiritual and physical renewal.

Reprinted and adapted with permission from Wiley-Blackwell Publishers. Kagan, P. N., Cowling, W. R., Smith, M., & Chinn, P. L. (2010). A nursing manifesto: An emancipatory call for knowledge development, conscience and praxis. *Nursing Philosophy, 11*, pp. 67–84.

Essential Theoretical Readings for Change Agents and Emancipatory Practice

Several authors outside of nursing have influenced how nurses think about power, empowerment, oppression, and emancipation. A good place to begin is with the writings of feminist scholar Patricia Hill Collins (1998, 2000, 2004, 2006, and with Anderson, 2007), critical race theorist bell hooks (1994, 1995, 2000), and other Black feminist scholars who in the 1960s initiated and established a way of analyzing social and cultural patterns, systems, and experiences that came to be known as *intersection-ality*. The anthology titled *Still Brave: The Evolution of Black Women's Studies* (James, Foster & Guy-Sheftall, 2009) offers a twenty-fifth anniversary revised edition of the foundational volume of early writings on intersectionality, *All the Women Are White, All the Blacks Are Men: But Some of Us Are Brave* (Hull, Scott, & Smith, 1982). Intersectionality offers a framework of analysis for examining interlocking systems of power and domination in social and cultural relationships at the interpersonal, community, corporate and nation-identity levels. Intersectionality posits that all intolerances and socially unjust systems, beliefs, rituals, habits, and behaviors are connected in the way persons experience prejudicial treatment and limited opportunity. Poor health and general life outcomes arise from interlocking systems of oppression, such as racism, classism, and homophobia. For the black women scholars who developed it, intersectionality was a way to understand how color and racism, gender and misogyny, poverty and classism, and being lesbian/queer and homophobia and heterosexism operate together to oppress. That is, racism, misogyny, classism, and homophobia do not operate in vacuums in isolation from one another. Intersectionality as a means to understanding challenges to safety and quality and practice derived from nursing values can lead nurses to a variety of choices and actions that they may not have otherwise known possible.

Intersectionality is especially relevant to nursing because it is congruent with professional codes such as that of the International Council of Nurses Statement on Human Rights (International Council of Nurses, 2011) that support equality, respect, and dignity for all persons as well as healthcare access as a human right with accountability and good outcomes. Discrimination and intolerance based on personal or group characteristics are anathema. People stay away from healthcare institutions and providers if they risk embarrassment, hatred, hostility, or harassment due to their gender, color, class, sexual orientation, or not having insurance. In addition to missing out on early detection and intervention, many people from marginalized groups receive fewer or inappropriate options for diagnoses and treatment. There is no safe care or quality of care in the presence of intolerance.

Reading nurse authors and their interpretations or applications of authors outside of nursing is helpful in informing and connecting nursing practice with the work of scholars across disciplines. A significant nursing scholar, Joan Anderson (Anderson & McCann, 2002), in one of numerous articles aimed at transformation and emancipation, explored post-colonial discourse and black feminist scholarship to suggest a methodology for nursing research and practice. Anderson stated that post-colonial feminist scholarship takes into account marginalized voices and experiences necessary to transform health care through the emergence of "transformative knowledge that guides transformative action" (p. 23); of points of departure of intellectual discourse from the dominant and traditional to perspectives of the silenced and hidden; of health systems based on the full range of human social locations; and of nursing's embrace of its social obligation toward social justice in theory and practice.

Michel Foucault (1994/1973), an influential French philosopher who examined and theorized about power relationships, is widely known for his work on power in medicine and clinical practice particularly in his book, *The Birth of the Clinic: An Archeology of Medical Perception.* Foucault used historical and theoretical methods to examine how social, political, and cultural ideas have influenced the history of medical knowledge.

Peter, Lunardi, and Macfarlane (2004) use the work of Foucault, who examined power relationships and feminist ethics, ethics specifically concerned with care, social justice, and emancipation, to evaluate empirical studies that show how nurses can challenge their feelings of powerlessness and ethical compromise through acts of resistance. Nurses can exercise positive power and resistance by acting on, and responding to, their concerns when framed as ethical issues. The authors also identify the backlash or counter-resistance that nurses who act on ethical concerns risk receiving, and argue that individual and systematic changes need to occur to prevent this in the future. Fahy (2002) wrote about women's empowerment using Foucault's concepts of disciplinary power, the power/knowledge construct, and the medical "gaze" among others. Cheek and Porter (1997) reviewed Foucault and offer a dialogue of scholarly difference between the two authors of the usefulness and relevance of Foucault's theory to nursing research and to health care.

Paolo Freire (2006/1970) wrote what for many is the handbook on praxis, *Pedagogy of the Oppressed*, in which he argued that education has the potential to promote either conformity to or change against oppressive economic, social, and political structures. Freire wrote in part from his experience of working with rural and urban, working and middle class people. He encouraged a critical consciousness and radicalization of teaching, research, and of creating change through community organization, input, and action not from institutional or establishment authority, but rather from the "grassroots." He also discussed community-based challenges to oppression through reflection and action toward transformation and enhancement of the human condition and the world.

Freire is a common foundation for several nurse scholars. Harden (1996) employed Freire's (2006/1970) model of education to support a more critical pedagogy within nursing, and demonstrated the serious necessity of promoting emancipation in nursing. A predominately women's field such as nursing that does not have required coursework in women's and gender studies is a key factor in the maintenance of health care that is unsafe, unsystematic, and biomedically dominated. There is presently not a focus on primary care and health promotion, which would lead to a consideration of family and community health and ultimately transformative and emancipatory nursing. Nurses in general have no framework to analyze their complicity with taking and implementing "doctors orders," practicing solely from medical model perspectives, and allowing themselves to be managed by those who do not have the very best interests of patients and nurses as their primary concern. Chinn (2012) also explicated Freire's concepts as congruent to the application of her *Peace and Power* processes, specifically in the definition of praxis as thoughtful reflection and action toward transformation and enhancement of the human condition and the condition or health of the world.

Putting It All Together: Praxis

In Table 4-1, praxis was defined as "professional practice that is explicitly guided and performed from social justice values and intentionally conducted for the good of persons and society." Power was defined as "a complex social process that constrains or enables human action." It is possible for nurses to marshal their power to make their professional practice one of *praxis* as opposed to just doing their jobs and feeling frustrated, unempowered, and immobilized. Initiating and implementing change can enhance the safety and quality of the workplace, and nurses

---

BOX 4-1   PRAXIS FOR CHANGE AGENTS

- Knowingly participate in change.
- Choose to practice emancipatory nursing.
- Recognize your moral obligation to praxis (see ICN Code of Ethics and Statement on Human Rights).
- Perform a self-power analysis. Perform a power analysis of your workplace.
- Practice calculated risk taking.
- SPEAK UP: Learn the art of considerate interruption.
- Find a mentor.
- Form coalitions with like-minded others at work. Start a proposal-writing group.
- Attend graduate school or further your certification—embrace lifelong learning.
- Read widely about health reform from critical perspectives, about nursing theory and philosophy, and about theory and philosophy across disciplines.
- Read liberation literature and that of oppressed and marginalized persons.
- Network widely throughout your workplace, within and outside your department.
- Join professional organizations and organizations focused on social justice.
- Network outside of nursing and the hospital to share your progressive and emancipatory view of nursing and health care.
- Change jobs when needed.

BOX 4-2   POWER ANALYSIS, RISK ASSESSMENT, AND BUILDING A NETWORK

It is important to conduct a self-evaluation of how power works in your own life. What are the policies, unspoken rules of conduct, or systems that structure your workplace? Who are the people that are dominant, and who is in more subordinate roles? Where are you in this schema? This is the *power analysis*. Write a list or create a table considering the ways you have experienced privilege, prejudice, and discrimination in your life. Utilize your new knowledge of intersectionality and consider the domains of gender, sexuality, race and ethnicity, social economic class, disability, age, and nation to organize your analysis. Consider your childhood as well as teenage or adult years, and note how some areas change over time. Specifically, recall times or events when you spoke up or made your ideas known even in the face of resistance to those ideas. Though a personal topic on some levels, discussing this with classmates and in class may be beneficial. Now, make a table that illustrates you in relation to your work and the people who you work with or who are influential to how your work is accomplished. In addition, identify areas of safety or quality in your workplace that you think need change.

At the same time, evaluate the types and level of risk if you choose to voice an unpopular or, as of yet unvoiced, idea. This is the *risk assessment*. You will want to be politically smart, be able to assess situations and people, build alliances with those who have obvious power (formal and informal power), and build a network of support. Find a mentor who is inclined toward social justice goals, respect for patients, and for nursing knowledge and expertise. Finding someone who has more formal power in the institution than you and establishing rapport is essential for moving new ideas forward and protecting yourself. Talk to your colleagues and form coalitions of like-minded people so that the possibility is strong that ideas for change can be formulated as a group and presented as such. Join committees such as the policy or governance committee at your hospital. Get to know as many people as you can at every level and in as many departments as possible.

EMBRACE LIFELONG LEARNING, EXCELLENCE, AND EXPERTISE

Further, establish yourself as a competent, knowledgeable, and skillful nursing professional. Obtain more education and credentials for two reasons: the most important is that for each educational experience in which you participate, you will develop in ways you cannot imagine, strengthening your knowledge, sense of self, and powers of analysis. The second reason to obtain more education and credentials is because those with formal power tend to respect formalized badges of experience and knowledge, even though there are informal ways that people learn and acquire expertise. Another reason to become educated at the graduate level is to be able to work in positions of formal power within the workplace and have a more viable chance to create change.

In addition, you want to read widely about change and power across disciplines, as mentioned earlier, and specifically how nurses have increased safety and quality across healthcare settings. Becoming aware of the theory and methodologies of emancipatory inquiry and action will assist you in speaking about the changes you wish to see take place. Take the ideas you have and write a two- to four-page proposal that consists of an introduction, a statement on the problem, why it is important (significance), statistics or demographics that illustrate the frequency and distribution of the problem, and your proposed solution that includes a timeline, and if needed, a budget. Be sure to include all the collaborators and stakeholders that are important to making the change happen. Take your proposal to your mentor and colleagues who are in management positions and work with them to create the change you want.

Be patient and realize that even the smallest change may take years or may be dismissed by administrators and/or peers. Keep going and remember, not every setting is right for every nurse. Sometimes the best change and contribution to safety and quality in health care is changing where you contribute, where you work. Working outside of hospital settings can also make a difference, and wherever you work, joining political and professional organizations is a must for the support you give to them and for the support you as a member can gain by being affiliated with a large network of nurses or others who also seek change.

can follow guidelines for putting their ideas to work to make this happen (see Box 4-1). The concept that nurses can be empowered by something or someone else is a myth. For the nurse to be empowered, the nurse has to understand and exercise his or her own power.

Systematic change is important and begins as personal change. The processes for power analysis and risk assessment are essential to create change. Keep in mind the dimensions of change specified by Barrett (2010) as knowingly participating in change were awareness, freedom, choice, and action. These concepts dovetail with Chinn and Kramer's (2010) ideas of praxis as the process of emancipatory knowing, which is becoming aware of injustice and underlying causes, choosing to create change, understanding one's power to act, and taking action.

Prepare Yourself

The goal of any nurse should be to become a nurse whose practice is emancipatory, based on social justice principles, and lived as action toward those principles, otherwise known as *praxis*. The difficult part for many nurses is realizing that they have the freedom to choose from myriad options. Many assume that the way things are conducted is the only way. The first step is to have resolve and intellectually and emotionally prepare for a commitment to promote change. Nurses have a moral obligation to actively analyze for unjust, unsafe, and poor quality health care and to act to correct the weaknesses in the system that they identify (International Council of Nurses, 2011). The first priority is to identify issues that affect quality and safety in the workplace, know the research, and understand the theory of the discipline of nursing.

Accessing and asserting freedom and choosing options that move the workplace toward safety, quality, and change is not without risk. Conducting a personal risk assessment can help nurses decide what kind and how much risk can be tolerated. One part of risk assessment is the willingness to walk away from a job, lose friends and colleagues, sustain a reprimand, and receive a cold shoulder, loss of anonymity, or disregard and silencing. Before choosing to act, nurses must understand the potential for risk and their ability to tolerate the repercussions of actions, should there be any. On the other hand, the response to nurses' voiced ideas could be overwhelmingly positive and welcome, and the nurses who spoke up and took action could become successful and sought after change agents.

Synthesis: Summary and Further Considerations

As nurses consider the concepts of power, empowerment, and change, they must think about their own power and ability to choose intentional action so that their practice becomes one of praxis, the goal of emancipatory nursing as described by Chinn and Kramer (2010). The disparity

CASE STUDY: *Nadine*

Nadine is a registered nurse with a BSN who has practiced for four years, two years in a critical care setting and two years in a community health center. She finds that the community practice allows her to engage in more patient teaching, support, and advocacy. Intuitively, Nadine understands the important role a professional nurse can have for people and families outside the hospital setting. She begins to feel a new urgency to change. This urgency was a result of the trends in health she observed during her community practice in different patient populations, as well as the social and political questions regarding patient resources that arose at the community center.

Nadine decides to seek out one of her professors from the BSN program who emphasized social justice and critical perspectives. This professor stood out to her because she recommended readings and films that spoke to the many ethical and policy related issues in nursing. The professor had emphasized personal power, professional networking, involvement in nursing associations and committees, and continuing higher education. Nadine did not think she was ready to do this when she was in school, but doing so made some sense to her now as she realized she was ready to take the next steps in her professional life. Nadine's professor also had emphasized that the more education Nadine had, the greater her knowledge, skills, and influence could be at multiple levels of health policy, law, and clinical decision making.

Within five years Nadine had a doctorate and was a nurse practitioner. She presided over the Policy Committee of the Nurses Association, participating with a group of nurses in researching and writing policy position papers that created the basis for healthcare legislation. Surprising herself, and going beyond her expectations, Nadine also published articles and spoke at conferences around the world regarding issues of quality of care and power. She also consulted on critical care and medical-surgical units on ways to enhance safety and quality by ensuring that nurses learn to utilize nursing science and theoretical perspectives to frame their practice methodology. Nadine also trained nurses to conduct power analyses of their practice and environment in order to change outcome patterns. In a short period of time, Nadine went from having a job in nursing to establishing herself as a sought-after educator, policy maker, and consultant on nursing practice that embraces safety, quality, and social justice.

between professional practice derived from nursing's core values and that derived from the biomedical and technologically driven practice expected of nurses in most hospital settings leads to an overall gap in addressing safety and quality from nursing perspectives. This leads to frustration and despair on the part of many nurses who may be immobilized by the challenge of creating change. To address this lack of capacity, theoretical perspectives can promote social justice goals and emancipatory practice methods. Readings within the discipline of nursing and across other disciplines can enhance nurses' knowledge of power, emancipation, and intersectionality. Ultimately, nurses are responsible for moving toward the changes they wish to accomplish in order to improve safety and quality in the hospital, as depicted in Box 4-2.

CHAPTER HIGHLIGHTS

- Many critical nurse feminists have paved the way for nurses to become more autonomous and powerful.

- The power structure and administrative structure in the healthcare setting affect all who work in the setting. Nurses need to be aware of the structure of the healthcare setting in their workplace and beyond.

- Nurses need to develop the vision for change and apply emancipatory practice principles to safety issues in their workplace to ensure the safe delivery of care.

- All healthcare providers should remain aware of political and ethical issues affecting their practice and develop a plan for lifelong learning.

Pearson Nursing Student Resources

Find additional review materials at
nursing.pearsonhighered.com

Prepare for success with additional NCLEX®-style practice questions, interactive assignments and activities, web links, animations and videos, and more!

REFERENCES

Aiken, L. H., Clarke, S. P., Cheung, R. B., Sloane, D. M., & Silber, J. H. (2003). Educational levels of hospital nurses and surgical patient mortality. *Journal of the American Medical Association, 290*(12), 1617–1623.

Aiken, L. H., Clarke, S. P., Sloane D. M., Sochalski, J., & Silber, J. (2002). Hospital nurse staffing and patient mortality, nurse burnout, and job dissatisfaction. *Journal of the American Medical Association, 288*(16), 1987–1993.

Aiken, L. H., Sloane, D. M., Cimiotti, J. P., Clarke, S. P., Flynn, L., Seago, J. A., Spetz, J., & Smith, H. L. (2010). Implications of the California nurse staffing mandate for other states. Health Research and Educational Trust. Doi: 10.1111/j.1475-6773.2010.01114.x

Aiken, L. H., Smith, H. L., & Lake, E. T. (1994). Lower Medicare mortality among a set of hospitals known for good nursing care. *Medical Care, 32*(8), 771–787.

Aiken, L. H., Xue, Y., Clarke, S. P., & Sloane, D. M. (2007). Supplemental nurse staffing in hospitals and quality of care. *Journal of Nursing Administration,* 37(7), 335–342.

Anderson, J. M. & McCann E. K. (2002). Toward a post-colonial feminist methodology in nursing research: Exploring the convergence of post-colonial and Black feminist scholarship. *Nurse Researcher 9*(3), 7–27.

Ashley, J. A. (1976). *Hospitals, paternalism, and the role of the nurse.* New York: Teacher's College Press.

Barrett, E. A. M. (1983). *An empirical investigation of Martha E. Rogers' principle of helicy: The relationship between human field motion and power.* Unpublished doctoral dissertation, New York University, New York.

Barrett, E. A. M. (2010). Power as knowing participation in change: What's new and what's next. *Nursing Science Quarterly, 23*(1), 47–54.

Beagan, B., & Ells, C. (2009). Values that matter, barriers that interfere: The struggle of Canadian nurses to enact their values. *Canadian Journal of Nursing Research, 41*(1), 86–107.

Cheek, J. & Porter, S. (1997). Reviewing Foucault: Possibilities and problems for nursing and health care. *Nursing Inquiry* 4(2), 108–119.

Chinn, P. L. (2012). *Peace and power: Creative leadership for building community* (8th ed.). Sudbury, MA: Jones & Bartlett.

Chinn, P. L., & Kramer, M. K. (2010). *Integrated theory and knowledge development in nursing* (8th ed.). Philadelphia: Mosby.

Collins, P. H. (1998). *Fighting words: Black women and the search for justice*. Minneapolis: University of Minnesota Press.

Collins, P. H. (2000). *Black feminist thought: Knowledge, consciousness, and the politics of empowerment* (2nd ed.). New York: Routledge.

Collins, P. H. (2004). *Black sexual politics: African Americans, gender, and the new racism.* New York: Routledge.

Collins, P. H. (2006). *From black power to hip hop: Essays on racism, nationalism, and feminism.* Philadelphia: Temple University Press.

Collins, P. H., & Anderson, M. (Eds.). (2007). *Race, class, and gender: An anthology* (6th ed.). Belmont, CA: Wadsworth Publishing.

Cornett, P. A., & O'Rourke, M. W. (2009). Building organizational capacity for a healthy work environment through role-based professional practice. *Critical Care Nursing Quarterly, 32*(3), 208–220.

Daniels, D. G. (1989). *Always a sister: The feminism of Lillian D. Wald.* New York: Feminist Press at the City University of New York.

Du Plat-Jones, J. D. (1999). Power and representation in nursing: A literature review. *Nursing Standard, 13*(49), 39–42.

Fahy, K. (2002). Reflecting on practice to theorize empowerment for women: Using Foucault's concepts. *Australian College of Midwives Incorporated 15*(1), 5–13.

Falk-Rafael, A. (2005a). Advancing nursing theory through theory-guided practice: The emergence of a critical caring perspective. *Advances in Nursing Science, 28*(1), 38–49.

Falk-Rafael, A. (2005b). Speaking truth to power: Nursing's legacy and moral imperative. *Advances in Nursing Sciences, 28*(3), 212–223.

Foucault, M. (1994/1973). *The birth of the clinic: An archaeology of medical perception.* New York: Vintage Books.

Freire, P. (2006/1970). *Pedagogy of the oppressed.* New York: Continuum.

Guidry, M., Vischi, T., Han, R. & Passons, O. (2010). *Healthy people in healthy communities: A community planning guide using.*

Harden, J. (1996). Enlightenment, empowerment, and emancipation: The case for critical pedagogy in nurse education. *Nurse Education Today, 16*, 32–37.

Hascup, V. A. (2003). Organizational silence: The threat to nurse empowerment. *Journal of Nursing Administration, 33*(11), 562.

Hawks, J. H. (1991). Power: A concept analysis. *Journal of Advanced Nursing, 16*, 754–762.

Heede, K. V. d.; Clarke, S.P.; Sermeus, W.; Vleugels, A.; & Aiken, L.H. (2007). International experts' perspectives on the state of the nurse staffing and patient outcomes literature. *Journal of Nursing Scholarship 39*(4), 290–297.

Hooks, b. (1994). *Teaching to transgress: Education as the practice of freedom.* New York, NY: Routledge.

Hooks, b. (1995). *Killing rage: Ending racism.* New York: H. Holt and Co.

Hooks, b. (2000). *Feminist theory: From margin to center* (2nd ed.). Cambridge, MA: South End Press.

Hull, G. T., Scott, P. B., & Smith, B. (Eds.). (1982). *All the women are white, all the blacks are men, but some of us are brave: Black women's studies.* New York: Feminist Press at the City University of New York.

International Council of Nurses. (2011). *The ICN position statement on nurses and human rights.* Geneva, Switzerland: Retrieved from http://www.icn.ch /policy.htm

James, S. M., Foster, F. S., & Guy-Sheftall, B. (Eds.). (2009). *Still brave: The evolution of black women's studies.* New York: Feminist Press at the City University of New York.

Kagan, P. N. (2006). Jo Ann Ashley 30 years later: Legacy for practice. *Nursing Science Quarterly, 19*, 317–327.

Kagan, P. N. (2009). Historical voices of resistance: Crossing boundaries to praxis through documentary filmmaking for the public. ANS. *Advances In Nursing Science* 32(1):19–32.

Kagan, P. N., & Chinn, P. L. (2010). We're all here for the good of the patient: A dialogue on power. *Nursing Science Quarterly, 23*(1), 41–46.

Kagan, P. N., Smith, M. C., Cowling, W. R., & Chinn, P. L. (2010). A nursing manifesto: An emancipatory call for knowledge development, conscience, and praxis. *Nursing Philosophy, 11*, 67–84.

Kalisch, P. A., & Kalisch, B. J. (1986). A comparative analysis of nurse and physician characters in the entertainment media. *Journal of Advanced Nursing, 11*, 179–195.

Kalisch, P. A., Kalisch, B. J., & Clinton, J. (1982). The world of nursing on prime time television: 1950 to 1980. *Nursing Resources, 31*, 358–363.

Kanter, R. M. (1977). *Men and women of the corporation.* New York: Basic Books.

Knol, J., & van Linge, R. V. (2009). Innovative behavior: The effect of structural and psychological empowerment on nurses. *Journal of Advanced Nursing, 65*(2), 359–370.

Koberg, C. S., Boss, R. W., Senjem, J. C., & Goodman, E. A. (1999). Antecedents and outcomes of empowerment: empirical evidence from the health care industry. *Group and Organizational Management, 24*(1), 71–91.

Kuokkanen, L., & Katajisto, J. (2003). Promoting or impeding empowerment? nurses' assessments of their work environment. *Journal of Nursing Administration, 33*(4), 209–215.

Kuokkanen, L., & Leino–Kilpi, H. (2000). Power and empowerment in nursing: Three theoretical approaches. *Journal of Advanced Nursing, 31*(1), 235–241.

Laschinger, H. K. S., Almost, J., & Tuer-Hodes, D. (2003). Workplace empowerment and Magnet hospital characteristics: Making the link. *Journal of Nursing Administration, 33*(7), 410–422.

Laschinger, H. K. S., & Finegan, J. (2005). Using empowerment to build trust and respect in the workplace: A strategy for addressing the nursing shortage. *Nursing Economics, 23*(1), 6–13.

Laschinger, H. K. S., Finegan, J., & Shamian, J. (2001). Promoting nurses' health: Effect of empowerment on job strain and work satisfaction. *Nursing Economics, 19*(2), 42–52.

Laschinger, H. K. S., & Sabiston, J. A. (2000). Staff nurse empowerment and workplace behaviors. *Canadian Nurse, 96*(2), 18–22.

Laschinger, H. K. S., Sabiston, J. A., & Kutszcher, L. (1997). Empowerment and staff nurse decision involvement in nursing work environments: Testing Kanter's Theory of Structural Power in organizations. *Research in Nursing and Health, 20*, 341–352.

Newman M. A., Smith M. C., Dexheimer-Pharris, M., & Jones, D. A. (2008). The focus of the discipline revisited. *(ANS) Advances in Nursing Science, 31*(1), E16–E27.

Parse, R. R. (1998). *The human becoming school of thought:* *A perspective for nurses and other health professionals.* Thousand Oaks, CA: Sage.

Peter, E., Lunardi, V. L., & Macfarlane, A. (2004). Nursing resistance as ethical action: Literature review. *Journal of Advanced Nursing, 46*(4), 403–416.

Rogers, M. E. (1970). *An introduction to the theoretical basis of nursing.* Philadelphia: F. A. Davis.

Scott, J. G., Sochalski, J., & Aiken, L. H. (1999). Review of Magnet hospital research: Findings and implications for professional nursing practice. *Journal of Nursing Administration, 29*(1), 9–19.

Smith, M. C. (2002). Health, healing, and the myth of the hero journey. *ANS. Advances in Nursing Science, 24*(2), 1–13.

Wald, L. D. (1915). *The house on Henry Street.* New York: Henry Holt and Company.

Wald, L. D. (1934). *Windows on Henry Street.* Boston: Little Brown and Company.

Wittmann-Price, R. A. (2004). Emancipation in decision making in women's health care. *Journal of Advanced Nursing, 47*(4), 437–445.

Wolf, K. A. (Ed.). (1997). *Jo Ann Ashley: Selected readings.* New York: National League for Nursing Press.

Zurmehly, J., Martin, P. A., & Fitzpatrick, J. J. (2009). Registered nurse empowerment and intent to leave current position and/or profession. *Journal of Nursing Management, 17*, 383–391.

QUALITY AND SAFETY EDUCATION STRATEGIES

Deborah Struth and Cheryl Carr

5
CHAPTER

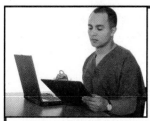

visi.stock/Shutterstock.com

Adam Smith, a junior nursing student, was taking care of his patient Ben, a 10-year-old with asthma, in the emergency department (ED). Ben had been admitted twice in the past year to the pediatric intensive care unit (PICU), where he had been intubated and placed on a ventilator each time. On this particular visit to the ED, he was complaining of having a bad cold for the past week. His vital signs were T 38.2°C, P 112, R 45, BP 122/80 with bilateral inspiratory and expiratory wheezing and poor aeration. The nursing instructor verified Adam's assessment, and they notified the nurse in charge, who asked them to call the physician on call. The physician called in a verbal order for 35 mg albuterol nebulizer in 30 mL of normal saline STAT. The nursing instructor grabbed the albuterol from the medication room, and she and Adam administered the nebulizer not at 2.5 to 3 mg per 3 mL, which would have been the correct dose, but at 10 times the recommended dose.

CORE COMPETENCY

Synthesize current recommendations for integration of safety and quality concepts in all levels of nursing school curriculum.

LEARNING OUTCOMES

1. Demonstrate awareness of safety and quality projects focused on minimizing harm through system effectiveness.
2. Identify knowledge, skills, and attitudes needed for every nurse in the context of core competencies in the Quality and Safety in Nursing Education (QSEN) program for nurse educators.
3. Apply quality improvement models to education strategies to decrease risk of harm.

As the famous German poet Johann Wolfgang von Goethe said, "Knowing is not enough; we must apply. Willing is not enough; we must do." The great challenge in transforming health care into an idealized, safe, patient-centered environment is in educating healthcare professionals both to know and to do. This education must include nurses, physicians, and pharmacists. The National League for Nursing (NLN), the American Academy of Colleges of Nursing (AACN), the Quality and Safety Education for Nurses (QSEN) project, and the American Nurses Association (ANA) all have statements and plans for enhancing nurse educators' focus on safety and quality in health care. They also have a unified goal to increase safety and quality awareness as well as provide a foundation for evaluation and continual process improvement in new nurses.

A newly graduated nurse who is transitioning into practice enters the patient care environment with a respectable knowledge of patient care gained from both classroom work and clinical experiences. This novice nurse has knowledge from many sources, including the traditional didactic lecture and book learning, clinical simulation scenarios and case studies, and student nurse clinical experiences that are added to real-world experience and evidence-based practices to guide patient care. Yet, in spite of this complex and high-level knowledge base, a significant gap exists between the new nurse's knowledge and his or her ability to practice safely. As in the preceding quotation by Goethe, the individual needs the ability *both to apply and to do.*

Efforts to Educate Nurses about Quality and Safety

High patient acuity, unrealistic assignments, constant interruptions of workflow (Biron, Lavoie-Tremblay & Loiselle, 2009), disruptive behaviors on the part of colleagues (JCAHO, 2008), and communication issues all collide in the care environment to create an overwhelming workplace for the novice nurse. The reality is that new nurses, even with a high-level knowledge base, have difficulty executing effective nursing practices related to quality and safety.

Transition to Practice

The National Council of State Boards of Nursing's Transition to Practice (TTP) model, described in Chapter 3, recommends a solution to this gap between knowledge and competent practice. The TTP model is based on several months of extensive orientation followed by many months of mentoring. Berkow, Virkstis, Steward, and Conway (2008) reported the satisfaction levels of nurse executives, managers, and educators with new graduate proficiency. They studied new nurses with a longer orientation and preceptored entry to practice in specific areas of 36 clinical and nonclinical skill sets (Berkow et al., 2008). Over 3,265 nurse leaders contributed to this assessment of new graduate performance. These researchers reported that the top five strengths that new nurses bring to the environment include:

- Use of informational technologies

- Rapport with patients and families

- Respect for diverse cultural perspectives

- Conducting thorough patient assessments (including physical exam, history, and vital signs)

- Customer service

The weakest areas of performance on the part of new nurses were identified as:

- Delegation of tasks

- Ability to identify patient risk

- Ability to prioritize

- Conflict resolution

- Completion of individual tasks within expected timeframes

- Understanding of quality improvement methodologies

These findings are similar to findings reported by the National Council of State Boards of Nursing (NCSBN). The NCSBN study asked students to identify what they perceived as the biggest gaps in their nursing education program content related to actual nursing practice (Suling & Kenward, 2006). Top gaps identified by the 7,497 new nurses who participated in the study were consistent with the weakest performance skills identified by the nurse leaders in assessing new nurse performance. The greatest perceived gaps in their nursing education were reported as:

- Opportunities to administer medicine to multiple groups of patients

- Ability to practice the delegation of tasks to others

- Opportunities to supervise care delivered by others

- Knowing when and how to call the physician

Common Stressors of Practicing Nurses

Whether novice or expert, the stressors of practicing nurses are similar and include feeling overwhelmed by unrealistic practice expectations and fears about harming patients (Suling & Kenward, 2006). Experienced nurses are often frustrated by the same unrealistic expectations placed on novice nurses. Both novice and expert nurses worry about patient safety. The difference between the new nurse and the experienced nurse may be the magnitude of these feelings. With increased experience the nurse may become frustrated with care systems and develop ineffective or negative coping mechanisms.

Defense mechanisms, which are not helpful for dealing with these stressors, include psychological defenses (poor communication approaches and disruptive behaviors) and system workarounds, that is, shortcuts that allow the nurse to get work done in spite of poor work processes. Neither coping approach addresses the underlying issues that create an undesirable work environment for the nurse and negatively affect patient care outcomes, but multiple efforts aimed at safety have been developed. These include Transforming Care at the Bedside (TCAB), Team Strategies to Enhance Performance and Patient Safety (STEPPS), QSEN, and Crew Resource Management, all of which will be discussed throughout this chapter.

Transforming Care at the Bedside (TCAB)

To focus on solutions for nursing, the Transforming Care at the Bedside (TCAB) national collaborative brought together 13 healthcare facilities, their nursing leadership, and bedside nurses with 14 academic partners. These collaborators took on the challenge of creating the ideal patient care environment for the nurse and developing educational strategies to teach new nurses quality improvement methods necessary for nurses to contribute to a workplace that can be vital and joyful and to keep patients safe (Rutherford, Lee, & Greiner, 2004).

A primary goal of TCAB was to highlight and improve medical–surgical nursing as a career destination for nurses and as a place where every patient received "the right care, at the right time, in the right way, every time" (Merryman, 2004). The quality improvement methods designed by TCAB allowed the bedside nurse to create meaningful changes to the work environment that improved patient outcomes. Using these methods, the nurse addressed poor work processes, eliminated wasted time, and as a result had more time to spend with patients and their families.

TCAB identified a framework for change in patient care environments built around improvements in four main categories (Rutherford et al., 2004):

- Safety and Reliability
- Care Team Vitality
- Patient-Centeredness
- Increased Value

Each design element will be discussed in this chapter to help address necessary nurse education topics, including activities designed to help the new nurse enter practice with specific knowledge, skills, and attitudes (KSAs) necessary for safe nursing practice with optimal patient outcomes. The four main TCAB categories are listed with definitions and examples in Table 5-1.

TABLE 5-1 ■ Transforming Care at the Bedside (TCAB): Four Goals, Definitions, Innovations, and Outcomes

	Safety and Reliability	Care Team Vitality	Patient-Centeredness	Increased Value
Definition	Care for patients who are hospitalized is safe, reliable, effective, and equitable (Rutherford et al., 2004)	Within a joyful and supportive environment that nurtures professional formation and career development, effective care teams continually strive for excellence (Rutherford et al., 2004).	All care processes are free of waste and promote continuous flow (Rutherford et al., 2004).	Truly patient-centered care on medical–surgical units honors the whole person and family, respects individual values and choices, and ensures continuity of care (Rutherford et al., 2004).
Examples of Innovations Aimed at Improvement	Time-out is held prior to surgery to review patient name, data, and surgical procedure.	Tranquility room is designated near break room to help nurses destress and maintain health (decrease burnout).	Units schedule quiet time to ensure patient rest time.	Patient and family plan of care developed on white board in patient's room.
Outcomes	Fewer adverse events such as wrong site surgery and fewer medication errors	Less nursing staff turnover occurs.	Increased patient satisfaction is measured.	Increased patient, family, nursing, and administrative satisfaction is measured.
Long-Term Measures	Tracking adverse events.	Staffing and turnover trends are analyzed.	Patient surveys and hospital admissions trends are administered.	Multiple data sources indicate positive trend toward patient and family satisfaction as well as cost savings.
Nursing Impact	Less shame and stressors related to adverse events and better quality of care.	Positive environment enhances overall well being and ultimately health.	Increasing nurse awareness of patient issues and patient perspective.	Cost and quality awareness and development of nurse-led benchmarking for future quality nursing care.

The KSAs represent QSEN competencies, which were developed from the Institute of Medicine (IOM) recommendations for health professions education reform (IOM, 2003). QSEN outlines the entry-level competencies necessary to "continuously improve the quality and safety of the healthcare systems in which [health professionals] work" (Cronenwett et al., 2007). New nurses graduating with an understanding of the TCAB Framework for Quality Improvement and QSEN competencies will become leaders in quality and safety, and they will adopt behaviors and practices of the KSAs that improve care, keep patients safe, and create vitality in the workplace (Cronenwett et al., 2007). By deliberately reflecting on how to use these educational strategies that aim to develop quality and safety competencies in student nurses, it may be possible to begin to bridge the education–practice gap.

TCAB Goal: Safety and Reliability

Care for patients who are hospitalized is safe, reliable, effective and equitable.

—Rutherford et al., 2004

Safety and reliability were not evident in the case of Adam Smith that began this chapter. Was there intent to cause harm? No. There were three mistakes: taking a verbal order from the physician with the wrong dose, not communicating with the nurse on duty regarding the administration of the drug, and not checking the safety of the dose. Each adverse event can be traced by root cause analysis to its source, which often turns out to be a simple miscommunication, a failure to check and double-check physician orders, or many other causes.

TCAB Goal: Care Team Vitality

Within a joyful and supportive environment that nurtures professional formation and career development, effective care teams continually strive for excellence.

—Rutherford et al., 2004

The ideal patient care environment aimed at safe, reliable, effective, and equitable care is one in which all members of the patient care team communicate effectively and collaborate to meet the needs of patients. In fact, teamwork and collaboration are paramount to both care team vitality and patient safety. While teamwork has been studied extensively over the past two decades, a focus on building skill sets around teamwork is only beginning to emerge in nursing education programs and staff development activities in healthcare organizations. The case study about Emily that appears later in this chapter is a good example of teamwork that is focused on safe, reliable, effective, and equitable care.

TCAB Goal: Value-Added Care Processes

All care processes are free of waste and promote continuous flow.

—Rutherford et al., 2004

When supply delivery is inconsistent and supply needs of the unit are not consistently monitored, nurses can spend hours doing non-nursing tasks. Nurses can spend up to 40% of their time traveling to central supply rooms, gathering bits of needed supplies for dressing changes or catherization, or simply tracking supplies. Systems must become more streamlined and consistent, using appropriate workers for appropriate tasks.

TCAB Goal: Patient-Centered Care

Truly patient-centered care on medical and surgical units honors the whole person and family, respects individual values and choices, and insures continuity of care.

—Rutherford et al., 2004

Muda is a Japanese word that describes activities that absorb resources but are not productive and create no value. The idea and lessons of muda have their roots based in "lean" organizations that classify the processes in their work as steps that add value and those that do not. Toyota is considered a lean organization. One of its organizational expectations is that waste, or muda, is eliminated during car manufacturing. Factors involved in the successful application of the Toyota Production System in healthcare are eliminating unnecessary daily activities associated with "overcomplicated processes, workaround and rework" (Printezis, 2007).

Keeping Patients Safe The Institute of Medicine's *Keeping Patients Safe* (2004) places the waste that occurs in hospitals into seven categories:

- Poor utilization of resources
- Excess motion
- Unnecessary waiting
- Transportation
- Process inefficiency
- Excess inventory
- Defects/quality control

Increasing value requires greater efficiency, not as an end in itself, but so that caregivers can provide more care. Increasing available nurse hours by 30 minutes per patient day is associated with a decrease of 4.5% in urinary tract infection, 4.2% in pneumonia, 2.6% in thrombosis, and 1.8% in pulmonary compromise (Kovner and Gergen, 1998).

Healthcare organizations that use the TCAB methodology have dissected the categories and are experiencing success as they tackle Tests of Change (TOC) to eliminate waste in their institutions. Hospital units have successfully embraced the redesign process, but it must continue if strides are to be made in eliminating waste and improving patient care. In his Rose Garden speech of July 15, 2009, President Barack Obama addressed the nonvalue-added but necessary activities of nurses. "If we modernize health records, we'll streamline the paperwork that can take up more than one-third of the average nurse's day, freeing them to spend more time with their patients" (Obama, B. Remarks by the President on Healthcare Reform. July 15, 2009).

Value-Added Care Process in Nursing Education

One problem identified by the IOM related to health professions education that speaks directly to nursing is the lack of standardized curriculum around quality and safety for every prelicensure program in the country (IOM, 2003). A recent focus of the NLN has been investigating clinical education via surveys of educators. The NLN Think Tank on Transforming Clinical Nursing Education, which convened in April 2008, constructed recommendations for improving clinical education, which included the following.

- Assess student clinical learning and time spent so that instructors can be most effective in helping them learn the practice.

- Ensure that there are connections between learning the classroom, clinical, and laboratory.

- Emphasize task completion less and increase the emphasis on communication and critical thinking as well as thinking on one's feet so that future nurses can practice independently and interdependently.

- Continue to integrate quality and safety in all courses (NLN, 2008).

With the above recommendations we have a clear path to improving education and thus improving the level of clinical practice in nursing.

The Nine Essentials for Baccalaureate Nursing Programs

The AACN has included safety, quality, a focus on critical thinking, communication, and continuity of care in their baccalaureate essentials and masters essentials for curriculum in nursing schools, shown in Box 5-1. The AACN list is an excellent source of the most current wisdom on today's nursing curriculum.

Once the critical curricular components are integrated into nursing programs, could nursing education be redesigned to eliminate the waste, or muda? Can education become lean? Customer need drives the process of lean, and the outcome is the elimination of nonvalue-added activities. In nursing education, there are many customers: students, faculty, patients, and the patient care service area in which graduate nurses will eventually work. To achieve the goal of developing a graduate nurse capable of successfully integrating into today's challenging healthcare arena, educators must take advantage of every opportunity to expose students to value-added, evidence-based processes during their time in school—especially time spent in the clinical setting. Therefore, time-consuming, nonvalue-added tasks must be identified and eliminated from the student nurse's clinical experience.

A structured clinical curriculum focused on value-adding activities is the goal. It is essential that students learn the methodology to carry the competencies of the IOM and QSEN into their chosen work setting. The redesign in nursing education must continue if progress is to be made in the achievement of the competencies recommended by the IOM in their report *Health Professions Education* (2003, p. 121): "All health professions should be educated to deliver patient-centered care as members of an interdisciplinary team, emphasizing evidence-based practice, quality improvement approaches, and informatics."

BOX 5-1 AACN's NINE ESSENTIALS FOR BACCALAUREATE NURSING PROGRAMS

The essentials pertaining to quality and safety in nursing are underlined.

ESSENTIAL I: LIBERAL EDUCATION FOR BACCALAUREATE GENERALIST NURSING PRACTICE

A solid base in liberal education provides the cornerstone for the practice and education of nurses.

ESSENTIAL II: BASIC ORGANIZATIONAL AND SYSTEMS LEADERSHIP FOR QUALITY CARE AND PATIENT SAFETY

Knowledge and skills in leadership, quality improvement, and patient safety are necessary to provide high-quality health care.

ESSENTIAL III: SCHOLARSHIP FOR EVIDENCE-BASED PRACTICE

Professional nursing practice is grounded in the translation of current evidence into one's practice.

ESSENTIAL IV: INFORMATION MANAGEMENT AND APPLICATION OF PATIENT CARE TECHNOLOGY

Knowledge and skills in information management and patient care technology are critical in the delivery of quality patient care.

ESSENTIAL V: HEALTHCARE POLICY, FINANCE, AND REGULATORY ENVIRONMENTS

Healthcare policies, including financial and regulatory, directly and indirectly influence the nature and functioning of the healthcare system and thereby are important considerations in professional nursing practice.

ESSENTIAL VI: INTERPROFESSIONAL COMMUNICATION AND COLLABORATION FOR IMPROVING PATIENT HEALTH OUTCOMES

Communication and collaboration among healthcare professionals are critical to delivering high quality and safe patient care.

ESSENTIAL VII: CLINICAL PREVENTION AND POPULATION HEALTH

Health promotion and disease prevention at the individual and population level are necessary to improve population health and are important components of baccalaureate generalist nursing practice.

ESSENTIAL VIII: PROFESSIONALISM AND PROFESSIONAL VALUES

Professionalism and the inherent values of altruism, autonomy, human dignity, integrity, and social justice are fundamental to the discipline of nursing.

ESSENTIAL IX: BACCALAUREATE GENERALIST NURSING PRACTICE

The baccalaureate graduate nurse is prepared to practice with patients, including individuals, families, groups, communities, and populations across the lifespan and across the continuum of healthcare environments. The baccalaureate graduate understands and respects the variations of care, the increased complexity, and the increased use of healthcare resources inherent in caring for patients.

American Association of Colleges of Nursing (AACN), 2008, *The essentials of baccalaureate education for professional nursing practice.*

TeamSTEPPS

The Agency for Healthcare Research and Quality (AHRQ, 2008) created the Team Strategies to Enhance Performance and Patient Safety (TeamSTEPPS) curriculum. The curriculum defines teamwork as "a set of interrelated knowledge, skills, and abilities (KSAs) that facilitate coordinated, adaptive performance, supporting one's teammates, objectives and missions" (AHRQ, 2008, p.1). Mastery of the teamwork KSAs is demonstrated by multidisciplinary work teams that share a clear vision of optimal care for the patient and expected outcomes. Effective teams are adaptive and constantly monitor individual and team performance against patient progress. They then adjust actions accordingly (AHRQ, 2008). Nurses who demonstrate mastery of the teamwork and collaboration competency are able to give and receive feedback from all members of the care delivery team to improve team performance and patient care outcomes.

Quality and Safety Education in Nursing (QSEN)

The QSEN project (Cronenwett et al., 2007) identified two competencies for nursing practice with KSAs that the nurse must master to function effectively on teams and contribute to the vision for care team vitality. The first competency is teamwork and collaboration, and the second is safety. A definition of each competency and select KSAs from these competencies are found in Tables 5-2 and 5-3. The KSAs are addressed by educational strategies presented in this section. One should carefully review the specific behaviors described within these tables that illustrate exemplary nursing performance of the first two QSEN competencies. These tables do not contain all KSAs for these competencies; rather they provide the specific behaviors that the activities, if practiced frequently and mastered by the student nurse, will help bridge the education–practice gap.

In achieving competency in these QSEN safety KSAs, the new nurse will be able to recognize changes in patient status quickly and effectively intervene or report changes to healthcare team members. The new nurse needs to identify high-risk situations for patients and anticipate strategies to keep patients safe. This includes the ability to complete and interpret assessment data, and use sound clinical judgment to select nursing interventions to care for an at-risk patient. In keeping the patient safe, the new nurse will quickly recognize unsafe practices while effectively utilizing communication tools to voice concerns to team members regarding perceptions of unsafe situations. Finally, a safe nurse should take time to reflect on his or her own care practices, recognize the need to alter behaviors and interventions, and know when to ask for clarification or assistance with patient care.

TABLE 5-2 ■ Achieving QSEN Competency: Teamwork and Collaboration

Function effectively within nursing and interprofessional teams, fostering open communication, mutual respect, and shared decision making to achieve quality patient care.

K (Knowledge)	• Describe own strengths, limitations, and values in functioning as a member of a team • Describe scopes of practice and roles of healthcare team members • Describe impact of own communication style on others • Discuss effective strategies for communicating and resolving conflict • Describe examples of the impact of team functioning on safety and quality of care • Explain how authority gradients influence teamwork and patient safety • Identify system barriers and facilitators of effective team functioning
S (Skill)	• Initiate plan for self-development as a team member • Function competently within own scope of practice as a member of the healthcare team • Initiate requests for help when appropriate to situation • Communicate with team members, adapting own style of communicating to needs of the team and situation • Demonstrate commitment to team goals • Solicit input from other team members to improve individual, as well as team, performance • Initiate actions to resolve conflict • Follow communication practices that minimize risks associated with handoffs among providers and across transitions in care • Choose communication styles that diminish the risks associated with authority gradients among team members
A (Attitude)	• Acknowledge own potential to contribute to effective team functioning • Value the perspectives and expertise of all health team members • Value teamwork and the relationships upon which it is based • Value different styles of communication used by patients, family, and healthcare providers • Contribute to resolution of conflict and disagreement • Appreciate the risk associated with handoffs among providers and across transitions in care

Cronenwett, L., Sherwood, G., Barnsteiner, J., Disch, J., Johnson, J., Mitchell, P., et al. (2007). Quality and safety education for nurses. *Nursing Outlook, 55*(3), 122–131.

TABLE 5-3 ■ Achieving QSEN Competency: Safety

Minimizes risk of harm to patients and providers through both system effectiveness and individual performance.

K (Knowledge)	• Examine human factors and other basic safety design principles. Identify commonly used unsafe practices (e.g., work-arounds and dangerous abbreviations) • Delineate general categories of error and hazards in care • Describe factors that create a culture of safety (e.g., open communication strategies and organizational error reporting systems) • Describe the benefits and limitations of selected safety-enhancing technologies (e.g., barcodes, computer provider order entry, medication pumps, and automatic alerts and alarms)
S (Skills)	• Demonstrate effective use of technology and standardized practices that support safety and quality • Communicate observations or concerns related to hazards and errors to patients, families, and the healthcare team • Use national patient safety resources for own professional development and to focus attention on safety in care settings
A (Attitude)	• Value the contributions of standardization and reliability to safety • Appreciate the cognitive and physical limitation of human performance • Value own role in preventing error • Value vigilance and monitoring (even of own performance of care activities) by patients, families, and other members of the healthcare team

Cronenwett, L., Sherwood, G., Barnsteiner, J., Disch, J., Johnson, J., Mitchell, P., et al. (2007). Quality and safety education for nurses. *Nursing Outlook, 55*(3), 122–131.

Crew Resource Management Principles

How does the new nurse or student nurse work to achieve QSEN competency in safety and teamwork collaboration? The TCAB design framework identifies two broad strategies to help nurses communicate effectively to keep patients safe and improve care team vitality. These strategies are embedded in a safety model referred to as Crew Resource Management (CRM) (Rutherford et al., 2004). Principles of CRM are illustrated in Figure 5-1.

CRM principles include effective communication skills and the willingness to speak up if something in the environment does not seem correct. CRM relies on identification of the role and value of every team member to safe patient care and the understanding that every team member, regardless of perceived rank or authority, must be able to lead the team to keep patients safe. Constant monitoring of the environment to look for indicators that errors may occur and increase patient risk is critical to effective CRM, along with correction of risk-producing situations.

Extensive research supports the effectiveness of these strategies in reducing communication failures and error (Leonard, Graham, & Bonacum, 2004). Model systems to ensure safety in nursing were adapted from techniques developed by the aviation industry to keep commercial airline travel safe for passengers. Consider that in the early 1980s, one in every 5,000 people receiving general anesthesia died as a result of human error during surgery. Today, as a result of incorporating CRM training into required education for anesthesiologists and nurse anesthetists, deaths from anesthesia are about one in 300,000 (Hallinan, 2009).

Clearly the nursing profession must have clear leadership in place with a focus on communication, collaboration, and error anticipation

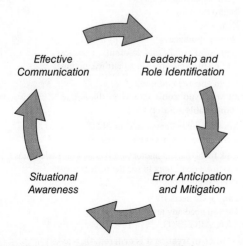

Figure 5-1 Crew Resource Management Principles
The cycle of effective communication, leadership and role identification, error anticipation and mitigation, and situational awareness is constantly evolving.

TABLE 5-4 ■ SBAR Reporting

BEFORE CALLING:
1. Assess the patient
2. Review the chart for the appropriate physician to call
3. Know the admitting diagnosis
4. Read the most recent Progress Notes and the assessment from the prior shift
5. Have **available** when speaking with the physician:
   Chart, allergies, meds, IV fluids, lab/other results, code status

S = SITUATION	State your **name and unit** you are calling about: **(Patient Name and Room Number)** The **problem I** am calling about is: Briefly state the problem, • What it is • When it happened or started • How severe
B = BACKGROUND	State the **admission diagnosis and date of admission.** State the pertinent **medical history.** A brief synopsis of the **treatment to date.**
A = ASSESSMENT	Most recent vital signs: BP _____ Pulse _____ Respirations _____ Temperature _____ The patient **IS** or **IS NOT** on oxygen **Any changes from prior assessments:** Mental status Respiratory rate and quality Retraction or use of accessory muscles Skin color Pulse, BP Cardiac Rhythm changes Neuro changes Pain Wound drainage Musculoskeletal (joint deformity, weakness) GI/GU (nausea, vomiting, diarrhea, output)
R = RECOMMENDATIONS	**What do you recommend?** **(State what you would like to see done. Use "CUS" words: Concern – Uncomfortable – Safety)** Transfer the patient to ICU or PICU? Come to see the patient at this time? Talk to the patient and/or family about the code status? Ask for a consultant to see the patient now? Other suggestions? **Are any tests needed?** Do you need any tests like: CXR, ABG, EKG, CBC, BNP, others? **If a change in treatment is ordered, then ask:** How often do you want vital signs? **If then the patient does not improve, when do you want us to call again?**

(JCAHO, 2008). As stated in Chapter 2, the models and definitions of quality improvement need to be a primary focus in the clinical setting and in nursing education. The QSEN safety KSAs regarding communication and collaboration shown in Table 5-2 serve to delineate and promote these principals.

Situation, Background, Assessment, and Recommendations (SBAR)

A consistent, easy-to-use communication and organization tool is SBAR, which is an acronym for Situation, Background, Assessment, and Recommendations. This tool is a situational briefing model developed to bridge differences in individual communication styles and rank (perceived authority or power gradient) of the people involved. The student nurse may use this format to deliver clear, concise, focused patient care information to faculty, nurses on the unit, and other healthcare team members. The nurse can reduce reliance on memory and utilize prompts on an SBAR reporting card, as shown in Table 5-4, to help develop what information needs to be communicated.

If a student nurse learns SBAR in the classroom but does not practice the technique frequently, this vital communication tool may not become a part of practice. Creating a concise patient statement in SBAR format also forces the student nurse to reflect on the patient, especially assessments and interventions. This type of reflection may be viewed as part of the new nurse's cognitive workload, helping with evaluation of his or her effectiveness and aiding in the prioritization of goals related to future interactions with the patient.

To demonstrate the effectiveness of SBAR in improving physician-nurse communications, two hospitals within a large, integrated healthcare system performed a quality improvement test of change evaluation. Prior to educating care teams about SBAR, they asked family practice residents and nurses two simple questions. To the resident physicians, they asked how often during a phone consultation concerning a specific patient did the nurse provide all the information needed for the physician to make a care decision. Resident physicians in training at both hospitals reported that 86% of the time they communicated with nurses about a patient, the nurse needed to interrupt the conversation to get additional information. The nurse did not have the essential information needed about the patient's situation to make a good decision about patient care. On the other side, nurses reported that 68% of the time they needed to interrupt the call to the physician to obtain additional information. The 18% difference may be perception or reality; it is not clear. After an hour-long educational session about SBAR that included coaching on the unit, both nurses and physicians reported that communication interruptions related to incomplete information decreased to less than 20% during phone consultations on these nursing units. This is a dramatic improvement in communication and less time wasted. Just as Tamara in the case study used the SBAR tool to describe the patient's condition in much more vivid detail, nurses can be more confident and competent in their practice by using SBAR.

CASE STUDY: *Tamara*

Tamara, a nurse who has worked on the respiratory medical–surgical unit for 5 years, recalls the first year she practiced on the unit. "I used to page the doctor on call in the middle of the night and tell her that the patient looked worse and was breathing heavier. Now it's much easier to focus on the most important details, and I like developing my own plan of care. It's easier using SBAR because I need to gather all the data, interpret the data, and plan the best solution."

An example of Tamara's statement can be seen in her care of David, an adult patient with an acute asthma exacerbation that did not respond to nebulizer treatments in the emergency department. Once David was placed on the bronchodilator and transferred to a patient room, his aeration improved, he grew calm, and his blood gases were back to near normal. David was settled in for the evening. During Tamara's first assessment at 3 p.m., David had end expiratory wheezing with good aeration, and he had a respiratory rate of 22 breaths per minute, heart rate of 64 beats per minute, blood pressure of 116/84 mmHg, and temperature of 99°F. Before her dinner break at 6:30 p.m., Tamara did another assessment and found David sitting bolt upright, and he was tachypenic with poor aeration and wheezes on inspiration and expiration. He had an increased respiratory rate of 54 breaths per minute, heart rate of 72 beats per minutes, blood pressure of 120/90 mmHg, and temperature of 102°F. She prepared the following SBAR report after administering a nebulizer treatment.

S (situation): David is much less comfortable and seems anxious. He is sitting up with a very labored breathing pattern. Breath sounds decreased since prior assessment with inspiratory and expiratory wheezes throughout, poor aeration, and circumoral cyanosis. T increased from 99°F to 102°F, respiratory rate increased to 54, heart rate increased to 72, and blood pressure 120/90.

B (background): Minimal improvement after nebulized treatment with bronchodilator.

A (assessment): Acute respiratory distress with worsening wheezing and poorer aeration. Temperature may be indicative of pneumonia. Increased respiratory rate is worrisome, and lack of response to nebulized treatment is concerning; may need acute care or intensive care admission.

R (recommendation): Need doctor to come to unit and assess patient for signs of pneumonia and possibly draw blood gas to determine oxygenation. Order needs to be done for possible chest film to rule out pneumonia. May need to be transferred to intensive care unit.

Practicing with the SBAR tool allows the student nurse to consider all critical pieces of information to communicate to a physician or other member of the care team, improving the accuracy and precision of this communication. The nurse's care team colleague has all patient information and data needed at the time the call is placed for patient care decisions to be made.

Leonard and colleagues (2004) suggest that utilizing SBAR facilitates the development of critical thinking skills in members of the healthcare team. While research supporting this assertion was not presented, faculty at one school of nursing who required student nurses to report patient status utilizing the SBAR format anecdotally reported finding a rich opportunity in SBAR. Faculty reported that this meta-cognitive exercise allowed the clinical educator to identify and correct errors in assessment, analysis, and evaluation of patient conditions, thus helping the student or novice nurse to correct errors of cognition regarding specific patient care situations (Struth, 2009).

Situation Monitoring, Situation Awareness, and Mutual Support

New nurses have difficulty identifying patient risk and knowing when to call for help. TeamSTEPPS defines situation monitoring as "the process of actively scanning and assessing elements of the situation to gain or maintain an accurate awareness or understanding of the situation in which the [patient care] team is functioning" (AHRQ, 2008, p. 11). Thus, situation monitoring implies that the student nurse is learning to actively and systematically scan the whole patient care environment as a member of the team delivering patient care. In fact, current clinical education practices often recommend that the student nurse focus on one skill set or task at a time, such as preparing medications for administration to one patient. An expert nurse completing the same task of medication preparation is also continually monitoring the care environment in general to anticipate the needs of patients and other team members on the unit. This vigilance allows early problem recognition and promotes flexibility and adaptability, thus keeping the care environment safer. Experts maintain that the skill of situation monitoring can be taught and that, with practice, individual team members will improve in the use of this skill (AHRQ, 2008).

A more focused form of situational monitoring is that of situation awareness. Situation awareness is the state of knowing the conditions that affect one's work (AHRQ, 2008). The often chaotic patient care environment requires the nurse to continually reassess the environment and update his or her own situation awareness. Every human contact, whether with patient, family, physician, or peer, is an opportunity for the new nurse to reassess the context and content of the care situation.

Sixty-Second Situation Assessment

One tool the student nurse can use to develop situation awareness is the Sixty-Second Situation Assessment (Box 5-2) (Struth, 2009). The tool

---

BOX 5-2   SIXTY-SECOND SITUATION ASSESSMENT TOOL

A teaching tool to help students learn quick patient observations.

Purpose: This exercise is designed to assist nurses in developing situation awareness. In the patient care area, situation awareness focuses on the art of patient observation. This includes routine use of general survey (observation) of the patient, family, and environment during every incidental encounter and periodically at planned intervals throughout the day, for example, regular rounds. Situation awareness promotes a safer patient care environment and helps the nurse develop care priorities and attention to clinical detail.

Directions: Enter the patient's room. Observe the patient, family, and environment for up to 60 seconds, while reviewing the following questions in your mind:

(continued)

BOX 5-2 **SIXTY-SECOND SITUATION ASSESSMENT TOOL (*continued*)**

ASSESS AIRWAY BREATHING CIRCULATION (ABCs) WITHOUT TOUCHING THE PATIENT

- What data lead you to believe there is a problem with airway, breathing, or circulation?

- Is the problem urgent or nonurgent?

- What clinical data would indicate that the situation needs immediate action, and why?

- Who needs to be contacted, and do you have any suggestions or recommendations?

ASSESS TUBES AND LINES

- Does the patient have any tubes or an IV?

- Is the IV solution the correct one at the correct rate?

- Does the patient need those tubes? If so, why?

- Do you note any complications?

- What further assessments need to be done?

ASSESS RESPIRATORY EQUIPMENT

- If the patient is using an oxygen delivery device, what do you need to continue to monitor to ensure safe and effective use of the system?

PATIENT SAFETY SURVEY

- What are your safety concerns with this patient?

- Do you need to report this problem and to whom?

ENVIRONMENTAL SURVEY

- What in the environment could lead to a problem for the patient?

- How would you manage the problem?

SENSORY ASSESSMENT

- What are your senses telling you?

- Do you hear, smell, see, or feel something that needs to be explored?

- Does the patient's situation seem "right"?

ADDITIONAL ASSESSMENT

- What additional information would be helpful for further clarification of the situation?

- What questions are unanswered? What answers are unquestioned?

AFTER YOUR ASSESSMENT

Meet with your fellow students and faculty. Review each student's patient. Decide which patient you would focus on first as a team, and why. Determine which elements of the team's work require continual situation monitoring.

Struth, D. (2009). TCAB in the curriculum. *American Journal of Nursing Supplement*, 55–58.

was created to assist nurses in developing situation awareness by practicing focused observation skills. It is recommended that this exercise be completed by each student nurse prior to receiving the handoff report at the beginning of the shift to promote dialogue about the care environment based on the situation monitoring completed by the students.

Without simple structures such as SDAR and the Sixty-Second Situation Assessment Tool, the nurse may lose track of priorities and become engaged in activities that distract from the most critical interventions. Research shows that when members of the patient care team lose situation awareness and fail to monitor what is going on around them, resultant feelings of "ambiguity, confusion and decreased communication" occur in the environment (AHRQ, 2008, p. 13). Simple tools can be implemented to decrease likelihood of errors.

Mutual Support

Mutual support is another key element of CRM and effective teamwork. It involves the "willingness and preparedness to assist other team members during operations" (AHRQ, 2008, p. 16). An experienced nurse depends on good situation monitoring skills to enhance the concept of mutual support in the patient care environment. Helping a team member complete a task (task assistance) is one example of mutual support. Embedded in this concept of mutual support and task assistance are two areas identified as problematic as the new nurse transitions into practice: delegation and asking for help.

Task assistance involves providing support to another team member by helping to complete an activity or solve a problem (AHRQ, 2008). The complexity of the relationship between a professional nurse and a patient care technician (PCT) is an example. Taking routine vital signs and meeting the hygiene needs of the patient is work that belongs to the PCT, yet an experienced nurse is continually monitoring the environment to be certain this important work is being completed. If the nurse identifies that the PCT is busy and unable to keep up with the workload, the experienced nurse would offer task assistance to the PCT. The language of task assistance often takes this form: "Jean, I notice you are very busy with your care responsibilities at the moment, and I have about 15 minutes before my new admission arrives from the emergency department. Can I finish taking vital signs on your patients so that you can finish bathing Mr. Smith?" Notice that in offering task assistance, the nurse clearly defines what he or she is able to assist with and for how long.

The student nurse can practice mutual support through task assistance on the clinical unit by using situation monitoring to identify peers or other team members who may need task assistance. Seeking out opportunities to help others creates stronger teamwork in the care environment. A nurse may also ask for task assistance. In an urgent situation, the nurse may ask a member of a rapid response team to help implement emergency orders given to treat a patient. The student nurse should identify opportunities related to mutual support and practice asking for task assistance while on the clinical unit or in the simulation lab.

Appropriate Assertion and Critical Language

For the new nurse, knowing how to ask for help, when to call a physician, or how to advocate for a patient can be difficult. Perceived or real authority can intimidate nurses and inhibit communication and feedback. What is commonly seen in the clinical environment is a more passive and indirect communication style, which can put patients at risk due to communication error. This approach has been referred to as the "hint and hope model" (Leonard et al., 2004). Student nurses may use the hint and hope approach with a co-assigned registered nurse (RN) or clinical instructor. Practicing nurses may use this approach when communicating with physicians.

Assertion Cycle

Leonard and colleagues (2004) created the assertion cycle as a means to effective, direct, and assertive communication. Their five-step cycle includes (1) Get the person's attention, (2) express your concern, (3) state the problem, (5) propose an action, and (6) reach a decision. Nurses can use the assertion cycle when advocating for a patient or in other clinical situations.

Critical Language, or CUS

Another communication strategy aimed at keeping patients safe is that of critical language, or CUS. Developed by commercial aviation as a part of crew resource management training, CUS stands for concerned, uncomfortable, and safety, as in "I'm concerned, I'm uncomfortable, this is unsafe or I'm scared" (Leonard et al., 2004). Healthcare organizations are working to agree on the critical language their organizations use to convey a message of extreme urgency in a clinical situation. The CUS agreed upon at the University of Pittsburgh Medical Center (UPMC) Health System is, "I need clarity." When an individual at any UPMC hospital asks for clarity, the receiver of this request must stop and listen attentively while the sender asserts the issues that need to be clarified.

Student nurses should be encouraged to discuss strategies with nurses at clinical sites. Instructors should encourage student nurses to observe nurses' assertion and critical language skills for evidence of teamwork and safety issues in the organization and to report findings at postclinical conferences. Students should practice identifying situations in which assertion and critical language were utilized by nurses on the clinical units and evaluate the effectiveness of the communication intervention. Additionally, students should identify ineffective communication or patient care issues that could have been corrected with appropriate assertion and the use of critical language. Clinical faculty should require students to practice using SBAR, the assertion cycle, and CUS language during clinical and simulation experiences.

Investigating Waste in Clinical Education

To facilitate change in clinical education, it is necessary to convince all participants that change is needed. As Donald Berwick, president of the Institute for Healthcare Improvement states, "An innovation must be perceived as beneficial and compatible with users' values, beliefs, history, and current needs" (Berwick, 2003, p. 1971). Rational-empirical strategy theory states that change occurs when we give the factual evidence to support the need (Marquis, 2003). Nursing education is charged with the task of discovering the areas of waste and eliminating them in order to get nursing back to the bedside.

Personal Digital Assistant (PDA) Pilot and Study

Worker productivity is a focus at many industrial workplaces. Other industries have utilized time and motion studies along with work sampling analysis to determine how workers spend their time during the workday. Hospitals in the TCAB project utilized a work sampling analysis of their professional nurses. The goal was to identify the amount of time nurses spent in value-added patient care activities versus nonvalue-added activities, which distract the nurse from patient care.

Work sampling methodology was explored as a pilot at one TCAB study site, Shadyside School of Nursing in Pittsburgh, Pennsylvania, to measure time spent in value-added patient care activities by student nurses and faculty during clinical training and to identify sources of muda. To determine the productive time versus wasted time, personal digital assistants (PDAs) were used to measure how the clinical instructor and students spent their time in the clinical setting (Carr, 2009). Carried during the clinical day, the PDAs with specially designed software allowed for data points to be captured and divided into value-added, nonvalue-added, and necessary categories, based on the TCAB study definitions (see Table 5-5). Value-added nurse activities included those that were reimbursed by payers and linked to positive patient outcomes. Nonvalue-added activities included additional steps for the nurse that did not add value to patient care and should have been avoided. Necessary activities represent unavoidable waste, such as steps that create no value but are unavoidably the work of the nurse in the current patient care system (Rutherford et al., 2004). The goal of the TCAB hospitals was to increase the amount of time nurses spend in value-added activities by eliminating muda (particularly waiting time and documentation). The goal of the pilot study was to identify how much valuable clinical education time was wasted on activities TCAB tries to eliminate from actual practice.

The results of data collected at Shadyside, a provider-based, precensure professional nursing program, confirmed suspicions regarding clinical instruction. Clinical instructors and students spent the greatest portion of their day on medication preparation and administration and on documenting in both paper and electronic health records. Almost 28% of

TABLE 5-5 ■ PDA Work Sampling

Value Added	Nonvalue Added	Necessary
Direct care bedside procedures	Waiting delay	Documentation
Vital signs	Other	Admission paperwork documentation
Wound and other skin care	Retrieve supplies	Daily assessment documentation
Incontinence	Retrieve equipment	Transcribing orders
ADLs	Personal time	Writing care plan
Admit/discharge	Look for patient	Meds paperwork
Assessment	Look for equipment	Teaching documentation
Communication with care team	Look for supplies	Discharge paperwork documentation
Communication with patient	Look for information	Other documentation
Patient services	Waiting for student	Computer data entry
Emergency	Waiting for instructor	Bed control
Family services		Paging caregiver
Care processes		Calling ancillary department
Admission		White board
Discharge		Copy or fax
Give meds		
Prepare meds		
Chart review		
Report		
Monitor patient		
Care rounds with team doctor		
Care conference		

Carr, C. A. (2009). *National study of clinical nursing education: Discovering opportunity for redesign.* Waynesburg University, Wilmington, PA: Unpublished doctoral dissertation.

student samples during the work sampling found the student nurse engaged in a nonvalue-adding nursing activity (Carr, 2009).

After completion of this pilot study, a national study utilizing work sampling methodology was undertaken to identify and analyze sources of waste in clinical education across program types but with a focus on medical–surgical nursing clinical experiences (Carr, 2009). The selected schools utilized PDAs in the medical–surgical portions of their clinical nursing programs for one semester each.

Analysis of Data

The eight participating schools collected 3,190 data points. Instructors collected 1,690 points, and 1,401 points were collected by students. Data points demonstrated a predictable outcome: Students and instructors spent the majority of their day performing the tasks of documentation and medication administration. Of the data points collected by instructors, 48% of them were attributed to value-added activities, 36% to necessary activities, and 16% to nonvalue-added activities, which included personal

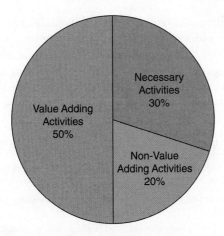

Figure 5-2 Work Sampling Analysis: All Students

Results of data collected at eight prelicensure professional nursing programs revealed that 30% of student nurses were engaged in a nonvalue-adding nursing activity during the work sampling.

Carr, C. A. (2009). *National study of clinical nursing education: Discovering opportunity for redesign.* Waynesburg University, Wilmington, PA: Unpublished doctoral dissertation.

time. Of the data points collected by students, 50% were attributed to value-added activities, 30% to necessary activities, and 20% to nonvalue-added activities. (See Figure 5-2.)

For students, the majority of value-added data points were attributed to medication administration. This accounted for 23.7% of the students' value-added activities, while patient assessment accounted for only 5.6% of the students' value-added activities. Yet the most critical data collection is the nurse's assessment of a patient. Not only the initial assessment but the frequent and comparative assessments that represent the first step in the nursing process are critical skills nurses use to keep patients safe. The student nurses in the study were almost five times more likely to be involved in documenting and medication administration-related activities as they were to be involved in assessing a patient during their clinical education.

While documentation and medication administration are important activities, patient assessment is arguably one of the most important activities and cannot be delegated to non-nurse workers. A switch to focused clinical activities related to patient assessment may strengthen student nurses' ability to identify patient risk, prioritize care, and identify rapidly declining health status that requires a rapid response team or a call to a physician.

The other top 10 value-added activities were bedside procedures, communication, chart review, vital signs, patient services, activities of daily living (ADLs), assessment, teaching, and care conferences. In the necessary category, 37% of the students' data points were collected during documentation. Students were engaged in a wide variety of necessary activities, including other aspects of medication administration and documentation along with teaching and delivering supplies.

These findings (Struth, 2009) further demonstrate that both students and instructors spent the majority of their day in passing medications and documenting patient care, either in paper charts or in the electronic health record. These statistics were not surprising, as staff nurses in the clinical

TABLE 5-6 ■ Quality Improvement QSEN Competency with Selected KSAs

Use data to monitor the outcomes of care processes and use improvement methods to design and test changes to continuously improve the quality and safety of healthcare systems.

K (Knowledge)	• Describe strategies for learning about the outcomes of care in the setting in which one is engaged in clinical practice
	• Engage in processes in nursing and other health professions focused on students as parts of systems of care and care processes that affect outcomes for patients and families
	• Explain the concepts of variation and measurement in assessing quality of care
	• Describe approaches for changing processes of care
S (Skills)	• Apply information about outcomes of care for populations served in care settings
	• Use information about quality improvement projects in care settings
	• Use tools (such as flow charts, cause-effect diagrams) to make processes of care explicit
	• Actively participate in a root cause analysis of a sentinel event
	• Practice aligning the aims, measures and changes involved in improving care
A (Attitude)	• Integrate continuous quality improvement as an essential work of all health professions
	• Value what individuals and teams can do to improve care

Cronenwett, L., Sherwood, G., Barnsteiner, J., Disch, J., Johnson, J., Mitchell, P., et al. (2007). Quality and safety education for nurses. *Nursing Outlook, 55*(3), 122–131.

TABLE 5-7 ■ Patient-Centered Care QSEN Competency with Selected KSAs

Recognize the patient or designee as the source of control and full partner in providing compassionate and coordinated care based on respect for the patient's preferences values and needs.

K (Knowledge)	• Integrate understanding of multiple dimensions of patient-centered care
	• Demonstrate comprehensive understanding of the concepts of pain and suffering, including physiological models of pain and comfort
	• Examine nursing roles in ensuring coordination, integration, and continuity of care
S (Skill)	• Assess presence and extent of pain and suffering
	• Assess levels of physical and emotional comfort
	• Elicit expectations of patient and family for relief of pain, discomfort, or suffering
	• Initiate effective treatments to relieve pain and suffering in light of patient values, preferences, and expressed needs
	• Provide patient-centered care with sensitivity and respect for the diversity of human experience
A (Attitude)	• Value seeing health care situations through the patient's eye
	• Appreciate the role of the nurse in relief of all types and sources of pain or suffering

Cronenwett, L., Sherwood, G., Barnsteiner, J., Disch, J., Johnson, J., Mitchell, P., et al. (2007). Quality and safety education for nurses. *Nursing Outlook, 55*(3), 122–131.

setting report similar issues. Allocating so much clinical time to performance of nonassessment duties removes the clinical staff nurse from the bedside. Allocating so much instructor and student time to performance of these tasks inhibits the development of other necessary skills, such as communication with the interdisciplinary team, assessment, and critical thinking.

After review and analysis of the results of the PDA pilot study, it was determined that while there was a need for change in the way students learn, it had to begin with a change in the way students were taught. The results of the study enabled the faculty to work as a team to design the best clinical experience.

Changing Clinical Education to Achieve QSEN Competency

With the determination of missed opportunities in clinical education, it is imperative that clinical education for nurses be altered to include a greater proportion of value-added processes, such as quality improvement and patient-centered care. QSEN has provided guidelines for improvement via the KSAs, as shown in Tables 5-6 and 5-7.

The following sections describe select changes that were made and met with success during the PDA study, and other initiatives whose efficacy will continue to be measured. Student nurses and faculty can work together to add value to clinical time utilizing many of these approaches.

Evidence for Best Practices: Grand Rounds for Evidence-Based Nursing

When a nagging clinical question emerges such as "What is the best way to treat pain in acute head trauma patients?" clinical rounds with an evidence-based interprofessional focus can promote healthy discussion and policy development on a specific unit. Evidence-based clinical rounds have been used very successfully as described by Melynk and Fineout-Overhold (2002) in the University of Rochester School of Nursing, Medical Center, and community model entitled Advancing Research and Clinical Practice through Close Collaboration (ARCC). Once a week one clinical provider from a group of nurses, physicians, pharmacists, and occupational or physical therapists follows the outline for leading the clinical rounds. The outline includes: first, identification of a clinical question; second, conducting a literature search for evidence to answer the question; third, appraisal and analysis then synthesis of the literature; and last, development of a recommendation for practice changed based on the evidence (Melynk & Fineout-Overhold, 2005). The recommendation is discussed and may become policy for the unit or adapted as a new best practice. This more focused clinical rounding can have more significance on the practice than traditional grand rounds lectures that are held in a formal auditorium with hundreds of doctors. The discussion and interaction in the more formal grand rounds is less immediate. The clinical rounds with evidence-based interprofessional focus used in the ARCC model may have a more significant safety and quality impact.

Clinical Timeline

In the world of quality improvement, reliability implies that once the proper procedure is defined through study and evaluation, it will be carried out the proper way every time. It should be replicated with precision. A clinical timeline that can track reliable procedure practice was developed to identify value-added concepts of quality and safe patient care for student nurses throughout their medical-surgical clinical experience. Use of a clinical timeline also had its impetus from the QSEN initiatives. Dr. Linda Cronenwett asked the question, "Why do we teach total patient care first and systems thinking last?" (Cronenwett et al., 2007). Unless tools that promote patient safety and effective teamwork are constantly used, they may be forgotten once students transition to the cultures of the organizations in which they work.

During the PDA study, students in one provider-based, prelicensure professional nursing program spent 24 weeks in medical–surgical didactic and clinical education. Through analysis of the teaching activities, it was determined that during these 24 weeks, there was a lack of standardization among clinical faculty regarding how to meet the IOM/QSEN recommended competencies. Clinical conference time was not structured, and learning opportunities were missed. A timeline was developed to take every advantage to introduce students to the QSEN competencies at the medical-surgical level. Various aspects of the QSEN competencies were addressed each week either on the clinical unit, in postclinical conference, or in the simulation lab.

Components of the Timeline

The timeline, objectives, and all forms and paperwork needed to meet the weekly objectives were posted on the electronic course management system for easy accessibility by students and faculty. The eight components of the 24-week timeline included the following points.

Incorporating Nurse-Sensitive Indicators into Patient Care In the early 1990s, the ANA initiated an effort to develop a database of Nurse-Sensitive Indicators (NSIs). Out of this came the National Database of Nursing Quality Indicators (NDNQI). This database is a quality measurement program that allows for a unit-based collection of performance reports and the opportunity for comparison to national averages. Some of the NSIs include pressure ulcers, patient falls, use of restraints, urinary catheter–associated infections, and ventilator-associated pneumonia.

During the PDA study students were instructed to have an NSI focus. During various weeks of the timeline, they were assigned an NSI to investigate on their floor during their clinical time in this setting. Nurse unit quality experts were frequently asked to speak to the students about their unit-specific indicators, their successes, and their failures, and student nurses were urged to seek information regarding unit-specific indicators. A bulletin board on the unit listed quality indicators, along with the progress being made.

Exposure to High-Risk, Error-Prone Medications During their clinical experience, students were assigned patients on high-risk medications, such as heparin and insulin. These two drugs have been identified as "high-alert medications that bear a heightened risk of causing significant patient harm when they are used in error" (Institute for Safe Medication Practices, 2003, p.1). On the clinical unit, the various sliding scales and weight-based nomograms associated with these medications were carefully investigated, along with the types of errors that can accompany administration of these medications. Clinical conferences consisted of focused discussions regarding these error-prone medications.

Reflective Journaling after Caring for the Patient Experiencing Pain Students were assigned patients with pain management orders (patients experiencing pain) during their clinical experience. Through reflective journaling, students were able to investigate their feelings regarding pain, risk for addiction, and pain control methodologies other than drugs. The students reflected on the frustration they felt if adequate pain control was difficult to achieve for their patients. This reflection allowed for a deeper introspection surrounding the care of the patient experiencing pain and self-contemplation of deeply held beliefs about pain. Some of the questions students addressed in this self-reflection include:

- Did the patient's pain contribute to his or her inability to perform ADLs?
- What was the patient's reaction to this issue?
- Did you encounter any barriers when trying to alleviate the patient's pain (e.g., no pain medication ordered, medications not on unit, patient's unwillingness to take pain medications)?

Integration of the Joint Commission Patient Safety Goals During preconference, the students discussed the current Joint Commission Patient Safety Goals. Each student chose one or two of the goals and investigated compliance and noncompliance with the goals in their various clinical settings. They shared their findings in postconference. If the issue of noncompliance was one that needed to be addressed immediately, the student was held responsible for reporting it to the appropriate person.

Exposure to Issues Surrounding Patient Literacy Over 30% of patient readmissions are linked directly back to the patient's poor understanding of discharge instructions. Students were given several articles to read regarding the high cost of healthcare illiteracy to both the patient and the healthcare system. These articles were designed to expose students to little-thought-of complications of healthcare illiteracy, followed by discussions of subsequent problems such as readmissions due to misunderstanding of discharge instructions.

Investigation of Medication Errors Students had access to a national publication that highlighted medication safety. Each student was assigned an article and was responsible for extrapolating the highlights and discussing the implications of the medication safety information in their personal practice.

Performing a Root Cause Analysis of a Sentinel Event Root cause analysis (RCA) is used extensively in engineering as a way to formalize investigations and to provide a problem-solving approach to identify and understand the underlying cause of an adverse event (AHRQ, 2007). Use of this technique can aid in understanding that often it is not a human factor that causes an error in the clinical setting, but rather a system failure.

Students were taught about root cause analysis and were given the opportunity to dissect either a witnessed or researched sentinel event (an event in which harm was done or could have been done to the patient). They drilled down to find the various factors that contributed to errors. The exercise provided the instructor and students the opportunity to discuss human factors, work-arounds, policies, and system breakdowns.

Self-Reflective Journaling Regarding Time Spent in Medical–Surgical Nursing At the end of each shift in medical-surgical nursing, students were expected to write a retrospective, self-reflective paper on their experience for the day. Students were encouraged to think about lessons learned from their experience. They were given general journaling guidelines to follow. Questions to explore included:

- What did I do well today in clinical?

- What assessments or interventions was I most confident with?

- Did I support the work of the care team?

- What did the care team do well in this situation?

- Where did the care provided fall short?

- What were the actual or anticipated outcomes of patient care?

- Did I advocate for the patient?

- Did I communicate my concerns to my instructor and ideas about patient care effectively to nursing team members?

Journaling was one way for each student nurse to work on defining his or her self-identity as a nurse and a member of a high-performing work team engaged in patient care.

Multipatient Simulation

Often, when students enter the medical–surgical portion of their nursing education, they have completed pharmacology lecture and labs. Most likely they have also completed a pharmacy competency where they are expected to simulate giving medications to a patient. Most of these students have never administered medications to a real patient at this point in their education. Clinical instructors often attempt to have each student administer medications every day while they attempt to discern the students' clinical awareness and ability to assess patients.

High fidelity multiple patient simulations were developed to introduce student nurses to the complexities of the medical–surgical nursing environment. Scenarios focused on receiving patient handoff reports, clarifying medication orders, and safely preparing and administering medications to two patients. Observation and evaluation of each student was performed by the faculty attending the student at the bedside utilizing a medication competency assessment tool, as well as faculty observers in the control room. These evaluations were then submitted to each student's clinical instructor for remediation throughout the 24-week medical–surgical rotation.

Focus on Assessment

Regardless of the model used to bring curricular improvement to clinical education, every clinical education initiative must begin with the original first step in the nursing process: assessment. The data points collected during the PDA study demonstrated that only 5.6% of the data points collected were captured as students assessed their patients. Before students can understand the concepts of pain and suffering and before they can describe the limits and boundaries of therapeutic patient-centered care, they must know how to carefully assess. With instructors and students spending the majority of their day involved with medication administration and documentation, how can educators be sure that students are capable of performing thorough assessments and effectively communicating findings? As stated earlier, the first four weeks of the clinical timeline were devoted to student mastery of physical assessment. Instructors were not challenged by frequent interruptions for medication administration, and they were available to assist and validate the students' assessment skills. Use of the Sixty-Second Situation Assessment Tool (Box 5-2) enhanced students' ability to identify pertinent information about each patient's situation. It enabled students to make inferences and prioritize patient care needs. Use of the tool helped students enhance their assessment technique and allowed for an organized approach.

Patient-Centered Care

"Patient-centered care is considered to be interrelated with both quality and safety. The role of patients as part of the 'team' can influence the quality of care they receive and their outcomes." (Hughes RG [ed.], 2008, Chapter 2, p. 9).

In the relationship-based care model, "all care practices visibly demonstrate the mission and values of the organization, including those of clinicians and staff members from all disciplines. The activities of care are organized around the needs and priorities of patients and families"

(Koloroutis, 2004, p. 15). In an environment of patient-centered care, the patient and family are at the center, that is, they are the foundation of the relationship. All systems and processes within the care environment are built around them.

Participating in interprofessional rounds at the patient's bedside with the goal of encouraging communication between patient, family, and care team is one important patient-centered care activity for students. The motto for the patient should be "Nothing about me, without me." In other words, the care team should not discuss any part of the patient's plan of care without the patient present and involved. Student nurses should seek out every opportunity to participate in rounds on patients with the interprofessional team. Strong teamwork develops as the disciplines discuss their perspectives of the patient's progress toward care goals. New nurses can begin to appreciate the role each member plays and begin to develop resources to facilitate care. The patient is involved in this dialogue, ideally clarifying his or her own goals for treatment. The outcomes of this activity include increased patient satisfaction with care, greater patient adherence to the treatment plan, and an opportunity for immediate educational interventions for the patient, directly from the discipline responsible.

Student Nurses' Perceptions of QSEN

Using a survey called the QSEN Student Evaluation Survey (SES), 17 schools of nursing assessed student nurses' perception of the effectiveness of these quality and safety education strategies in their schools of nursing (Sullivan, Hirst, & Cronenwett, 2009). Students across all programs reported that quality and safety competencies were very important as they entered practice. This instrument asks the student to consider selected QSEN competency KSAs and assess (1) their knowledge of the KSA (whether it was addressed in their program), (2) their preparation to perform that skill, and (3) the importance of that skill for nursing practice.

One school of nursing involved in the QSEN study assessed students' perceptions of quality and safety education effectiveness using the QSEN SES with the graduating classes in 2008 and 2009. This school of nursing utilized all the quality and safety education strategies outlined in this chapter. Over these three years, the faculty worked to incorporate quality and safety education strategies in the classroom, clinical, skills lab, and high-fidelity simulation theatre. As students' exposure to the KSAs through varied educational activities in class, clinical, and simulation increased, they reported greater understanding and skill performing the competency. They also reported that these competencies were extremely important for professional practice.

Mastery of quality and safety competencies is not a journey new nurses will take alone. All nurses need to engage in reflective practices to gain mastery of these quality and safety strategies to keep patients safe and improve care outcomes.

CASE STUDY: *Emily*

Emily, a new nurse, began her career on the pediatric hematology unit. She loved the children, and she was good at working with families. She started on the night shift, the youngest nurse and the only one with a bachelor's degree in nursing. She quickly became the night charge nurse. The other nurses on the night shift were resentful of her power and her early advancement related to her degree. The nurses began to talk about her and make fun of her. They told her that they would not abide by her rules because they had so many more years of experience.

Emily tried to work out the situation by asking for the other nurses' opinions when complicated situations arose. When she asked their opinion, it only heightened their criticism. The unit coordinator, Jessica, responded to Emily's concerns by telling her to work it out on her own. Jessica was not going to intervene and did not want to take sides.

After four months of working in a hostile environment, Emily put in a request to work in the emergency department (ED). Once she began working in the ED, her mood and her outlook for the future improved. The nurses and doctors were supportive and collaborative. She felt that she was listened to. When an interesting patient was admitted, the doctors would find her and make sure she observed the patient's symptoms and treatment.

One patient was really interesting to Emily. A 10-year-old boy was hit by a car while riding his bike. He did not have a helmet on, and he had an open skull fracture. The ED head, Dr. Reynolds, called her into the room to observe the trauma protocol. She watched as the nurses reacted immediately and called the neurosurgeons, the pediatric surgery team, the intensive care staff, and the operating room. The three nurses started the intravenous (IV) line, took vital signs every five minutes, and were in charge of the situation. They asked the doctor if the child needed more IV fluids. Then when the child started to become less aware, the nurses began doing neurological assessment every two to three minutes. The child was rushed to the operating room and had a four-hour surgery to stop the epidural bleeding and swelling. He recovered in the intensive care unit (ICU) and went home two weeks later.

After seeing the ED nurses in action, Emily knew she had found the right environment. The positive teamwork was incredible. She felt like she was a vital member of a great healthcare team.

1. What other steps might Emily have taken to address the hostile environment on the pediatric hematology unit?

2. Contrast the safety implications of the teamwork on the pediatric hematology unit with the teamwork in the ED.

CHAPTER HIGHLIGHTS

- Multiple projects and efforts have focused on safety and quality in nursing, including Transforming Care at the Bedside (TCAB), Quality and Safety Education in Nursing (QSEN), Crew Resource Management (CRM), and Situation, Background, Assessment, and Recommendations (SBAR).

- Nursing education must focus on integration of safety and quality concepts and initiatives so that new nurses are experts in ensuring safe care and measuring quality in nursing and health care.

- Nursing and health care can improve dramatically if collaboration, communication, and teamwork are developed with a unified goal of excellent safe nursing and health care.

Pearson Nursing Student Resources
Find additional review materials at
nursing.pearsonhighered.com
Prepare for success with additional NCLEX®-style practice questions, interactive assignments and activities, web links, animations and videos, and more!

REFERENCES

Agency for Healthcare Research and Quality (AHRQ). (2008). *TeamSTEPPS: Strategies and tools to enhance performance and patient safety*. Rockville, MD: AHRQ. Publication No. 06-0020-2.

American Association of Colleges of Nursing (AACN). (2008). *The essentials of baccalaureate education for professional nursing practice*. Retrieved from http://www.aacn.nche.edu/education/pdf/BaccEssentials08.pdf.

Berkow, S., Virkstis, K., Steward, J., & Conway, L. (2008). Assessing new graduate nurse performance. *Journal of Nursing Administration, 38*(11), 468–474.

Berwick, D.M. (2003). Disseminating innovations in health care. *Journal of the American Medical Association*, 289(15), 1969-1975.

Biron, A. D., Lavoie-Tremblay, M. N., & Loiselle, C. G. (2009). Characteristics of work interruptions during medication administration. *Journal of Nursing Scholarship, 41*(4), 330–336.

Carr, C. A. (2009). *National study of clinical nursing education: Discovering opportunity for redesign*. Waynesburg University, Wilmington, PA: Unpublished doctoral dissertation.

Cronenwett, L., Sherwood, G., Barnsteiner, J., Disch, J., Johnson, J., Mitchell, P., et al. (2007). Quality and safety education for nurses. *Nursing Outlook*, 55(3), 122–131.

Hallinan, J. T. (2009). *Why we make mistakes*. New York: Random House.

Hughes, RG (ed.). (2008). Patient safety and quality: An evidence-based handbook for nurses. (Prepared with support from the Robert Wood Johnson Foundation). AHRQ Publication No. 08-0043. Rockville, MD: Agency for Healthcare Research and Quality.

Institute of Medicine (IOM). (2003). *Health professions education: A bridge to quality*. Washington, DC: National Academies Press.

Institute of Medicine (IOM). (2004). *Keeping patients safe: Transforming the work environment of nurses*. Washington, DC: National Academies Press.

Institute for Safe Medication Practices (ISMP). (2003). *ISMP's list of high-alert medications*. Horsham, PA: ISMP.

Joint Commission on Accrediditation of Healthcare Organizations (JCAHO). (2008). *Sentinal event statistics: Behaviors that undermine a culture of safety*. Retrieved from http://www.jointcommission.org/assets/1/18/SEA_40.PDF.

Koloroutis, M. (2004). *Relationship-based care: A model for transforming practice*. Minneapolis, MN: Creative Healthcare Management.

Kovner, C. T., & Gergen, P. J. (1998). Nurse staffing levels and adverse events following surgery in U. S. Hospitals. *Image: The Journal of Nursing Scholarship, 30*, 315–321.

Leonard, M., Graham, S., & Bonacum, D. (2004). The human factor: The critical importance of effective teamwork and communication in providing safe care. *Quality and Safety in Health Care, 13(Supplement)*, 85–90.

Marquis, B. & Huston, C. (2003). *Leadership roles and management functions for nursing: Theory and application* (4th ed.) Philadelphia: Lippincott, Williams and Wilkins.

Melynk, B.M., & Fineout-Overholt, E. (2002). Putting research into practice. Rochester: ARCC. *Reflections on Nursing Leadership, 28*(2), 22–25.

Melynk, B.M., & Fineout-Overholt, E. (2005). *Evidence-based practice in nursing & healthcare: A guide to best practice*. Lippincott, Williams & Wilkins. Philadelphia, PA.

Merryman, T. (2004). The story of Transforming Care at the Bedside. *Robert Wood Johnson Foundation Nurse Leaders Meeting* (pp. 1–7). Princeton, NJ: Robert Wood Johnson Foundation (RWJF).

National League for Nursing (NLN). (2008). *Think tank on transforming clinical nursing education*. Indianapolis, IN. Retrieved April 30, 2012 from http://www.nln.org/facultyprograms/pdf/think_tank.pdf.

Printezis, A. G. (2007). Current pulse: Can a production system reduce medical errors in healthcare? *Quality Manage Health Care, 13*(3), 226–238.

Rutherford, P., Lee, B., & Greiner, A. (2004). *Transforming Care at the Bedside whitepaper*. Cambridge, MA: Institute for Healthcare Improvement.

Struth, D. (2009). TCAB in the curriculum. *American Journal of Nursing Supplement*, 55–58.

Suling, L., & Kenward, K. (2006). A national survey of nursing education and practice of newly licensed nurses. *JONA's Healthcare Law, Ethics, and Regulation, 8*(4), 110–115.

Sullivan, D. T., Hirst, D., & Cronenwett, L. (2009). Assessing quality and safety competencies of graduating pre-licensure nursing students. *Nursing Outlook, 57*(6), 323–331.

EVALUATING A PROGRAM: METRICS AND STAKEHOLDERS

Matthew Sorenson

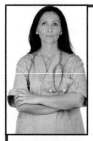

Lillianna was working her 12-hour night shift and trying to document her initial assessments in the computer. She had just sat down at the computer when she heard a loud scream and a thud. She thought it was her 83-year-old patient Louis who was healing following a prostatectomy. She had just given him his pain medication an hour earlier. The charge nurse ran to the bedside with Lillianna to assess the situation.

Gelpi/Shutterstock.com

CORE COMPETENCY

Construct and implement evidence-based metric measures to track safety and quality outcomes.

LEARNING OUTCOMES

1. Define the terms "metric" and "stakeholders" in the context of nursing practice and quality improvement methods.
2. Integrate metric measurement concepts into a healthcare delivery system.

3. Apply quality improvement metrics to a high-risk care situation and assess appropriate formative and summative measures.

Falls are one of the major safety issues encountered in hospital and long-term care settings. Hospitals and long-term care facilities have devised numerous fall prevention programs designed to prevent the incidence of falls and minimize patient injury. These programs include interventions designed to prevent falls and an educational component designed to teach staff how to incorporate these changes. Evaluating the effectiveness of these programs requires an understanding of metrics.

An Overview of Evaluation

When planning an educational or interventional program, significant amounts of time and effort are spent on decisions related to course content and delivery. At times, evaluating the effectiveness of a given program may be an afterthought, with little consideration paid to it. However, without an effective evaluation plan, there is no way of determining whether the program achieved its desired effect.

Establishing an evaluation plan with measurable outcomes is just as important as any other aspect of educational planning, if not more important. To effectively evaluate an educational program requires serious thought regarding not only what is to be evaluated and how, but from what viewpoint the program should be evaluated. The previous chapters of this book provided information regarding risks to quality and safe care and explored how nursing can help identify risks to enhance patient care. This chapter turns toward the programming created by nursing professionals and how it can be evaluated effectively. A particular focus should be on how different viewpoints influence not only the outcomes that need to be considered in educational planning, but also how differing views can influence measurement of those outcomes.

In terms of establishing an evaluation plan for any educational offering, regardless of how formal (e.g., an educational program focusing on management of hypertension) or informal (e.g., discharge instructions on the use of anticoagulants), it helps to reflect on a means of program evaluation that all nurses are already familiar with, namely the nursing process. The nursing process with its steps of assessment, identification (diagnosis), planning, implementation, and evaluation resembles the elements of the process used in program evaluation.

To determine the effectiveness of any nursing or healthcare action, a process of evaluation needs to occur. This follows the process of quality improvement. First, the nurse needs to identify or diagnose the potential problem or educational need. This process of assessment requires careful consideration of what issues, or gaps, in nursing care exist on a particular unit. Assessing for knowledge gaps in a particular care setting and identifying those gaps then leads to the development of an educational plan to meet the existent or future educational needs of the staff and the implementation of the plan. Evaluation of the project then leads to the start of a circular process all over again. As Cronenwett and colleagues (2007) define the process of quality improvement, it "is the use of data to monitor the outcomes of care processes and the use of improvement methods to design and test changes" (Cronenwett et al., 2007, p. 127).

Program evaluation is a process of collecting information regarding the conduct or effectiveness of any program or activity. The first step is deciding what outcomes or programmatic elements are going to be evaluated, or what are the goals for the program. This process is greatly enhanced when a program has established outcomes or goals. To measure a particular outcome, there needs to be a clearly identified outcome along with a clear procedure as to how the information needs to be collected. Aiding in the completion of this process are metrics. Several forms of metrics for program evaluation exist, but all forms require a careful evaluation of the perspective of stakeholders, or those who have an interest in the program (Worthen, Sanders, & Fitzpatrick, 2004).

What Is a Metric?

The word "metric" can be defined either as a noun or an adjective. The term "metric," defined by the Oxford English Dictionary, is "the principle system of measurement" ("Metric," 2012). The term "benchmark" can also stand for a metric and is a term that may be familiar to nurses. In this chapter, the term "metric" will refer to a set of measurable criteria that is defined in advance of a project. A metric can be a specific measurable goal, or a cluster or group of goals. In terms of single goal, an example could be a specific benchmark or score of patient satisfaction with the hospital.

Evidence for Best Practices: Preventing Falls

Can falls really be prevented, and how do we measure fall prevention? The metric all nurses aim for is zero falls during a specific time frame. The metric is the number of recorded incidents of falls on a specific unit. Screening and prevention programs have recently been associated with decreased risk for falls. However, the metric measured could be the number of patients screened for falls in addition to the total number of falls. When patients who are at risk for falling, such as sedated or elderly patients, are identified by wearing brightly colored socks, vests, or wristbands, nurses and nurse aides can be alerted to high-risk patients even if they are not assigned to the patient. When a patient is in the hall or when a nurse aide comes in to help a patient with whom he or she is not familiar the alert-for-fall-risk item can help providers be extra vigilant to help reduce the risk for falls.

Shever, Titler, Lehan Mackin, and Kueny (2011) identified nurse practices in 51 hospitals as reported by nurse managers. The state of safe nursing practice, according to Shever and colleagues, remains inconsistent as is. Only 40% of units used a screening tool to assess risk for falls, 90% used bed alarms, and 68% used sitters for patients. The study found that alarms and sitters are not effective in fall prevention. Many also reported using restraints for patients at risk for falls. The most effective fall prevention approach is good screening and risk assessment, as reported by Graf (2011). Fall prevention should be included in data gathering.

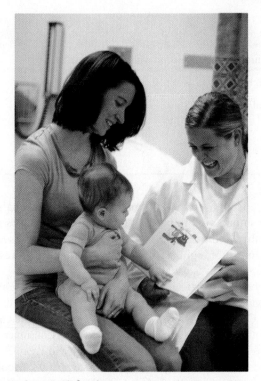

Figure 6-1   Patient Satisfaction
Quality nursing skills are essential to patient satisfaction.
Shots by Shelley

A hospital or other care setting may have a desired target score, and patient satisfaction scores can then be compared to the target. From an administrative perspective, using an example of a fall prevention program, a metric could be a set of the following outcomes or data: (1) the number of falls on a particular unit, (2) the number of falls in a particular group of patients, (3) the number of falls that occur in patients on fall precautions, and (4) the perceptions of staff members regarding the effectiveness of the fall prevention program. Also included is (5) the perspective of patients regarding the intrusiveness of these precautions. These five sources of information then provide a better idea of the overall effectiveness of a fall prevention program rather than simply asking if there is a difference in the number of falls after the implementation of a program. Having a clearly established metric can help determine when a goal has been met and can facilitate communication with other members of the healthcare team.

Another metric that is used commonly is the patient satisfaction survey. Hospital administrators are interested in the results of patient satisfaction indicators. The most common assessments of patient satisfaction use a zero to five or zero to seven scale and ask questions related to how the patient rates the nursing care, including how quickly

---

BOX 6-1   PATIENT SATISFACTION METRICS

A wide range of metrics can be used to measure patient satisfaction with care. Examples are:

- How quickly the nurse answered the call light

- The quality of the food while in the hospital

- The loudness of the unit staff

- How well the nurse communicated with the patient

---

the call light is answered. As Figure 6-1 illustrates, quality nursing care instills satisfaction in patients. Other question topics range from the food quality to the cleanliness of the patient's room (see Box 6-1). When the scores are high, staff may be rewarded. If scores are low, a plan for improvement is usually created.

A brief review of articles that address patient satisfaction with nursing care provides a great range of measures. These instruments include the following; a Caring Behavior Inventory (CBI) that measures nurse caring behaviors, Patient Satisfaction Scale (PSS), Hospital Consumer Assessment of Healthcare Providers and Systems (HCAHPS), and Press Gainey ratings of patient satisfaction with hospital stay (Goldstein, 2008; Brooks-Carthon, Kutney-Lee, Sloane, Cimiotti, & Aiken, 2011). In the past, patient satisfaction measures were used to determine nursing pay increases, even though measures included unrelated items such as rankings of food quality and television functionality. Current patient satisfaction measures are more closely aligned with the nursing care being evaluated; however, a wide range of surveys is still used. The most important issue is that the choice and summary of a patient satisfaction tool should be aligned with the issue that was intended. Nursing should be evaluated on specific nursing care, not food quality.

Another critical issue is the validity of the survey questions. To evaluate the patient's satisfaction with the postoperative nursing care, one of these two questions should be included:

1. Were all your postoperative needs met while recovering from surgery?

2. Did the nursing care provided after surgery meet your expectations?

These two questions will most probably get very different responses. Number 1 will rarely be answered with a "yes," but it includes all staff involved in the postoperative care, whereas number 2 asks only about nursing case. For that reason, number 2 results in a more valid assessment of nursing care provision and patient satisfaction.

Nurses should be aware of the measures being used to assess the level of safety, quality care, and patient perceptions of their care. When measures to evaluate nursing care are being chosen by hospital administrators, nurses should be present at the discussions and understand the strengths of each measurement survey or tool. When a nurse's pay raise

BOX 6-2	KEY LINKS AND RESOURCES

The following material will be of benefit to those interested in reading further on metrics and their evaluation.

- Preskill, H., & Jones, N. (2009). *A practical guide for engaging stakeholders in developing evaluation questions.* Princeton, NJ: Robert Wood Johnson Foundation (RWJF). Available at http://www.rwjf.org/pr/product.jsp?id=49951.

- Rutherford, P., Phillips, J., Coughlan, P., Lee, B., Moen, R., Peck, C., & Taylor, J. (2008). *Transforming Care at the Bedside how-to guide: Engaging front-line staff in innovation and quality improvement.* Cambridge, MA: Institute for Healthcare Improvement. Available at www.IHI.org.

- *A toolkit for redesign in health care.* Final Report (Prepared by Denver Health under Contract No. 290-00-0014). AHRQ Publication No. 05-0108-EF, September 2002. Rockville, MD: Agency for Healthcare Research and Quality (AHRQ). Available at http://www.ahrq.gov/qual/toolkit/.

and job security are being reviewed, the nurse should be comfortable with the metrics being used. Box 6-2 provides resources for learning more about metrics used for evaluations.

Establishing metrics for healthcare settings can involve the perspectives of several groups or individuals with differing interests and goals. These groups or individuals are referred to as stakeholders. The Institute of Medicine goals shown in Table 6-1 exemplify an approach that focuses on the patient as stakeholder. Determining which outcomes will be measured depends on the positions of the stakeholders. In brief, the term refers to those who have a stake, or concern, about a particular process or organization. For the purposes of this chapter, a working definition is someone who can affect, or be affected by, the nursing care provided. How, then, can the stakeholder's viewpoint influence the type of measurement criteria, or metric, that is used?

TABLE 6-1 ■ Institute of Medicine Goals

Patient Care Goals	• Safe
	• Efficient
	• Equitable
Framework to Measure	• Structure
	• Process
	• Outcome
Safety Measures and Predictors	• Number of staff
	• Length of stay
	• Morbidity and mortality
Patient Satisfaction	• Space around bed
	• Wound care
	• Food, call light response, and bedside manner

(Adapted from QSEN presentation by Jean Johnson, PhD, RN, FAAN on 3/16/11)

Stakeholders and Evaluation

Stakeholders' perspectives should be considered carefully when establishing metrics and when evaluating the ability of a program to accomplish goals. Setting up outcomes without identifying what is important to the groups involved can lead to wasted time and effort spent in collecting unimportant information. Stakeholders may share select common goals but may also have goals unique to their role or group. Nursing administrators may be more interested in performance goals in terms of shift coverage or nurse role performance, while individual staff nurses may be more concerned with patient acuity or care. Yet each of these groups has a shared interest in patient outcomes.

Many nursing metrics reflect the relative contributions of several different stakeholders, not those of just one person (Schalock, 2001). In the patient satisfaction example, the stakeholders are the patient, the nurses, and the administrators. If a nursing unit is using a metric that measures the number of falls on the unit, then performance involves the monitoring program set up by the staff members, the cognitive and functional capability of the patients on the unit, the training programs that have been developed to train the staff on fall precautions, and the hospital administration in terms of making a commitment to reduce the number of falls and provide adaptive devices such as bed alarms, modified call lights, adequate lighting, and appropriate footwear for patients. Evaluating nursing care on one parameter such as the number of falls can then involve several pieces of data and points of view.

To illustrate how the stakeholder's point of view influences what is measured, consider the example of a study that surveyed several key stakeholders within a medical institution on their perceptions of control on the part of each stakeholder group. The study posed the same set of questions to nurses, physicians, unit or department managers, patients, and the board of directors. The findings revealed that even when the same questions are asked of diverse stakeholder groups, the answers can be very different from one group to the next (Daake & Anthony, 2000). While the perspective of stakeholders may differ, there is room for agreement. A study of various stakeholder groups in long-term care facilities found agreement among three preeminent areas: quality of care, quality of life, and the rights of patients (Harrington et al., 1999).

Hospitals frequently evaluate response times to call lights, number of falls, nosocomial infection rates, and other outcomes of patient care. While nursing managers and staff nurses may consider these important indicators of patient care and outcomes, the patient may value other factors. Studies on the patient perspective tend to show that patients value the caring demeanor of nurses and other caregivers more than other clinical expertise (Attree, 2001). In others words, patients often place higher value on a caring demeanor than the quality of the physical care provided. However, it should be considered whether a measurement of patient satisfaction with a particular dimension is truly an indicator of unit quality. Satisfaction with care may not necessarily reflect quality of care.

The Collaborative Alliance for Nursing Outcomes (CALNOC) provides excellent resources for identifying appropriate outcome measures. The use of a metric that has a measure of patient satisfaction along with a measure of falls and perhaps infection rates may provide a better representation of unit quality.

An additional consideration is who is collecting the feedback from the stakeholders. The perspective of the listener, or data collector, will influence the type of information collected from various stakeholders. For instance, returning to the example of a fall prevention program, a nursing administrator and staff nurses may be interested in different factors and variables. If a nursing administrator is interviewing or collecting data from a patient, the questions asked may not be the same as the questions asked by a physician, for example, and the interpretation of the patient's responses may also be different. This is not to imply that nursing administration cannot effectively assess the needs of stakeholders; the point is that the reason information is being gathered can influence the information collected. The nursing administrator may be more concerned with the time that it took for staff members to respond to a fall, or the mix of unit personnel on the shift. The staff nurse may be more concerned with the reasons the patient may have attempted to exit a bed, whether obstacles were present, or the cognitive state of the patient at the time.

Stakeholder interests may then vary based on administrative level and whether there is direct patient contact. The interests of direct nursing staff and patients will also vary based on the type of unit the patient is on. Different nursing units have different needs and can have different metrics. The AACN Synergy Model for Patient Care described by Curley (2007) helps illustrate how different nursing units can have different aggregate goals. Curley was able to utilize the AACN Synergy Model for Patient Care to differentiate nursing goals between nursing units. Unit nursing staff were asked to identify patient-focused outcomes specific to the care provided on that unit. These conversations served as a basis for establishing metrics, which were defined as measurable standards of care based on the needs of the patient population served by the unit. Thus, the metrics established by nurses on the pediatric intensive care unit were different from the metrics set up by nurses working on the cardiac intensive care unit. The majority of the metrics were defined as process indicators evaluating nursing care through patient indicators, for example, the number of patients who had pain assessments completed and documented every four hours. Select system indicators were also incorporated to evaluate part of the nurse staff system, such as unit continuity of care (Curley, 2007). This example demonstrates how a set of outcomes can help staff evaluate different elements of nursing care: patient-centered outcomes and staff assignments. This set of outcomes is then a metric. It could then be said that metrics are means of determining the relative contributions of nursing care to patient outcomes.

CASE STUDY: *Evaluating Falls*

Over the past six months, the number of falls has been gradually increasing in the hospital. A policy and procedure has been prepared that documents measures that should be recorded by nursing personnel. In the eyes of nursing administration, the total number of hospital falls over the period of one month is established as an outcome metric (hospital administration as stakeholder). On a particular unit, the manager (unit manager as stakeholder) is more concerned about the number of falls that occur on the unit. This then becomes an outcome metric for the unit—the number of falls on the unit during a given month. This number would then be compared to other months of the year to determine if the policy change is effective. An individual nurse may not be as concerned with the total number of falls on the unit over the period of a month as he may be concerned with whether a fall occurs during his shift (nurse as stakeholder). The patient may not be overly concerned about the number of falls over a shift; instead, the patient is concerned about whether she falls (patient and family as stakeholder). Ultimately, the hospital may need to report this metric to the organization that oversees accreditation of the facility (accrediting organization as stakeholder).

Consider the situation presented in the evaluating falls case study. What are the determining issues in terms of deciding on a metric for evaluation? First, the institution and staff must determine what defines a patient fall. If a staff member is present in the room and catches a patient who is off balance, has a fall occurred? In some institutions, this would constitute a fall, and in others it may not. In the eyes of administration, the outcomes of the policy and procedure could be: (1) the number of falls in the hospital for a given time period, (2) the number of patients identified as at risk and provided fall precaution wristbands, and (3) the number of incident reports filed documenting a fall. In each of these situations, a clear outcome is provided, but each measures a different situation. For the unit staff, a patient might lose his balance, be caught, and be helped to the floor. This would be defined as a fall by the hospital but may not be considered a true fall by the staff member or even the patient. Another element is the degree of inconvenience the patient and family may perceive as a result of the intervention. If patients feel the intervention is too intrusive, their level of satisfaction may be affected and the score on another metric affected.

Goals, Process, and Outcome Evaluation

In the evaluating falls case study, the question of what is being evaluated was raised. The manner in which a situation is defined influences the measurement as well as the consequences of the program or study. By defining a fall as any situation in which the patient loses balance, the hospital will have a higher reporting rate of incidents. In turn, the higher reporting rate may lead to more attention paid to situations that could potentially place an individual at risk for fall. This could contribute to staff training and educational programs targeting patients that are at increased risk of fall. On the other hand, the hospital could then be reporting a higher rate of falls to accrediting bodies or other stakeholders. In choosing an outcome for evaluation, the definition of what is to be measured is then important.

If a nursing unit or facility is interested in determining the number of medication errors, then a definition of medication error needs to be provided. Is an error the provision of an inappropriate dosage of medication by the pharmacy, even if the mistake is caught by the nurse prior to the medication being given to the patient? Or does a medication error imply that a degree of harm has occurred to the patient? Some definitions of medication error incorporate an element of use or harm to the patient that occurs through inappropriate administration on the part of a healthcare professional (Classen & Metzger, 2003). Using such a definition begins to suggest measurement of outcomes. In this case, outcome measurement would focus on the degree of harm to the patient. So, in the process of laying out a set of criteria, definitions and terms are being provided that begin to suggest measurement. Ultimately then, a metric could be considered an outcome of nursing practice, one that is measured. Each healthcare unit or setting can then have different metrics. Once a decision is made regarding what is to be measured, an equally important question is how it will be measured.

After considering who the stakeholders are and the differing outcomes that may emerge, additional considerations start to appear. In terms of the outcomes or metrics that may be evaluated, one should also consider what kind of evaluation may be employed. A means of classifying evaluations breaks them down into goal, process, or outcome based (Worthen et al., 2004). Each of these evaluation methods would examine different metrics and collect stakeholder feedback regarding different elements of a program.

A goal-based evaluation examines how a program is performing related to meeting outcomes. In other words, it tries to provide a sense of how a program is doing in terms of meeting the established metrics. Going back to the example of a fall prevention program, the goal-based evaluation would seek to identify how well the unit is doing in terms of meeting this goal. Does the rate of falls fluctuate over time? Is there an overall reduction in the number of falls? Does the unit have the appropriate resources to implement a fall prevention program? Could the unit meet a target timeline? These are all questions that would be considered as part of a goal-based evaluation.

The process-based evaluation looks more at the system or pieces involved. An example would be to look at who is present on the night shift that may influence the number of falls. Are there adequate levels of staffing? Are any environmental factors contributing to the falls, such as loud noises from heart monitor alarms or beeping call lights that may wake a patient who could then be confused and somewhat uncoordinated while trying to walk into the bathroom? Are there any patient expectations that need to be considered?

Outcome-based evaluation tends to focus more on learning-centered activities or factors. If a program has been set up to teach patients about the risk of falls and means of avoiding them, do patients demonstrate an understanding of the information? Do different teaching methods need to be employed? Ultimately, the outcome-based evaluation is measuring the change that was supposed to result from the program, while the process evaluation is measuring the intervention itself. Did falls decrease, and did they decrease because of the fall prevention program? Or was there another factor that was not considered in the first place?

Timing the Evaluation

An important assumption of healthcare programs and interventions is that a change will occur. Whether the change is in the level of knowledge on the part of unit nurses after an educational program or a reduction in the number of falls, it is presumed that change will occur. When the measurement is made can also influence measurement of any change. If a fall prevention program is designed and implemented on a nursing unit, a reduction in the number of falls may not be expected in the first few days, but in a week or two. The process should be collaborative and supportive of everyone involved.

With an educational program, evaluation often follows immediately. Every nurse is familiar with cardiopulmonary resuscitation (CPR) classes, in which evaluation occurs immediately after the class in terms of a repeated performance of CPR procedure and a course test out and evaluation. Is this an adequate measurement? For the nurse who does not perform CPR on a regular basis, will the necessary pieces be retained if CPR needs to be performed four or five months later? To ensure readiness, many hospitals have begun to require yearly competency programs and reviews.

When evaluating any program, then, consideration should be given to when the evaluation of the program will occur. Perhaps more than one evaluation is necessary, depending on the goals of the program. A survey evaluating satisfaction with the educational program itself may be appropriate after a program, but an additional survey assessing the retention of knowledge two months after the program could provide an indication of whether the program has achieved the desired effect.

The Method of Measurement

Traditionally, an educational program may have a brief checklist that immediately follows the program. Those readers who have completed online educational programs or attended conferences will be familiar with these checklists. A general questionnaire asks whether the viewer was satisfied with the program, the means of delivering the content, the level of depth covered by content, and sometimes whether the presented information will influence clinical practice. Evaluation of an educational program can be helpful in determining whether the information was presented in an understandable manner. What an evaluation of this type does not do is evaluate whether any of the information presented actually changes clinical practice. After a metric is selected, and the input of stakeholder groups obtained, then attention is turned to the means of collecting the necessary data or information.

Measurement of Outcomes

When a safety issue is identified, the team must determine how to monitor the progress or changes to decrease the risk. The way that the safety issue is measured will be critical. The measure must be reliable and valid. To be reliable, it must measure what is intended to be measured. As an example, consider a recipe that calls for a tablespoon of oil. The cook, instead, uses a teaspoon of oil every time she makes the recipe. The results will be reliable and consistent because the cook uses a teaspoon of oil every time. However, the results will not be valid because the cook always prepares the recipe using an incorrect measurement. Validity is the concept of *truly* measuring what it is intended to be measured. A teaspoon will be measuring the same amount over and over, but it is not a tablespoon and thus it is not valid. The teaspoon is not a valid measure of a tablespoon of oil. Once a decision is made regarding what is to be measured, an equally important question is how it will be measured.

Patient satisfaction with nursing care, as discussed earlier, also has a variety of reliability and validity issues. The measure must be accurately representing the nursing care that should be evaluated. Once the accuracy, or reliability, is established, then the validity should be assessed. Patient satisfaction with nursing care must be measured in a manner that fits the nursing standards and the expectations. There is much value to measuring performance of nursing care, and the most important focus is on continually improving care. The balance that needs to be achieved is between the right survey or instrument, the proven validity of the instrument, and using the instrument in a non punitive way. The spirit should be one of learning how to be the best possible nurse.

Collecting the Data

Data can be collected retrospectively from computer systems within the hospital, or methods could be used to examine the attitudes and perceptions of members of the healthcare staff. Metrics can be set that focus on the frequency of documentation, the number of cases that a hospital or care setting serves with a particular diagnosis or condition, or the number of referrals that were made to a particular service. Data on all these situations can be collected retrospectively. Metrics that have a component of patient satisfaction, patient learning, patient understanding, or even patient participation and adherence need to have a means for gathering information apart from the hospital computer system. These methods should give the patient or other stakeholders a chance to share their concerns and beliefs. Some of the common approaches include questionnaires, satisfaction surveys, interviews or focus groups, and even observation of a particular group.

Questionnaires Questionnaires are a common means of assessing program effectiveness. Healthcare institutions often send patients postdischarge questionnaires to determine satisfaction with several dimensions of the facility during the hospitalization. Pre- and post-test measures are common in the evaluation of knowledge on nursing units. Examples include medication tests given at the point of hire or post-tests given after training sessions.

For the nurse determining whether to use a questionnaire to evaluate any program, there are several points to consider. A pre-established questionnaire may be employed. If so, information regarding the reliability and validity of the questionnaire should be determined. The reliability of information retrieved from a questionnaire refers to the consistency with which an individual answers the same questions on more than one occasion. If the same test is used on two occasions, and the answers that are given match one another to a high degree, the test could be said to have test-retest reliability. Validity concerns whether the questions on the test actually reflect the material they are intended to measure. One of the main means to determine the validity of questions that could be used to measure the taught concepts is to show the questionnaire to other nurses, those that might be considered experts in the area. The continuing education department of an institution could be consulted in the development of a questionnaire. In this case, content validity could be determined through the consultation of content experts who could clarify whether the questions are appropriate (Nunnally, 1978).

Other means of determining reliability include using a spreadsheet application or statistical program to examine how each item correlates, or relates, to other items. If all the questions seem to be asking related questions, the test could be said to have a high degree of internal consistency. Using a statistical procedure performed by Cronbach to examine the consistency of repeated findings is a common way of measuring this aspect of reliability (Cronbach, 1978).

Interviews and Focus Groups Interviews and focus groups allow for the collection of information that may not have been considered during the development of a questionnaire. The use of such data collection procedures can also help ensure that the concerns of stakeholders are truly heard.

Using an interview allows for more exploration of a topic and provides a better sense of the concerns and issues that a patient or nurse may have regarding an educational or procedural program. The interview could use either open- or closed-ended questions to collect information. In either case, the questions should be reviewed by other stakeholders

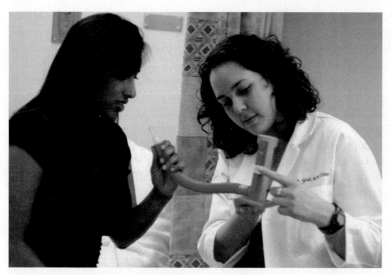

Figure 6-2   Evaluation Education
Patient interviews can help to evaluate educational instruction
provided prior to or following discharge
Shots by Shelley

prior to implementation. A trial run with a few nurses or patients can help resolve any problems or issues.

A focus group could be five or six nurses brought together to discuss the unit's educational needs. The intent behind a focus group is to have a process of dialogue between the group members that helps bring out thoughts or ideas that may not emerge otherwise.

Either of these approaches could also be used to help identify the perspectives of stakeholders or to evaluate educational offerings. An example of the former would be using a short series of select patient interviews to identify concerns or perceived educational gaps prior to or following discharge (see Figure 6-2). A postdischarge evaluation may be of more benefit, for after having navigated the community and home environments, the former patient may be able to identify additional areas for education.

Using a focus group of discharged patients, or patients attending a support group at the facility, can also help identify and summarize problems and needs. The disadvantage to each of these approaches is the necessary participant time and effort. In addition, if the questions are not phrased properly or the interviewer is not neutral, the response may be biased.

Observation of Behavior Another way of collecting data is via observation. Several studies have been done on hand washing procedures, and the rate of adherence on the part of several different healthcare providers. Most of these studies have employed an observational approach (Khan & Siddiqui, 2008; Surgeoner, Chapman, & Powell, 2009). Someone monitors staff members to determine whether hands are washed and to what degree.

In such studies, if more than one observer rates or scores the behaviors, then a means of ensuring consistency between observers is necessary. If two nurses are observing another nurse or a patient's behavior and scoring that behavior, the recorded scores can be compared to determine the degree of accuracy between the two scorers. This inter-rater reliability is a common procedure and is often referred to statistically as kappa. This provides a means of determining what the staff or patients are actually doing, rather than what is reported.

Global Trigger Tool Ensuring quality nursing care is the primary focus of this book, and how quality nursing care is measured is changing. A recent study (Classen et al., 2011) using a Global Trigger Tool (GTT) developed by the Institute of Healthcare Improvement revealed 10 times greater adverse events than previously reported.

The GTT used in the study included patient chart reviews by two or three employees, including nurses and pharmacists, who identified discharge codes, discharge summaries, medications, lab results, and narrative documentation. Triggers could include a stop medication order or an antidote medication such as naxolene (Narcan). Once identified, the trigger led to further investigation of whether an adverse event actually occurred. The GTT was much more sensitive than voluntary reporting of adverse events and more sensitive than the Agency for Healthcare Research and Quality's Patient Safety Indicators. In the study, 795 patient records were reviewed, and the GTT identified 354 out of 393 events. The self-reported events were only 4 (1%) out of 393, and the Patient Safety Indicators detected 35 adverse events (8.99%).

The GTT is more sensitive in measuring events that may not absolutely be defined as adverse, but clearly a middle ground needs to be identified to continue to measure adverse events. Future measures should be designed within electronic health records to highlight and alert healthcare providers regarding triggers that may indicate adverse events.

Utilizing the Obtained Information: Returning to the Stakeholders
After the evaluation process has occurred and data has been collected, time has to be spent in reviewing the findings and determining what they mean. If data related to satisfaction is collected on an educational program, then analyzing and interpreting the data could be fairly straightforward. If there have been a number of open-ended questions and the collection of several different pieces of information, analysis will take longer and may require the assistance of individuals familiar with statistics and other aspects of data analysis. One thing to keep in mind is what the original metrics were trying to measure and whether the data is reflective of the goals behind the choice of those outcomes and measures.

CASE STUDY: *Pressure Ulcer Study*

One of the nursing coordinators has noted an increase in pressure ulcers over the last three months on a critical care unit. A program is developed with a series of standardized turning protocols combined with skin checks every shift. The program is to be implemented on one of the critical care units as a pilot prior to implementation across the other units.

The educational coordinator develops a series of teaching materials and arranges a series of unit-based workshops to familiarize unit staff with the bedside-based training program. The remaining issue is identifying the outcomes to be measured. The outcome measure chosen needs to represent the individual and organization's definition of safety and quality. To begin to identify the best outcome indicator, or metric, answer the following questions:

1. Who are the potential stakeholders? What is the perspective of each in relation to evaluating program effectiveness?

2. What are some different techniques that can be used in gathering the perspectives of stakeholders?

3. How could the timing of follow-up influence the metrics established for evaluation of the program?

4. What types of instruments can be used to collect data on the effectiveness of the program?

5. Can the same metric be used across all units?

Data collected through the use of open-ended questions or interviews will most likely be qualitative in nature. This set of information will most likely address how someone feels about a particular program and can provide additional information regarding concerns and issues. This data is generally not presented in the form of numbers, but in terms of general themes and overall statements as to the meaning of the data. Data collected through the use of surveys and questionnaires will most likely be quantitative in nature, with the data presented in terms of a score or number.

To ensure that the data is truly representative of stakeholders' opinions, it should be presented to a representative group to make sure that the findings are easily comprehended by the stakeholder group. This means the preliminary data should be summarized and presented in a way that is easy to understand. Stakeholder input can help to contextualize the findings and determine how to implement necessary changes. As mentioned at the beginning of this discussion, program evaluation is an ongoing circular process.

Once the changes are put in place, then the process of evaluation starts again. Having clear metrics that reflect the outcomes aids greatly in this process.

CHAPTER HIGHLIGHTS

- To determine if nursing care has improved because of an initiative, there needs to be a process of evaluation.

- To facilitate the process of evaluation, metrics need to be established that provide a clear means of identifying whether the desired changes have occurred. A metric is a set of measurable criteria that is defined in advance of a project.

- During the process of both developing metrics and evaluating their effectiveness, the input of stakeholders—the primary people who benefit from measuring the outcomes—needs to be considered. Without an understanding of the perspective of stakeholders, the established metric may not encompass the necessary dimensions of care, and the evaluation will be truncated.

- Data can be collected by using questionnaires, interviews, focus groups, and observation. The Global Trigger Tool (GTT) is a reliable way to collect information about adverse events.

Pearson Nursing Student Resources

Find additional review materials at
nursing.pearsonhighered.com

Prepare for success with additional NCLEX®-style practice questions, interactive assignments and activities, web links, animations and videos, and more!

REFERENCES

Attree, M. (2001). Patients' and relatives' experiences and perspectives of 'good' and 'not so good' quality care. *Journal of Advanced Nursing*, 33(4), 456-466.

Brooks-Carthon, J. M., Kutney-Lee, A., Sloane, D. M., Cimiotti, J. P., & Aiken, L. H. (2011). Quality of care and patient satisfaction in hospitals with high concentrations of black patients. *Journal of Nursing Scholarship, 43*(3), 301–310. doi 10.1111/j .1547–5069.2011.01403.x

Classen, D. C., & Metzger, J. (2003). Improving medication safety: The measurement conundrum and where to start. *International Journal for Quality in Health Care, 15*(Supplement 1), 41–47.

Classen, D. C., Resar, R., Griffin, F., Federico, F., Frankel, T., Kimmel, N., et al. (2011). Global Trigger Tool shows that adverse events in hospitals may be ten times greater than previously measured. *Health Affairs,* 30, 4581–45589. i:10.1377/hlthaff.2011.0190

Cronbach, L. J. (1978). Test validation. In R. L. Thorndike (ed.). *Educational measurement* (2nd ed.). Washington, DC: American Council of Education.

Cronenwett, L., Sherwood, G., Barnsteiner, J., Disch, J., Johnson, J., Mitchell, P., Sullivan, D. T., & Warren, J. (2007). Quality and safety education for nurses. *Nursing Outlook,* 55(3),122–131.

Curley, M.A.Q. (2007). Synergy: The unique relationship between nurses and patients.

Indianapolis: Sigma Theta Tau International.

Daake, D., & Anthony, W. P. (2000). Understanding stakeholder power and influence gaps in a health care organization: An empirical study. *Health Care Management Review, 25*(3), 94–107.

Goldstein, M. (2008). *How hospitals rate sing HCAHPS: The first national, standardized survey of patients' perspectives of hospital care.* Paper presented at Academy Health Annual Research Meeting, Washington, DC. Presented June 10, 2008.

Graf, E. (2011). Magnet children's hospitals: Leading knowledge development and quality standards for inpatient pediatric fall prevention programs. *Journal of Pediatric Nursing, 26,* 112–127.

Harrington, C., Mullan, J., Woodruff, L. C., Burger, S. G., Carrillo, H., & Bedney, B. (1999). Stakeholders' opinions regarding important measures of nursing home quality for consumers. *American Journal of Medical Quality, 14*(3), 124–132.

Khan, M. U., & Siddiqui, K. M. (2008). Hand washing and gloving practices among anaesthetists. *Journal of the Pakistan Medical Association, 58*(1), 27–29.

"Metric." (2012). OED Online. Oxford University Press. http://www.oed.com/viewdictionaryentry/Entry/117658 (accessed April 26, 2012).

Nunnally, J.C. (1978). *Psychometric theory* (2nd ed.) New York: McGraw-Hill Publishing Company.

Schalock, R. L. (2001). *Outcome-based evaluation* (2nd ed.). New York: Kluwer Academic/Plenum Publishers.

Shever, L. L., Titler, M. G., Lehan Mackin, M., & Kueny, A. (2011). Fall prevention practices in adult medical–surgical nursing units described by nurse managers. *Western Journal of Nursing Research, 33,* 385–397.

Surgeoner, B. V., Chapman, B. J., & Powell, D. A. (2009). University students' hand hygiene practice during a gastrointestinal outbreak in residence: What they say they do and what they actually do. *Journal of Environmental Health, 72*(2), 24–28.

Worthen, B. R., Sanders, J. R., & Fitzpatrick, J. L. (2004). *Program evaluation: Alternative approaches and practical guidelines* (3rd ed.). Boston: Allyn and Bacon.

INTERPROFESSIONAL TEAM BUILDING

Kim Siarkowski Amer

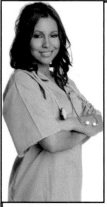

CHAPTER 7

R. Gino Santa Maria/
Shutterstock.com

Celina, a new nurse on the renal pediatrics floor, is in the nurses' station charting as the attending physician, Dr. Cone, arrives "Who has Jorge?" he asks.

Celina replies, "I do," as she looks up from her charting.

"How much prednisone, Aldactone, and Tylenol has he had today?"

Celina, very flustered says, "I gave him five milligrams of prednisone this morning, but I don't know about the rest."

The doctor responds, "You are his nurse and don't know his medications? How can you not know all the doses and schedule of what he's on?" Dr. Cone slams the chart down and walks away with a disgusted look on his face. Celina walks into the bathroom and tries to compose herself as tears stream down her face. This is *not* what she expected her nursing career to be.

Two months later, the unit tries daily huddles to help foster communication with all healthcare team members. All nurses and doctors on the unit convene at 8 a.m. daily. The nurses prepare all pertinent data on their flow sheets, and each nurse presents the patient and family data, social and medical history, and the past 24-hour status report. Doctors, pharmacists, dietitians, medical students, and residents discuss the lab data, revise the plan with the collaborative team, and make sure all team members have an opportunity to provide input.

Dr. Cone has now become an ally, and the nursing and medical teams have a good working rapport. With planning and a positive team approach, Celina is now a member of a team focused on the universal goal of providing the best patient care possible.

CORE COMPETENCY

Acknowledge the positive effect of interprofessional team communication and collaboration on safety outcomes.

LEARNING OUTCOMES

1. Describe positive and negative communication and collaboration between nurses and doctors.

2. Discuss the use of morbidity and mortality conferences to promote safety and transparency.

3. Examine the benefit of collaborative care teams to nursing.

4. Explore research on outcomes with and without interprofessional teams.

5. Identify a collaborative care strategy that can improve quality healthcare delivery.

This chapter describes the challenges and the benefits of being part of an interprofessional team. Being part of a team can promote efficient, safe, and quality care, but building an interprofessional team requires a unique nursing professional equipped to manage multiple demands. A typical interprofessional team includes multiple health providers who focus on specific populations of patients. Regular meetings that include all providers are critical pieces for the team approach to patient care. Nurses are a central part of interprofessional teams and bring their unique mastery of physiological, psychological, social, developmental, and community health knowledge to the team. Nurses are frequently the hub of communication and have a variety of roles such as case manager, discharge planner, advance practice nurse, or coordinator of care. Nurses must have excellent communication skills, mastery of information systems, and a collaborative care-focused decision-making ability, as well as a focus on patient- and family-centered care that incorporates elements of all aspects of physical, social, spiritual, and cultural health. All providers and consultants who interact with patients must become skilled at creating collaborative partnerships through regular team meetings, collaborative education, and excellent communication integrated in their daily routines.

Effective Communication for Collaboration and Interprofessional Team Building

Communication between nurses and other members of the healthcare team is the most important means to provide efficient and adequate care for an individual in a healthcare setting. The roles of nurses, dietitians, physical therapists, pharmacists, and physicians are different but overlapping. Depending on how power is perceived and the quality of communication among team members, the separation of roles may have positive or negative implications for the provision of care. Authoritative attitudes of physicians toward nurses, minimization of nurses' roles in patient care, and poor communication prevent providers from reaching their desired goal of quality and safe care for patients and families. Communication is the critical tool healthcare professionals must use in collaboration to expedite the delivery of healthcare services. Collaboration is a complex phenomenon that brings together two or more individuals, often from different professional disciplines, who work to achieve shared aims and objectives (Houldin, Naylor, & Haller, 2004). Sharing information that can increase the awareness of a healthcare issue, problem, or solution is a core use of communication in the healthcare arena. It affects attitudes by creating support for individuals or collective action, demonstrating skills, increasing the demand for health services, and reinforcing knowledge (Dochterman & Grace, 2001).

Over the past 20 years, good communication skills have been identified as important in nursing and healthcare. As a result of the attention paid to this issue, there has been a positive effect on patient care and provider satisfaction (McMahan, Hoffman, & McGee, 2002). Christensen and colleagues (2000) describe communication between nurses and physicians as a way to maximize the sharing of information unique to different professional participants. This allows the opportunity for each to learn more about the other's knowledge and talents. With the disciplines of medicine and nursing working in close proximity, communication is not just practicing together, but individually interacting to achieve a common good: the health and well-being of patients.

Historical Perspective on the Nurse's Role

The primary source of conflict in the nurse–physician relationship is physicians not recognizing nurses' value and the quality of their patient care. Some physicians still view a nurse's role as simply carrying out their orders and reporting the patient's progress to them. According to Miccolo and Spanier (1993), when physicians were asked for suggestions to improve nursing care, they typically compared good nursing care with fulfillment of their orders and demands. A more complete view of the scope of nursing practice can help with mutual understanding and support. The 2011 Institute of Medicine (IOM) report *The Future Of Nursing: Leading Change, Advancing Health* targets the roles, responsibilities, and education that should be recognized in nursing. More than three million nurses in the United States have the potential to strengthen the health and well-being of our country. The engagement of nursing with other providers will help the profession assume the status needed to redesign health care and provide improved quality and safer nursing care. Current interprofessional team structures are based on equal partnerships, with all members having invaluable roles within the team. The shared power structure is aimed at equal voice and equal stature.

The "doctor–nurse game," first described in the 1960s (Stein, 1967), is a stereotypical pattern of interaction in which female nurses, deferring to the doctor's authority (in past scenarios, usually male), learn to show initiative and offer advice. In this "game," nurses would often be forced to attempt to convince a physician that a suggestion being posed was actually the doctor's idea in the first place. Historically, physicians were described as "freely conferring" with other colleagues, but consultation with a nurse seemed inappropriate (Stein, 1967). Many doctors felt threatened if they were not completely independent and totally in control of the management of "their" patients.

Nursing as a profession accepted the position of deference to physicians. The nurse, who traditionally was expected to be a female, was described as "docile, subordinate, and deferent, with a traditional reputation of fulfilling a role of blind obedience rather than one of autonomous professionalism" (Stein, 1967, p. 701).

In playing the game, nurses were expected to be responsible for making significant recommendations while at the same time appearing passive. Their contributions were to appear as if they had been initiated by the physician rather than by the nurse (Stein, 1967). In an update of that classic article on the doctor–nurse game, Stein, Watts, and Howell (1990) believed that since the beginning of the 1980s, nurses have become more highly educated with a defined area of expertise. This expertise allows nurses to function as more autonomous healthcare professionals. These authors characterize the new relationship between physicians and nurses as one of "mutual interdependency" and cite movement toward collaboration and collegiality, with a less hierarchical and more open relationship than in the past.

Contributing Factors to Roles

Contributing factors to the development of these roles were that most physicians were male and most nurses female; physicians generally attained a higher level of education than nurses; and the striking salary differences between the two groups (Stein, 1967). These factors greatly contributed to the lack of mutual respect for each profession.

Medical and Nursing School Curricula

Often the root of communication problems between nurses and physicians is the physician's lack of adequate understanding of the functions and goals that the nurse has set forth. Similarly, the nurse may lack insight into the scope of the physician's responsibilities (McMahan et al., 2002). Nurses and physicians place different values on specific parts of the healthcare process. Nursing and medical students do not receive the same education and training, nor are they aware of the level of studies of the other group. A common understanding has not been established between the two professions, yet both are expected to work together for the well-being of the patient (McMahan et al., 2002).

The wide range of nursing education can be confusing to physicians and may pose significant issues that affect the nurse–physician relationship. With the addition of the advance practice degree in various specialties, nursing's role may appear threatening to some physicians. A 2005 survey study researching the role of licensed nurse midwives found that the advanced practice nurses sought from their physician colleagues increased communication, respect, and appreciation (Brown, Chetty, Grimes, & Harmon, 2005).

A simple solution to enhance collaboration is to socialize both nurses and doctors early in their program of studies by implementing various communication elements and techniques into nursing and medical student curricula. This would allow students to use a collaborative approach to communicate and learn early in their respective careers (Shumaker & Goss, 1980; Prescott & Bowen, 2000). Such interprofessional programs will assist professionals in better understanding each other's roles, supporting communication and cooperation, and promoting respect for assertion of the individual professional perspective in patient care. The knowledge of potential problems and issues regarding communication between nurses and physicians can prepare both parties to efficiently deal with them when they arise in the future.

Nursing Degrees

Another issue that must change to raise the status of nursing as a profession is the minimum degree to practice. In 1979, a white paper was issued calling for the bachelor of science degree to be the entry level for practice. Now, more than 30 years later, there has been no definitive action taken to ensure that nursing has a standard level of education that constitutes the basic level of practice. This change is essential to elevate the status of the profession and increase credibility of nurses as competent providers of care. The IOM's report *The Future of Nursing: Leading Change, Advancing Health* (2011) focused on the need for nurses to achieve higher levels of education and training, and it includes the goal of increasing the proportion of baccalaureate-prepared nurses to 80% by 2020. Presently, fewer than 50% of nurses in most states are baccalaureate prepared. Another goal of doubling the number of nurses with a doctorate by 2020 would help to fill the gap of qualified nursing educators. There should be a personal, professional, and organizational commitment for all nurses to engage in lifelong learning. The best way to ensure lifelong learning is a strong foundational education.

Related Ethical Issues

Ethical issues in nurse–physician communication patterns can range from physicians not answering nurses' pages or phone calls to nurses refusing to carry out physicians' orders. In general, both disciplines focus on the physiological issues of the patient, but nurses place greater emphasis on the patient's psychosocial needs. Conversely, nurses believe that physicians do not recognize the patient as a whole person. This can result in major ethical misunderstandings between nurses and physicians.

Power in an organization may be defined based on salary and earning potential. In most hospital settings, staff nurses are paid on an hourly basis while physicians are salaried. Nurses with higher education—for example, masters-prepared nurses—are salaried. Nurse practitioners and nurse anesthetists are paid in a similar structure to physicians. When nurses have a salaried position, the "punching the time clock" mentality

CASE STUDY: *Arnold*

Arnold, the nurse caring for Billy, an 8-year-old boy dying of end-stage leukemia with sepsis, was at the bedside with the family. The patient was slowly fading, and his breathing became irregular. The family had decided to withhold ventilator support and let Billy die peacefully. Billy's family also had some questions regarding the amount of morphine being given. The nurse paged Dr. Carlito. The nurse knew that Dr. Carlito, the pediatric hematologist, was not with another patient and on call for the hematology and oncology service. With no response after 15 minutes, Arnold paged the doctor again. After an hour of waiting and three more pages, Arnold notified the chief resident. Arnold was informed that this pattern of behavior was not new from Dr. Carlito, as in the past he was not available when his patients were dying. The chief resident, Dr. Lamb, took care to ensure that all of the family's questions were answered, and Billy died that evening. The family's disappointment was dramatic. Their primary contact—the person who provided the most consistent care of Billy—was gone. The family was left feeling abandoned.

becomes less of an issue, and they have greater sense of professional commitment. Measuring six adverse patient event measures, Teng and colleagues (2009) reported that nurses' professional commitment positively influenced overall patient safety and elevated patients' perceptions that they had received quality care. It is logical that nurses who practice in a positive interprofessional environment along with supportive colleagues inside and outside of nursing are happier and safer.

Communication and Collaboration

For nurses to successfully collaborate with the rest of the healthcare team and provide quality patient care, shared interests and open lines of communication are required. Goals, objectives, roles, processes, and outcomes must be explicitly articulated and agreed on by members of the collaborating team. Details about when and how to collaborate, how to structure interactions, and how to evaluate outcomes must be established in advance. Well-articulated and deliberate strategies ought to be in place to navigate unavoidable and sometimes ideological differences between nurses and physicians (Houldin et al., 2004).

There are indications that the old hierarchical ways of communicating between nurses and physicians are changing. Physicians are increasingly depending on nurses' expertise and skill in critical care settings and emergency departments, as well as in community settings, residential care facilities, and home care services (Altman et al., 2001; Whale, 1993). It is crucial for both nurses and physicians to realize the potential problems, and most importantly harm, that their lack of adequate communication patterns can cause. Good communication should be an ultimate means for providing improved patient care.

Good Communication Saves Lives

Certain characteristics of nurse–physician relationships correlate directly with patient care quality (Kramer & Schmalenberg, 2003). Research carried out at 14 hospitals that had achieved Magnet status from the American Nurses Credentialing Center (ANCC) indicated that healthy collaborative relationships between nurses and physicians were not only possible but were directly linked to optimal patient outcomes (Kramer & Schmalenberg, 2003). The results of this ANCC study indicated a positive correlation between the qualities of the nurse–physician relationships (as evidenced by measures of collegiality and collaboration) and the quality of patient care outcomes.

Resolving Barriers to Communication

Several approaches have been proposed and described in the literature to promote good communication and collaboration between nurses and physicians. Kramer and Schmalenberg (2003) proposed different approaches to promote effective communication that include awareness of gender role, utilization of basic communication techniques, and recognition of the unique contributions of each healthcare provider in the professional interchange of the nurse–physician relationship. The authors emphasize that individuals participating in communicative roles must be aware of the role that gender plays in communication. In the traditional nurse–physician relationship, the male physician may take the dominant role; the female nurse, recognizing this, can attempt to equalize the communication through assertiveness, accentuating the patient's well-being as the center of the interaction.

With the expanded role of nursing, the balance of power should be equal in a collaborative relationship. The physician needs to recognize the strengths of working with an expert nurse with extensive knowledge and autonomy. The physician may view nurse practitioners as a means for assistance in primary care responsibilities, while the bedside nurse may view nurse practitioners as advocates for a more holistic approach to patient care (Brown & Grimes, 1995). The expanded role of the nurse practitioner can aid nurses and physicians in understanding each other's role. But first the role of the nurse practitioner must be viewed by all healthcare providers as that of an independent practitioner who makes decisions related to diagnosing and treating patients and families.

When a doctor is on rounds and wishes to know information about the status of the patient, he or she may ask for the nurse caring for the patient. If the nurse is on break or busy with another patient, the nurse may not be able to speak with the physician. This can cause frustration for both the nurse and physician. Later, when the nurse is back on the unit and needs to contact the physician, the physician may be unavailable. Using Six Sigma technique, the nurse and doctor can identify the communication gap first (define) and the time wasted trying to contact one another (measure), then analyze the time and pattern and why it is not working (analyze), find a better way to communicate (improve), and structure a set goal for better communication (control). With simple structural changes and team members with good will, a unit or even an entire hospital can enhance teamwork, communication, and attitudes toward safety.

Models for Interprofessional Care Programs

Szekendi, Barnard, Creamer, and Noskin (2010) described regular morbidity and mortality conferences with nursing, pharmacy, and medicine as a means to support safe systems, share information to develop safer care, increase openness among members of all involved groups, and minimize the hierarchy of institutions. The focus of such conferences is on promoting learning and not placing blame on those who were involved in safety breaches.

The quality program at Northwestern Memorial Hospital in Chicago, Illinois, is held every month. After the quality improvement conferences began at Northwestern Memorial, the primary change noted was that staff perceptions of the safety culture became more positive as goals were focused on improvements and not on punitive action. This improvement process carried out at Northwestern Memorial describes a model program for developing an interprofessional quality care program.

To help nurture knowledge about such collaborations, several collaborative programs have been established. New programs of study such as the Arizona State University College of Nursing and Health Innovation integrate education of pharmacists, physicians, and nurses. The integration of disciplines includes learning about common concepts such as physiology and healthcare budgeting. Healthcare professionals who learn to rely on one another, including those from other disciplines, are more open to innovations in care delivery. Such interprofessional education develops openness to collaboration, which will continue onward, influencing attitudes in other workers (Szekendi et al., 2010).

Research on Outcomes With and Without Interprofessional Teams

Few prospective controlled studies assess the effect of interprofessional teams and differential patient outcomes. However, a few studies have evaluated patient outcomes after the implementation of interprofessional teams. Risk-adjusted health outcomes in frail elderly were improved when the Program of All-Inclusive Care for the Elderly (PACE) involving 2,401 patients was implemented in 26 different facilities (Mukamel et al., 2005). The study based on the PACE model provided good empirical evidence for the benefit of team performance and functional outcomes in the elderly patients including functional and mental status, short and long-term improvements in perceived health, and management of urinary incontinence. Prior to the PACE study, the team members involved also evaluated leadership, communication, coordination, and conflict management as positive and predictive of team cohesion and team effectiveness (Temkin-Greener, Gross, Kunitz, and Dnan, 2004). The benefits of interprofessional teams appear to be excellent for both patients and providers.

To accomplish new goals for collaboration and better outcomes, all persons involved need to be open to innovation. One example of this openness was described by Regina Herzlinger (2006) in the article, "Why Innovation in Health Care Is So Hard: Six Forces That Can Drive It or Kill It." The list of potential supports or barriers are: the ability to be friends or foes, getting support for the collaboration, showing a revenue stream, making sure that you adhere to policies and standards in the profession, using the best technology, and having satisfied customers who are interested in the success of the innovation.

Research consistently links better outcomes to hospital units that use effective communication and collaboration between disciplines. Interprofessional collaboration can help to keep patient well-being central in spite of economic pressures. Mature, motivated healthcare professionals must work together to thrive by fostering self-awareness and preventing burnout.

Innovations in Interprofessional Collaboration

The Robert Wood Johnson Foundation (RWJF) has supported initiatives to accelerate the monumental task of educating nursing faculty and student nurses to prepare them to provide high levels of patient care. Innovations are being created and tested by nurses in distance learning and expansion of nursing schools. However, to advance such healthcare improvements, an interprofessional approach is needed. Collaboration and communication with physicians is critical to delivering a high level of health care along with safety innovations and education.

Transforming Care at the Bedside (TCAB), which is discussed at length in Chapter 8, includes elements to integrate interprofessional quality and safety initiatives. From 2004 to 2006, Children's Memorial Hospital in Chicago, Illinois, developed several innovations and tested the strategies on special TCAB units. The focus on the process of change is referred to as a test of change, which involves identifying a problem and immediately developing a potential solution. The solution is the test of change, which is monitored for a short time (e.g., a week), and the outcome is immediately evaluated. If the plan worked, it becomes an initiative. If the plan failed, it is filed away as a "dud." The innovations at Children's Memorial Hospital were integrated into existing programs and support structures. The primary goal was to attempt an innovation, evaluate the outcome, and either accept the new policy or discard the failed attempt. Please see chapters 5 and 8 for more discussion about TCAB. Among the innovative methods for improving patient care through heightened collaboration and effective communication were interprofessional rounds, daily huddles (informal meetings to share information between team members), and the "heads up" approach to insure that potential issues are discussed in a proactive manner.

Interprofessional Rounds and Quality Outcomes

New approaches to collaborative practice can have a significant impact on outcomes. When nurse case managers, pharmacists, dieticians, and physicians in Connecticut collaborated in two-hour interprofessional rounds three times a week, length of stay was decreased and standard quality care measures improved (O'Mahoney, Mazur, Charney, Wang, & Fine, 2007). The data revealed that overall performance increased with interprofessional rounds, and core measure success was higher than expected. Many studies have reported similar results. There is a clear need for interprofessional rounds.

Daily Huddles

Prior to beginning the clinic at Children's Memorial Hospital for children with diabetes and growth disorders, Dr. William Patrick assembled his team of residents, nurse coordinator, dietitian, pharmacist, and social worker. The team went through the full patient list to update all team members about new family psychological, social, and physical issues that had emerged since the last visit. This 15-minute "huddle" provided all team members with a more informed approach to providing comprehensive and holistic care to the children and their families. The cohesion and consistency among the providers was clear to the patients and families, and they were very satisfied with the care they received.

During the TCAB experience at the Children's Memorial Hospital in Chicago, physicians, nurses, respiratory therapists, and other staff involved with patient care would meet for 30 minutes on the 7 p.m. to 7 a.m. night shift for a daily huddle. The assembled care providers discussed the patients who were on the floor that day. Current plans of care were reviewed, and all members focused on the most important priorities for the day, such as discharging patients or preparing patients who needed new treatments such as surgery or new medication. Huddles can easily be built into the schedule of all providers (see Figure 7-1). Use of huddles facilitates excellent communication and enhances patient safety (Payson, Currier, & Streelman, 2011). Such rounds are well worth the 30-minute investment in time and can prevent adverse events as well as increase efficiency and productive time. When all persons involved in patient care agree on a scheduled time to communicate, a stronger collaborative process is nurtured. Chapter 8 includes an example of a unit that benefited from daily huddles.

Most adverse events can be prevented when nursing staff work in a supportive environment that emphasizes collaborative care. Using huddles and consistent communication models that are situation based, such as SBAR (situation, background, assessment, and recommendation), can reduce medical errors and save lives.

Interprofessional "Heads Up" Meetings

A model that focuses on quality initiatives, interprofessional communication, and collaboration is the 30-minute "hot topics" or "heads up" miniconferences. This model is built on the premise that both nurses and physicians can learn from one another. The collaborative process includes

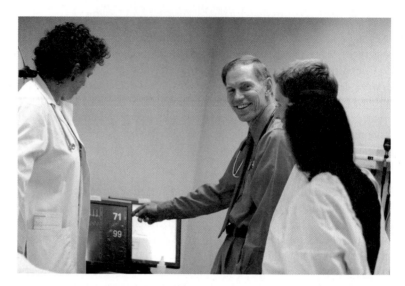

Figure 7-1 Interprofessional teams improve patient outcomes.
Shots by Shelley

communication, compassionate caring, and conciliatory interactions to solve problems.

During the weekly heads up meetings at Children's Memorial Hospital in Chicago, both physicians and nurses identify issues or hot topics, as depicted in Table 7-1. After the brief meeting, the group decides on an action plan for the coming week. Each week, the action plan is evaluated and a new plan is developed.

Goals of the Heads Up Meetings The heads up meetings focus on generating new solutions to issues that the providers identify. The charge nurse or nurse educator facilitates the team process at the unit level to include performance evaluation, communication needs, staff development, and individual performance improvement. Nurses are reminded about their professional development and yearly performance review criteria, and progress is discussed. The continuing education focus is guided by a senior nursing or medical faculty member who monitors data on the number of regular (weekly or monthly) heads up meetings that are held. Qualitative information is gathered in an attempt to provide regular research updates in an easily visible format on the floor. Suggested research topics are written on a white board on the unit. The selected research articles to be discussed are posted one week before the meeting to allow staff to become familiar with the material that will be discussed.

Collaborative Care Teams and Nursing

Collaborative care in nursing includes intra- and interprofessional communication as well as supportive, patient-centered goal setting. At the minimum, collaborative care includes a mutual respect among healthcare

TABLE 7-1 ■ Example of a "Heads Up" Debriefing

Date	Meeting Time and Attendees	Issue #1 Respiratory Therapy Late for Treatments for CF Children	Action Plan for Issue #1	Issue #2 Teen with Asthma Will Not Keep O$_2$ Mask On	Action Plan for Issue #2
March 3rd	8:00 p.m. AB, TP, CH, JL	4 Reports of Late Treatments	RT, MD, and RN staff discuss implications for late treatment Goal: No more than 30-minute delay with treatment	SpO$_2$ monitor indicated saturations of less than 80% twice one evening	Team explores possible solutions and barriers to using oxygen therapy
March 10th	9:00 p.m. AB, TP, CH, JL	1 Treatment Late	Kudos to RT	Patient shown different options for oxygen masks	Less desaturations noted
March 17th	8:30 p.m. AB, TP, JL, WH	Resolved		New options presented for flexible nasal cannula	Patient states that the new equipment is much more comfortable
March 24th	8:45 p.m. TP, JL, CS, WH	No reports of late treatments; Issue Resolved			

workers. Collaborative care can include interprofessional rounds, morning huddles at shift change, or electronic care planning with input from all providers (see Table 7-2). Interprofessional teams require a much more intensively planned process with more equal provider input. In past decades, student nurses were used to staff all shifts in the hospital, and they were boarded in dormitories nearby. Today, professional nurses are paid staff members, but the ability to collaborate as a member of an interprofessional team is still no better in many settings. The ultimate goal of the interprofessional team is to have patient care as the primary focus and then to treat physicians, administrators, and staff nurses as equal members of the team.

Collaborative practice saves lives when mutual respect of all healthcare providers transcends any status or ego issues. The 15-minute daily interprofessional huddle or patient care rounds can enable all team members to work in a more cohesive and coordinated manner.

Joint Commission Sentinel Event Alert 40: Behaviors That Undermine a Culture of Safety

Behaviors that undermine any healthcare worker can lead to mistakes and poor outcomes (Joint Commission, 2008). Multiple sources of research are cited in the Joint Commission's sentinel alert describing the pattern of intimidating and disruptive behavior that fosters a poor environment and results in poor patient satisfaction, preventable adverse events, and

TABLE 7-2 ■ Examples of Collaborative Healthcare

	TCAB	American Board of Pediatrics Continuing Medical Education Guidelines	IOM
Mechanisms	"Huddle"	Residents must be able to demonstrate interpersonal and communication skills that result in effective information exchange and teaming with patients, patient families, and professional associates. Expectations include: ■ Creating and sustaining a therapeutic and ethically sound relationship with patients ■ Use of effective listening skills and elicit and provide information using effective nonverbal, explanatory, questioning, and writing skills ■ Working effectively with others as a member or leader of a healthcare team or other professional group	Panel to respond to 10,000 lives
Results	Less frustration and less adverse events	Good standard Need good role models in senior physicians	"Quality Chasm" series was published and a media campaign begins
Grade	+++	++	+
Drawbacks	Not always sustained after the first implementation	Good in theory, but still lagging in practice	General knowledge regarding risk of adverse events is lacking

increased cost of care. The traditional physician–nurse conflict is not the only source of disruptive behavior. Administrators, pharmacists, therapists, and support staff also report behaviors that are intimidating and inappropriate. The Joint Commission has suggested actions that focus on preventing such behavior. First, there must be a zero tolerance attitude toward intimidating or inappropriate behavior. There must be education for all team members regarding the proper etiquette for communication. When problems arise, team members need to have a clear organizational process to follow to report those problems. When a reporting system and surveillance system are in place (possibly with anonymous reporting), the general culture of the unit should improve with the assurance of support from colleagues and supervisors.

Review of Literature on Physician–Nurse Collaboration

Few physicians realize the fear new nurses feel when they must communicate with physicians. Too little time is spent in nursing school preparing students to communicate with physicians. Simple role-playing practice can boost confidence. Some clinical instructors perform mock physician contacts and case studies to increase critical thinking and practice communicating with physicians.

Collaboration is a multifaceted process that requires a cooperative spirit and the need to share knowledge and the responsibility for patient

Evidence for Best Practices: What Is SBAR and Does It Work?

SBAR is the new acronym used in charting and reporting off on patients. SBAR, or **S**ituation, **B**ackground, **A**ssessment, and **R**ecommendations, helps nurses remember the most important parts of giving a report on a patient. SBAR has been proven to help communication and outcomes in health care whether it is used for a change in status, such as reporting worsening pain in a surgery patient to a physician or the transfer of a patient from nurse to nurse en route from surgery to the recovery room. The evidence is clear. Better communication between nurses and doctors prevents adverse events. This means that nurse-to-nurse communication and physician-to-nurse communication are all beneficial to the patient and affect their outcomes (Bello, Quinn, & Horrell, 2011).

care. Sometimes it occurs between longtime colleagues that have built mutual trust. However, there must be a model in place so that the professionals have an established expectation of collaboration. Whether they have a familiar pattern of communication or are new to one another, the team needs to establish an expectation of regular dialogue that is a standard for the group (LeTourneau, 2004). Each healthcare professional has information the other needs for safe practice and to accomplish their mutual goals. In the interest of safe patient care, neither profession can stand alone. Excellent collaboration skills are needed to ensure patient safety.

Collaboration has many facets, and it is not supervision or simply a one-way or even two-way information exchange. Effective professional collaborative relationships require mutual respect (Kramer & Schmalenberg, 2003). Even in our sophisticated healthcare systems, collaboration is too often difficult. To become good partners and collaborators, both nurses and physicians need excellent role models who portray mutual respect and interdependence, not ego. Kramer and Schmalenberg (2003) state that collaborative partnerships are worth the effort because they result in better outcomes for patients as well as professional growth.

Despite the challenge of resistance to collaborative habits, true collaboration is vital not only for the benefit of patients, but also for the satisfaction of healthcare providers. Collaboration between physicians and nurses is rewarding when responsibility for patient well-being is shared. Professionalism is strengthened when all members take credit for group successes. Physicians have often been viewed as the primary generators of income for a hospital. Nurses are often overlooked as revenue producers, and thus awareness is needed to view nurses as valued workers (Fagin, 1992).

Strategies for Team Building

An interprofessional team approach can be used as a method for open communication between nurses and physicians. Nurses, physicians, and other team members work together in the best interest of the patient. The

CASE STUDY: *Edith*

Edith has been working in labor and delivery for one year and is highly engaged in patient care. John is a first year resident who has just begun his family medicine residency. John is excited to be delivering babies based on his interest in this field during medical school. As a resident, John is doing vaginal exams and managing the care of the patients on the maternity unit today. John likes to be independent and feels confident in his abilities. Edith notices that John has missed some of the important lab draws that need to be ordered for the new patient she has just admitted due to the patient's medical history. Edith hates to correct a resident; however, she is confident that this order, neglecting lab draws, must be changed. Edith approaches John and says, "You might not agree with me, but some of the required lab orders for the new patient admission were missed and the orders should be changed." John immediately gets frustrated with Edith and responds, "I do not feel that those labs are necessary for this patient." Edith decides that it is best for her to use chain-of-command and calls the attending physician. The attending physician agrees with Edith and changes the orders appropriately. The attending then approaches John and says, "John, it may be best if you listen to the recommendations of our colleagues in the future."

advantages of the multiprofessional team are better service, easier workload management, and collegial support. Whether the team meets daily for walking rounds or gathers for tea in the afternoon to discuss patients, the benefits of communication and collaboration are many. The teams must respect the confidentiality of patient and family information and provide a venue that does not violate that confidentiality.

Physicians and nurses bring different perspectives to patient care. When unique disciplinary perspectives are valued, the uniqueness of each profession can be seen as an asset rather than a detriment to patient care (Pike, 1991). Interprofessional collaboration among individuals with different skill sets and knowledge bases may result in creative and practical solutions that would not otherwise occur. For these creative solutions to occur, professionals must avoid making assumptions about other professionals and take the time and effort to learn the other's perspective. Through intentional discovery of what motivates others as professionals, all healthcare workers can discover their common goals.

Team Development Strategies

Team development is one of the most popular organizational concepts. Collaboration is essential for team development and ongoing positive performance. Larson and LaFasto (1989) included a collaborative climate as one of their eight essential characteristics of team excellence. Their later work demonstrated that collaborative climates embody safe communication of rewards for collaboration, problem-solving behaviors, and management of negative behaviors (LaFasto & Larson, 1989). Team development includes the following tasks: team building, respectful negotiation, conflict management, containment of negative behaviors, and workplace design to facilitate collaboration.

Build the Team

Collaboration requires intentional team building. Collaborative practice is not a process involving side-by-side efforts; rather, it is a drawing together of the valued contributions of all team members to reach the best possible solutions.

Collaboration involves developing shared meanings. These meanings should not simply be information exchanges. Building trust takes much time and patience. Through the competence and commitment of collaborative group members, valuable partnerships are created. Developing a shared language between team members that reflects the diversity of contributing disciplines helps to build the team. The common goal of patient well-being greatly enhances team unity. First, collaborators must agree on a definition of patient well-being (Zwarenstein & Reeves, 2002). This definition may vary from patient to patient. Patients (and their families when feasible) must be viewed as full participants in the group process so that they can articulate what well-being means to them. Maintaining a patient focus creates common ground between team members.

Negotiate Respectfully

The manner in which collaborative relationships are negotiated has a direct impact on outcomes. Unequal power and authority negatively influences interprofessional collaboration. One way to balance power and authority is to drop titles and use given names to neutralize the deleterious effects of an unequal playing field. Additionally, nurses must learn to contribute to teams from positions of strength. Beck-Kritek (1994) describes this as "negotiating at an uneven table." Nurses need not strive for dominance on teams. In fact, such striving can be counterproductive. Rather, they can exude strength, innovation, and integrity in collaboration (Beck-Kritek, 1994). Nurses negotiate from a position of strength when they recognize the substantial power they do possess, remain confident in their expertise, and create their own freedom to make meaningful contributions (Eisenhardt, Kahwajy, & Burgeois, 1997a).

From the start, team members must define which tasks can be done individually, which must be worked on together, and what the expectations are for joint interactions (Zwarenstein & Reeves, 2002). It is best to function and negotiate within hierarchical structures and to respect the chain of command. It is never wise to jump over levels of authority to be expedient. When mutual goals and respect are woven into the fabric of a workplace, issues of hierarchy become secondary to the sharing of knowledge by competent group members.

Manage Conflict Wisely

Cohesiveness and joint problem solving are the desired results of collaborative teamwork. However, nurses and physicians will not always agree. In fact when managed correctly, conflict is actually a desired element of collaboration. Without it, the trap of groupthink may occur. In a groupthink situation, creative and contradictory solutions are suppressed in the interest of maintaining consensus and peaceful relationships.

Healthy conflict is a sign that diverse ideas are welcome at the table. Trying to force agreement can impede the group process due to haggling among group members (Eisenhardt, Kahwajy, & Bourgeois, 1997a). It is critical to keep in mind that conflict can be beneficial (Eisenhardt, Kahwajy, & Bourgeois, 1997b). Without it, relationships may become anemic and ineffective. When conflict is acceptable, multiple solutions emerge. Solutions not limited to those produced or endorsed by individuals with the greatest political clout are allowed to be voiced and acted upon.

It is important to quickly identify when achieving consensus has become unrealistic. When this occurs, communication difficulties must be analyzed, openness fostered, and inclusive language incorporated. Focusing on the facts as opposed to opinions helps to preserve unity. Often the best strategy is for the most senior member to receive group input and then make a decision. Encouraging productive conflict without destroying group cohesiveness requires mature team members and humble leadership.

Avoid Negative Behaviors

It takes only one difficult personality to cast a pall of dominance, negativity, or distraction that derails collaborative efforts. Fortunately, productivity and positivity can counteract debilitating influences and restore team productivity if there is a consistent, courageous, and deliberate leadership. Team leaders must be mature, value consensus, and be unwilling to settle for less than productive dialogue.

One strategy to encourage positive teamwork is to avoid the "blame game." Nurses must stop blaming others for problems that exist in nursing (Easson-Bruno, 2003). It is counterproductive and unprofessional to blame physicians, administrators, organizations, or other nurses for the frustrating and disappointing aspects of present-day nursing. Acting as victims will not encourage others to respect and trust nurses (Roberts, 1999). Willingness and courage to share the load of responsibility for patient outcomes will infuse the collaborative process with trust and respect. Nurses create momentum when they are confident in their contributions and secure in their identities. To project strength and competence, nurses can emulate nurse heroes, utilize nurse mentors, and become skilled role models themselves who can effectively lead the next generation of nurses. They can be frank while remaining flexible and open-minded.

What Do You Do When You Disagree and Need to Make Your Case? Assertiveness is a great asset in situations where a case has to be made contrary to popular belief (Blickensderfer, 1996). Nurses should use objective information such as SBAR as a means of communication. They should question care decisions calmly and directly when necessary. Also, they should refuse to play the doctor–nurse game; that is, they should refuse to use disclaimers that rob nurses of due credit for their contributions (Stein et al., 1990; Blickensderfer, 1996). It is important to avoid phrases with tag questions, such as, "You might think differently, but . . . ", "Sorry to bother you, but . . . ", "I know you are busy, but . . . ." These statements open the door to disagreement and erode the respect of others.

Design Facilities for Collaboration

Comfortable and inviting spaces facilitate team discussion. Facility design can directly impact teamwork. Research has shown that space allotment in the practice site influences productivity, work attitudes, confidentiality, and the professional image of health care (Lindeke, Hauck, & Tanner, 1998). Facility design improves collaboration when space is allotted to enhance formal and informal interaction between professionals.

Optimal design factors to consider include privacy, noise control, seating space, and convenience. The following suggestions help to ensure the space needed for effective teamwork. First, one must anticipate space and equipment needs. Priority must not be given just to patient and family space. Areas are also needed for interprofessional interaction, including conferencing and consulting. Second, articulate space needs clearly. Ambiguity is an obstacle for timely change. By enhancing a current unit, comfortable and inviting spaces can be created. This will facilitate team discussions as well as conferences with patients and families.

Communicate Effectively in Emergencies

Collaborative interactions are most effective and rewarding when they are efficient. When information is exchanged in emergency situations, it is critical to prioritize, leave out peripheral data, and provide current information. Henry (2000) offers tips for communicating in emergencies. These tips include getting the facts from informed sources, not blowing issues out of proportion, responding promptly, and remaining calm. In addition, divulging only information that others need and are ethically allowed to know will allow for the best possible communication in an emergent situation. Finally, following up on issues and highlighting positive aspects of an emergent situation will also enhance collaborative relationships.

Use Electronic Communication Thoughtfully

Much communication, whether it be social or professional, now is electronic via e-mail, voicemail, and fax. When using electronic communication it is important to remember the following tips in order to communicate effectively:

- Project openness in a collaborative manner.

- Do not insist on being right.

- Do not overanalyze the intended emotion of message.

- Be clear and concise.

- Do not use slang, symbols, abbreviations, or jargon.

Mature, motivated healthcare professional teams must work together to thrive. Effective, collaborative partnerships will waste little time posturing and will instead focus attention on issues of importance (Eisenhardt et at., 1997a). Leaders of collaborative teams will be optimistic and positive, inspiring hope in others when change is unsettling. Using the variety of strategies presented in this chapter can enhance interprofessional collaboration and promote quality patient care in an era of decreased resources and enhanced expectations.

CHAPTER HIGHLIGHTS

- A significant communication gap exists between nurses and physicians.
- Physicians' historical role of dominance and the devaluation of nursing have contributed to the lack of nurse–physician communication.
- Both groups of professionals are obstructed by a wide range of education, differences in billing structure, and gender biases.
- Communication will continue to be challenging for nurses and physicians until they take some time and explore their strengths and weaknesses amidst similarities and differences.
- The quality of care can only be enhanced through effective communication.

Pearson Nursing Student Resources

Find additional review materials at
nursing.pearsonhighered.com

Prepare for success with additional NCLEX®-style practice questions, interactive assignments and activities, web links, animations and videos, and more!

REFERENCES

Altman, D. G., Schulz, K. F., Moher, D., Egger, M., Davidoff, F., et al. (2001). The revised CONSORT statement for reporting randomized trials: Explanation and elaboration. *Annals of Internal Medicine, 134,* 663–694.

Beck-Kritek, P. (1994). *Negotiating at an uneven table.* Indianapolis, IN: John Wiley & Sons, Inc.

Bello, J., Quinn, P., & Horrell, L. (2011). Maintaining patient safety through innovation: An electronic SBAR communication tool. *Computer Informatics Nursing.* 29(9), 481–483.

Blickensderfer, L. (1996). Nurses and physicians: Creating a collaborative environment. *Journal of Intravenous Nursing, 19*(3), 127–131.

Brown, B., Chetty, M., Grimes, A., & Harmon, E. (2005). *Effortless monitoring of diet and exercise for students.* Poster presented at the Atlanta Student Research Competition.

Brown S. A., & Grimes D. E. (1995). A meta-analysis of nurse practitioners and nurse midwives in primary care. *Nurse Research. 44,* 332–338.

Christensen, C., Larson, J. R., Jr., Abbott, A., Ardolino, A., Franz, T. M., & Pfeiffer, C. (2000). Decision making of clinical teams: Communication patterns and diagnostic error. *Medical Decision Making, 20,* 45–50.

Dochterman, J., & Grace, H. Y. (2001). *Current issues in nursing.* St. Louis: Mosby, 125–132.

Easson-Bruno, S. (2003). Don't blame Florence. *Nursing Leadership, 16*(4), 8–9.

Eisenhardt, K., Kahwajy, J., & Bourgeois, L. (1997a). Conflict and strategic choice: How top management teams disagree. *California Management Review, 39*(2), 42–62.

Eisenhardt, K., Kahwajy, J., & Bourgeois, L. (1997b). How management teams can have a good fight. *Harvard Business Review, 75*(4), 77–85.

Fagin, C. (1992). Collaboration between nurses and physicians: No longer a choice. *Academic Medicine, 67*(5), 295–303.

Henry, R. (2000). *You'd better have a hose if you want to put out the fire.* Windsor, CA: Gollywobbler Productions.

Herzlinger, R. (2006). Why innovation in healthcare is so hard: Six forces that can drive it or kill it. *Harvard Business Review, 84*(5), 58–66.

Houldin, A. D., Naylor, M. D., & Haller, D. (2004). Physician-nurse collaboration on research in the 21st century. *Journal of Clinical Oncology Nursing, 22*(5), 1–3.

Institute of Medicine. (2011). *The future of nursing: Leading change and advancing health.* Washington, DC: The National Academies Press.

Joint Commission. (2008). *Sentinel event alert 40: Behaviors that undermine a culture of safety.* Retrieved from http://www.jcrinc.com /Sentinel-Event-Alert-40/.

Kramer, M., & Schmalenberg, C. (2003). Securing a "good" nurse physician relationship. *Nursing Management, 34*(7), 34–38.

LeTourneau, B. (2004). Physicians and nurses: Friends or foes? *Journal of Healthcare Management, 49*(1), 12–14.

Lindeke, L., Hauck, M., & Tanner, M. (1998). Creating spaces that enhance nurse practitioner practice. *Journal of Pediatric Health Care, 12*(3), 125–129.

McMahan, E. V., Hoffman, K., & McGee, G. W. (2002). Physician–nurse relationships in clinical settings: A review and critique of the literature, 1966–1992. *Medical Care Review. 51*(1), 83–112.

Miccolo, M. A., & Spanier, A. H. (1993). Critical management in the 1990s: Making collaborative practice work. *Critical Care Clinics, 9,* 443–453.

Mukamel, D. B., Temkin-Greener, H., Delavan, R., Peterson, D. R., Gross, D., Kunitz, S., &

Williams, T. F. (2005). Team performance and risk-adjusted health outcomes in the Program of All-Inclusive Care for the Elderly (PACE). *Gerontologist* 46(2), 227–237.

O'Mahoney, S., Mazur, E., Charney, P., Wang, Y., & Fine, J. (2007). Use of interdisciplinary rounds to simultaneously improve quality outcomes, enhance resident education, and shorten length of stay. *Journal of General Internal Medicine, 22*(8), 1073–1079.

Payson, C., Currier, A., & Streelman, M. (2011). Focusing on staff awareness and accountability in reducing falls. *American Nurse Today, 6*(3), 8–10.

Pike, A. (1991). Moral outrage and moral discourse in nurse–physician collaboration. *Journal of Professional Collaboration, 7*(6), 351–363.

Prescott, P. A., & Bowen, S. A. (2000). Physician–nurse relationships. *Annals Internal Medicine, 103,* 127–133.

Shumaker D., & Goss V. (1980). Toward collaboration: One small step. *Nursing and health care: Official publication of the National League for Nursing, 1*(4), 183–185.

Stein, L. (1967). The doctor–nurse game. *Archives of General Psychiatry, 16*(6), 699–703.

Stein, L. I., Watts, D. T., & Howell, T. (1990). The doctor–nurse game revisited. *New England Journal of Medicine, 322,* 546–549.

Szekendi, M. K., Barnard, C., Creamer, J., & Noskin, G. A. (2010). Using patient safety morbidity and mortality conferences to promote transparency and a culture of safety. *Joint Commission Journal Quality Patient Safety,* 36(1), 3.

Temkin-Greener, H., Gorss, D., Kunitz, S. J., & Dnan, M. (2004). Measuring interdisciplinary team performance in a long-term care setting. *Medical Care, 42*(5), 472–481.

Teng, C., Dai, Y., Shyu, Y. L., Wong, M., Chu, T., & Tsai, Y. (2009). Professional commitment, patient safety, and patient perceived care quality. *Journal of Nursing Scholarship, 41*(3), 301–309.

Whale, Zoe. (1993). Shiftwork and quality of care. *Journal of Clinical Nursing. 2*(5), 269–272.

Zwarenstein, M., & Reeves, S. (2002). Working together but apart: Barriers and routes to nurse–physician collaboration. *Joint Commission Journal on Quality Improvement, 28,* 242–247.

TRANSFORMING CARE AT THE BEDSIDE (TCAB) EXPERIENCE: INNOVATIONS, IMPROVEMENTS, AND QUALITY

Transforming Care at the Bedside Team:
Kim Siarkowski Amer, Sherri Ewing, Yvonne Bilak Krause, Constance Hill, Karen Richey,
and Michelle Stephenson

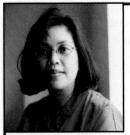

Blend Images /
Shutterstock.com

Martha transferred to the hematology oncology unit after working in the emergency department for three years following her graduation from nursing school. After two months on the hematology oncology unit, she felt a lack of support from the other nurses and a general shortage of team spirit. Some of the nurses seemed to exist in their own little worlds or bubbles with no vitality and without noticing Martha or other nurses. When she asked a few of the staff nurses how long they had worked on the unit, she discovered that during the past year, six nurses had transferred out of the unit. She realized that the difference between the emergency department and the hematology oncology unit was vitality.

CORE COMPETENCY

Integrate knowledge of past projects and models focused on quality, such as Transforming Care at the Bedside (TCAB), into a plan for future clinical innovations.

LEARNING OUTCOMES

1. Describe the benefits of the innovations that were used in Transforming Care at the Bedside (TCAB) at Children's Memorial Hospital in Chicago, Illinois.

2. Discuss the rapid cycle change process used to improve quality.

3. Articulate the implications of TCAB on nursing practice and nursing education.

Healthcare delivery is embarking on a new era of high-technology, cost-efficient, outcome-driven provision of care. This new era will require nursing professionals to be equipped to manage multiple aspects of health care, such as information systems, collaborative care decision making, patient and family integration into health provision, and environmental and cultural health. Information systems require the skills of using institutional software to access and input electronic health records and navigate institutional systems and Internet-based information. Interdisciplinary coordination between and among all healthcare providers is also critical to improving care delivery. Practice will be guided by clear, evidence-based standards. But the hallmarks of this new era will be safety and accountability.

An innovative model focused on this new phase in health care has been designed to infuse nursing practice and education with a quality and safety curriculum. The project, Transforming Care at the Bedside (TCAB), was established by the Robert Wood Johnson Foundation (RWJF) and the Institute for Healthcare Improvement (IHI) in response to the Institute of Medicine (IOM) report in 1999 that addressed the thousands of lives lost due to adverse events or preventable errors (RWJF & IHI, 2006). The first clinical sites throughout the United States initially participated in the program from 2004 to 2008, which at its core involved a method of developing quality nursing care that includes efficient use of time, evidence-based practice, and multiple strategies to improve processes in health care. Many projects based on the foundational work of the original TCAB project are continuing. Using TCAB as a model for ensuring quality nursing care, RWJF continues to provide funding for spreading TCAB innovations.

TCAB was designed to provide an opportunity for clinicians to look "outside the box" for solutions to seemingly simple problems in the hospital. While such problems may appear to be small on the surface, they often translate into wasted time and money for nurses and the hospital. How does a nurse gain the tools to initiate and implement seemingly simple innovations on the unit? TCAB is a program that helps empower nurses and provides the guidance needed to improve care while remaining responsible with finances at the same time.

Understanding TCAB

TCAB was created to support nurse-driven solutions designed to develop quality nursing care. It began on the medical–surgical units in the participating hospitals, since the highest rates of adverse events generally occur on those units (IHI, 2006). The focus of the TCAB process was on decreasing the nonclinical demands on nurses, eliminating inefficiencies, and preventing staff turnover.

TCAB was a grassroots effort. The selected hospitals and staff members who participated met quarterly at various locations in the United States and discussed common issues and solutions that each had tried. They shared successes and failures, and encouraged one another to try the most successful efforts at their own hospitals. The beneficial process of learning and solving problems together across institutions was effective. As more hospitals exchanged information, more units within each hospital adopted the innovations. The involvement of direct care providers and staff nurses to identify problems and generate unique solutions was the reason for the program's success. A top-down process of administrators imposing changes upon the staff would not have been successful.

TCAB Four Focus Areas

TCAB focused on four areas: safe and reliable care, vitality and teamwork, patient-centered care, and value-added processes. Each focus area was adapted to the unique issues or problems of each hospital or unit. The direct care nurses decided how to develop each of the four areas to address the specific weaknesses or problems in their institutions.

Safe and Reliable Care

Care for hospitalized patients that is safe, reliable, effective, and equitable is the trademark of TCAB. Safe and reliable care hinges on a culture of safety where people are encouraged not just to work toward change but to take action whenever necessary. A hospital is able to improve safety only when the leadership is visibly committed to change and when staff is empowered to openly share safety information. Organizations that do not have such an open culture often find staff members unwilling to report adverse events or unsafe conditions because of concerns of reprisal. Because of their proximity to patients and the direct care they provide, nurses and other front line staff are uniquely capable of identifying and implementing process improvements that could result in safer, more reliable care. Examples of safe and reliable care include:

- Reducing medication errors and adverse drug events

- Establishing rapid response teams

- Preventing inpatient falls

Vitality and Teamwork

Effective care teams continually strive for excellence when they work in a joyful and supportive environment that nurtures professional training and career development. Vitality can be facilitated by formal and informal leadership. Team vitality starts when teams are allowed to work on issues relevant to their success. Effective teams work together and get great results. The mindset of effective teams is that they must act in ways that make excellent work possible, sustainable, and satisfying. They are always looking for ways to improve their work. Teams with strong vitality strive to reduce or eliminate blame, name-calling, cynicism, conflict, and apathy. Developing a process for improving care and teamwork greatly increases team vitality by improving how the team acts and interacts. Examples of vitality and teamwork include:

- Optimizing communication among team members

- Engaging front line staff

- Providing personal and team recognition

- Incorporating management training and professional development programs for staff

Patient-Centered Care

Truly patient-centered care on medical–surgical units honors the whole person and family, respects individual values and choices, and ensures continuity of care. Patients often say of such institutions, "They give me exactly the help I want and need exactly when I want and need it."

Patient- and family-centered care is essential to cultivating a partnership at the bedside in making decisions, healing relationships, and facilitating interactions between the individual patient and professional. A key aspect of patient- and family-centered care includes healthcare practitioners listening to and honoring patient and family perspectives and choices, including beliefs and cultural backgrounds. Sharing complete, unbiased information between healthcare providers, patients, and families should be affirming and useful. Encouraging patients and families to participate in care and decision making is important.

Because patients and their families spend most of their time with nurses and other front line staff—and often express their preferences, expectations, and frustrations to them—nurses are in a great position to help ensure that the care a hospital provides is as patient-centered as possible. Examples of patient-centered care include:

- Involving the patient in the discharge process

- Adjusting medications to the patient's schedule

- Sitting for a few minutes with each patient at each shift

- Ensuring the patient is free of pain and has daily information regarding plan of care, schedule of tests, and prognosis

Value-Added Processes

Ensuring that all care processes are free of waste and promote continuous flow is an underlying goal of TCAB, but developing lean operations first requires distinguishing between value-added and nonvalue-added steps in every process. Commitment to a lean organization must begin with leadership and become part of a culture that is receptive to and rewarding of lean ideas. Staff should be involved in helping to redesign processes to improve flow and reduce waste.

Because nurses and other front line staff spend so much time in activities that take away from the amount of time they have to spend on direct patient care, they are well suited to identify processes that increase leanness in a unit. Examples of value-added processes include:

- Applying lean strategies such as space redesign and having all needed equipment at the bedside at all times

- Using cell phones to reach staff throughout hospital system

- Streamlined medication ordering, processing in pharmacy, delivery to unit, and administration

Rapid Cycle Change

Rapid cycle change is the process of direct care providers identifying problems that affect safety and finding solutions to them. The providers, who are staff nurses, analyze the problems by discussing the various causes and the people who are affected or influence the issue. Next, they brainstorm to think of possible solutions. Solutions are discussed, and a single solution is chosen. The solution is the test of change and is piloted for a short period of time. If it works, the change is adopted. If it is not effective, the rapid cycle change process begins again.

Test of Change

Specific individual change in TCAB is called test of change. The implementation of the solution agreed upon in the rapid cycle change process is the test of change, which is monitored for a short time (e.g., a week or two). The outcome is immediately evaluated. If it worked, it becomes an initiative. If the plan failed, it is filed away as a "dud."

Presently, ongoing efforts to improve the TCAB process continue with the IOM and its dedication to improving quality and safety in health care. Martin and colleagues (2006) identified strategies to decrease the estimated 1.5 million adverse drug events and unexpected deaths every year in the United States. The recommendations were integrated into the TCAB model. RWJF and IHI joined forces with multiple clinical sites throughout the country in the first two phases and added schools of nursing as partners in the third phase of TCAB. Several second stage efforts were spawned by the project, such as the American Organization of Nurse Executives (AONE) project TCAB 2 (Hudson Thrall, 2010), which moved beyond the 67 hospitals that had already adopted TCAB strategies.

AONE funded a two-year initiative for 50 hospitals to continue the TCAB process. Fewer missing medications between shifts, better reported vitality in nurses, and a decrease in falls are just a few of the results of the innovations adopted.

TCAB Project at Children's Memorial Hospital

From 2004 to 2006, Children's Memorial Hospital (CMH) of Chicago, Illinois, developed several innovations and tested the innovations on special TCAB units. Some of the innovations and efforts worked, and some did not. The TCAB team in Chicago at CMH teamed with DePaul University School of Nursing's Dr. Kim Amer in 2006 to enhance the dissemination of TCAB efforts into curriculum. Since CMH is designated by the American Nurses Credentialing Center as a Magnet hospital, the structure of the institution is supportive of nursing innovation. At CMH, nurses are encouraged to develop as clinical experts and scholars. The collaborative care environment encourages a rich dialogue with medical practitioners, dietitians, physical therapists, respiratory therapists, and other healthcare professionals. There is also a strong presence of advance practice nursing, with over 100 advance practice nurses in the hospital.

A slow-spread strategy was used for TCAB at CMH. The first unit tried various innovations and then shared results with other units. Presently, many units are in the process of adopting the innovations.

Evidence for Best Practices: A Framework for Spread

What happens to a good idea or innovation on a unit once it has proven to be effective? How do other units or other hospitals and nurses know that it is a good idea?

A framework for the "spread" or execution of a plan throughout an institution (Massoud, Nielsen, Nolan, Schall, & Seven, 2006) describes the method used for implementing effective innovations to broader units and hospitals. The primary components needed to implement effective innovations are:

- Preparation for each unit to ensure buy in
- Established goals or aims for the innovations
- Development from all people who will be involved

When the new innovation is implemented in a staged manner, there is more acceptance by staff. The ability to spread the innovations—or make sure that other units and hospitals use the new, effective methods—depends on the step-by-step leadership of an educated administrator who will make sure that all front line staff nurses are aware and engaged in the process (Schall, Chappell, & Nielsen, 2008). Without staff involvement in decision making, the new innovation will not be adopted.

A strategic method was used to select a small group of units to begin the process. Each unit integrated the innovations that matched its unique safety and quality needs. After the innovations were adopted, the units came together and discussed the successes and failures. The participants also met at least twice yearly at national meetings to discuss all effective innovations at TCAB institutions.

Process of Implementation in the Pediatric Setting

The only pediatric setting in TCAB teamed with DePaul University School of Nursing in 2006. The goal of the collaboration was to ensure that the TCAB process was documented and disseminated in nursing literature and textbooks.

The pediatric setting is one of the most patient- and family-focused settings. The family-focused interdisciplinary team communication and regular rounding grew out of the need for limiting disruptions of the child and family, and the benefit of parents having a consistent time when they could talk with the whole team of nurse, doctor, pharmacist, and dietitian. Before TCAB, a family could be overwhelmed with unpredictable schedules, uncertain health outcomes, and the disruption of normal family operations. A simple solution such as regularly scheduled rounds helped decrease one stressor for families.

TCAB Nurse-Guided Innovations

The implementation of the TCAB project focused on the front line nurse directing care at the bedside. An overarching framework was used for all sites, with universal baseline data measured. Goals for all TCAB sites were:

- Increase staff involvement in decision making

- Decrease voluntary turnover

- Decrease time spent in non-nursing activities

- Help to identify simple solutions to everyday issues, test the solutions, and adopt the solutions or drop the ideas

- Empower nurses to be more satisfied with their practice and increase patient and family satisfaction

After the goals were developed, many innovations were proposed, and from those several were adopted. The following descriptions of the adopted innovations include the initial identification of the problem, the proposed solution, the test of change, and the evaluation. The innovations at CMH were integrated into the unit and then spread to other units if applicable. All staff nurse team members on TCAB units were involved in the process of tests of change, implementation on the unit, and spread of the innovation to other units in the hospital.

The Morning Huddle to Enhance Collaborative Communication

On the surgical unit for the first test of change process, nurses wanted to improve communication with the night charge nurse, nurse administrator, and physicians who were rarely in the same place at the same time. The solution was a daily ten to fifteen-minute "huddle" at shift change, during which the charge nurses from the night shift and the day shift, head of the unit, physicians, and staff nurses took 10 minutes to walk around to each patient's bedside and discuss the patient, potential safety issues (such as patients with the same or similar names), or communication issues. The huddle was adopted on two units and resulted in enhanced daily communication, as reported by nurse participants in qualitative reviews.

The huddle is an excellent example of collaborative patient-centered care. It increases the efficiency of work and decreases frustrations about fragmented care planning between caregivers. The investment of 10 to 15 minutes per day is well worth the benefit of more cohesive care. For the huddle to work, all team members must be present and must value the collaboration. If one team member is late or fails to show up consistently, the strength of the team is weakened. The time invested saves time spent on paging physicians, calling physical or occupational therapists, and questioning orders. Huddles have improved the safety and quality of care in multiple settings (Griffin & Madigan, 2007).

The piloting of the huddle is an excellent example of the simple but effective innovations of the TCAB project. Because of the initial pilot success, many other units have adopted the huddle or a variation on the theme. There are also many hospitals throughout the country that anecdotally report using the huddle.

Acuity-Adaptable Pulmonary Unit Pilot

At CMH, the pulmonary unit admits children with cystic fibrosis, asthma, respiratory syncytial virus (RSV), and other chronic pulmonary problems. Patients are often transferred from less acute care beds on the unit to the more intensive care area, and if needed to the pediatric intensive care unit (PICU). This frequent moving from location to location used many nursing care hours, was frustrating to families and children, and increased the risk of confusion and error among all caregivers. Since evidence-based research (Brown & Gallant, 2006; Hennon, Kothari, Maloney & Weigel, 2011) has determined that morbidity and mortality increase with multiple transfers between units, the pediatric pulmonary unit decided to try to keep patients in one location throughout their hospitalization regardless of acuity. The shared governance unit had multiple discussions with all involved physicians, administrators, and staff, and decided to design a 17-bed acute care unit that the patients would be admitted to and discharged from. Each room was acuity adaptable and staffed with nurses at expert level with mastery of intensive care. A corner of the unit was transformed into an eight-bed unit with the facilities necessary to accommodate the sickest patients. The process was inclusive, and the unit functioned well. The efficiency of nursing time was increased on the acuity adaptable respiratory unit since there was less time transferring patients to other beds or other units (see Table 8-1).

Quiet Time at Shift Change and a Tranquility Room

Another initiative at CMH during the TCAB program stemmed from a concern about the level of noise on a unit. The high level of noise from nurses, physicians, and other staff was identified by patients and some nurses as very distracting. This was solved by an hour of quiet time. Nurses and physicians adopted the respect for quiet time between 2:30 and 3:30 every afternoon. Patients and families commented on how lovely it was to have a predictable quiet time to relax and nap. The main barrier to implementation was the need for constant reminders for physicians and respiratory therapists who spent little time on the unit and simply came to the unit to round for a few minutes. The dimmed lights provided a good reminder, and within a few weeks everyone understood the benefit.

Another initiative that helped to calm the environment on a unit was aimed at nurses who did long and stressful shift work. To help decrease stress and manage the physical and psychological wear, a tranquility room was piloted on two units. The room had a massage chair and private headphones to listen to music of the individual's choosing. This was a good solution to the stress of 12-hour shifts, intense demands, and frustrating fatigue. Many nurses work 8- to12-hour shifts with no off-unit break time. Since the tranquility room was just steps away from the unit, it was more accessible than going off the unit for a break. Retention on the unit was not statistically impacted for the short time measured; however, the quality of work life was anecdotally reported to be improved.

TABLE 8-1 ■ Transfers at Children's Memorial Hospital, Chicago

Transfers in the acuity adaptable unit and pulmonary unit at Children's Memorial Hospital, Chicago, decreased during the TCAB project.

Patient Population	Outcome Measures	Time Frame	Transfers
Acute Asthma, pneumonia, Respiratory Syncitial Virus (RSV)	Patient, family, and staff satisfaction	March 2006	40
Chronic Cystic fibrosis, tracheotomy, ventilator dependent	Fewer medication errors (51% reduced wrong patient warnings)	May 2006	25
Critical Care Continuous nebulizer, high oxygen requirements	Improved continuity of care and increased nurse, patient, and family satisfaction	Post transitional care unit (TCU) July August	 6 2

Nursing Implications of TCAB

TCAB revolved around a process of change that increased efficiency in caregiving and developed simple changes that have significant impact. The project included a clear process for empowering nurses to identify system issues, assume responsibility for generating a solution, and deciding on whether the solution should be adopted. The impact on nurse practice and administrative costs was great. Ten hospitals tested 426 different initiatives and innovations, and they implemented and sustained about 284 of them (Buerhaus, 2010). During the TCAB project, the number of falls declined, and there were better outcomes when codes were called (Buerhaus, 2010).

The cost of replacing a registered nurse who leaves an employer is as much as $60,000, so nursing retention can improve an institution's profitability (Martin et al., 2007). In focus groups conducted after the TCAB project, nurses stated that if they could name one work incentive for staying on their unit for the next five years, it would be "Being respected," "Having my boss listen to our issues," or "Having the support to design a solution."

The focus groups with staff nurses who were involved in TCAB teams revealed the following comments:

- "People complain less because if they do complain, we all say, do a test of change to see what will help!"

- "It is good to know that your opinions are valued and that the administration will give you a chance to address the issues."

- "Some of the TCAB stuff done was already started on our unit. But the way we looked at whether it worked or not was a good thing."

- "At first it was like, here is this other thing that you need to do. Then I realized that it wasn't the charge nurse that was helped. It was the nurses who were able to help make it a better unit."

- "Since TCAB started, I feel much more connected to everyone on my unit. I feel like we all have a voice, and we listen to each other more. I know I am more involved and actually see changes through innovations that I helped develop."

Thanks to the TCAB program, nurses were able to work more efficiently with safer quality interventions and were less likely to leave. The units that participated had low voluntary turnover. The turnover on one unit was high due to multiple maternity leaves and moves to other states.

Nursing professionals should be able to adopt TCAB principles so that their work environments improve. Nursing schools must integrate TCAB concepts into the curriculum to prepare students for a future full of demands and unique opportunities. Content that keeps pace with current safety and quality needs in the high-technology healthcare industry must be included in nursing education. The first step is to establish content that increases awareness of safety and quality nursing practice (Viney, Batcheler, Houston, & Belcik, 2006). After the knowledge is acquired, new nursing graduates should practice innovations, and improvements in safety should follow.

The experience of collaborating with this extraordinary group of nurse scholars and RWJF and IHI provided Dr. Amer's team with a new and fresh outlook on the possibilities of the future of nursing.

CHAPTER HIGHLIGHTS

- Transforming Care at the Bedside (TCAB) brought together multiple sites with several support agencies with the shared goal of improving safety and quality nursing care.
- The TCAB process of instituting changes and innovations focused on safe quality care sets the standard for all hospitals to follow.
- Nurses need to be knowledgeable about the TCAB project and its successes to be able to integrate the concepts into day-to-day clinical care.

Pearson Nursing Student Resources

Find additional review materials at
nursing.pearsonhighered.com

Prepare for success with additional NCLEX®-style practice questions, interactive assignments and activities, web links, animations and videos, and more!

REFERENCES

Brown, K. K., & Gallant, D. (2006). Impacting patient outcomes through design: Acuity adaptable care/universal room design. *Critical Care Nursing Quarterly, 29*(4), 326–341.

Buerhaus, P. (2010). Lessons from TCAB, and more: An interview with health economist and quality researcher Jack Needleman. *Nursing Economics, 28*(4), 276–279.

Griffin, V., & Madigan, C. (2007). Incorporating patient safety initiatives into nursing practice. Nurse Leader, 5(6), 34–37.

Hennon, M. W., Kothari, A., Maloney, J. D., & Weigel, T. (2011). Implementation of an acuity adaptable patient care unit is associated with improved outcomes after major pulmonary resections. *Journal of Surgical Residency, 170*(1) 17–21.

Hudson Thrall, T. (2010). AONE helps hospitals improve care through second TCAB effort. *AONE Resource Case Study*. Retrieved from www.AONE .org.

Institute for Healthcare Improvement (IHI). *Transforming Care at the Bedside*. Retrieved from http://www.ihi .org/HH/Programs/TransformingCareAtTheBedside.htm on 9/2010

Martin, S. C., Greenhouse, P. K., Merryman, T., Shovel, J., Liberi, C., & Konzier, J. (2007). Transforming Care at the Bedside: Implementation and spread model for single-hospital and multihospital systems. *Journal of Nursing Administration*. 37(10), 444-51.

Massoud, M. R., Nielsen, G. A., Nolan, K., Schall, M. W., & Seven, C. (2006). A framework for spread: From local improvements to system-wide change. *IHI Innovation Series white paper*. Cambridge, MA: Institute for Healthcare Improvement.

Schall, M. W., Chappell, C., & Nielsen, G. A. (2008). Transforming Care at the Bedside how-to guide: Spreading innovations to improve care on medical surgical units. Cambridge, MA: Institute for Healthcare Improvement.

Viney, M., Batcheller, J., Houston, S, & Belcik, K. (2006). Transforming Care at the Bedside: Designing new care systems in an age of complexity. *Journal of Nursing Care Quality, 21*(2), 143–150.

CHAPTER 9

INFORMATICS AND NURSING: USING TECHNOLOGY TO IMPROVE QUALITY

Kim Siarkowski Amer

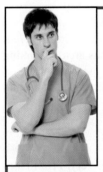

konstantynov/
Shutterstock.com

Dennis entered the break room at 10:30 p.m. just having finished a long day in the medical intensive care unit (MICU). He had a snack and chatted with the charge nurse. He had two patients who coded, and almost died, and a new patient with colon cancer who had unstable blood pressures and irregular heartbeat. The new patient, Irvin, had a central venous catheter inserted in surgery. At 74 years of age, he was a high risk with two bypass surgeries in the past. Dennis had been on duty when Irvin returned from surgery a few hours earlier. He noticed that the new ICU intern seemed overwhelmed with monitoring the two unstable patients. Irvin looked alert and calm, and his vital signs were stable, but he was coughing and complaining of pain. His intravenous (IV) infusion of normal saline was running at 45 mL/hour into his new central line. Irvin had some facial edema but no other problems.

Before Dennis signed off for the day, he logged on to the hospital system, checked the current vital signs of all his patients, and pulled up the chest x-ray and initial radiology reading to check the placement of Irvin's catheter. The x-ray revealed the tip of the catheter was 1 mm from the superior vena cava and looked like it was ready to fall back out of the chamber. If the tip migrated to an axillary vein, it could cause a serious pulmonary event.

Dennis called the radiologist and discussed the film. The radiologist had been busy doing a head computed tomography (CT) scan on a trauma patient. The radiologist agreed that the catheter was about to be dislodged. Dennis paged the surgeon on call, and she immediately came to examine Irvin. She then advanced the catheter in the MICU. The surgeon, Dr. Brown, was relieved that Dennis had checked the x-ray remotely. A few more hours could have been fatal if Irvin had pulmonary infiltration.

CORE COMPETENCY

Imagine ideal information systems to ensure the delivery of safe quality nursing care and meet client health needs.

LEARNING OUTCOMES

1. Describe current and emerging technologies that are available for use in health care, including the concept and function of electronic health records (EHRs).

2. Understand the impact of technology on nurse safety and quality issues.

3. Discuss the role of technology on nurse education.

Technology has transformed every area of contemporary life, and that is also true of nursing and health care. A recent focus area of nursing education is called informatics. The term refers to the use of information systems technology in specific environments, in this case, health care and nursing.

Trends in Technology

Information systems are transforming healthcare delivery. From electronic health records (EHRs) to bar coding for medication administration to advances in telemedicine, new systems of technology have been created and implemented to improve the level of safe care delivery. New systems can also improve the quality of patient- and family-centered care, providing health care that is culturally competent, accessible, and easy to use. Technology is moving health care beyond the days when entire medical record rooms were filled solely with patients' charts. The transition is still in progress, leaving some patients with paper charts and records at several different hospitals and clinics, which limits the ability to cross-reference. New patient record systems are improving the use of space by compressing electronic files, using less space, and allowing for greater access by all providers. Nurses adapting to technology that is integrated with clinical care may resist at first. However, the benefit is soon realized as nurses gain the ability to touch a button and access years of patient data, and the safety of patients improve.

The primary issue with technology is whether the systems that are being designed and purchased are congruent with the needs and abilities of the users, including healthcare providers, patients, and families. The new systems must be designed by nurses, providers, and other users, and they must be accessible and easy to use; otherwise, the systems will not be used or will be used suboptimally.

Focus on Electronic Health Records (EHRs)

In the past, all patients in hospitals had paper charts exclusively. To search the medical history of a patient, the provider needed to call the medical records department, which were large rooms full of thick paper charts, and have the paper chart delivered to the unit. Alternatively, the nurse could go to the basement of the hospital to view the record. Presently, EHR systems are being designed, upgraded, and implemented throughout the United States. Soon all patient information will be documented and stored electronically.

Health Policy

The U.S. federal government committed to the use of EHRs when Congress passed the Health Information Technology for Economic and Clinical Health (HITECH) Act, which was enacted as part of the American Recovery and Reinvestment Act of 2009. HITECH provides incentives to using EHRs in outpatient and inpatient settings for Medicare providers. Doctors and hospitals also receive grant funds through the act for the implementation of EHR systems.

Individual providers and hospitals using EHRs must meet specific criteria to receive the federal funding. One criterion is the requirement for certified EHR systems that are fully integrated into care delivery. This means patient information in a clinic across the city must be available and easily accessible to an emergency department across town or in another location. The second criterion is having technical, financial, and legal support so that information can flow securely and ensure that safe, confidential care is provided. Last, the healthcare workforce needs to be well-educated users of EHRs (Gartee & Beal, 2012).

The HITECH act was developed in part in response to the Institute of Medicine (IOM) report *To Err Is Human: Building a Safer Health System* (IOM, 1999), which outlined the dramatic impact of adverse events and medical errors on the public, including an estimated 44,000 to 98,000 deaths and a loss of $17 to $29 billion per year due to lost income and disability. Several technological efforts emerged as a result of the report. In addition to HITECH, an Office of National Coordinator for Health Information Technology (ONC) was established to develop a framework for the adoption of health information technology (Gartee & Beal, 2012). The framework included four goals:

1. Inform clinical practice by incentives for use of EHR and dissemination throughout the country

2. Interconnect clinicians and encourage regional and national collaborations and networks

3. Personalize care and encourage patients and families to use technology

4. Improve population health through streamlined technological systems that can track health data over time globally

The HITECH Act heightened the legislative emphasis and continued the ONC's emphasis on EHRs. The primary barriers to implementation of EHR systems universally to date include limitations in the knowledge base of healthcare providers regarding use of basic information systems, limited systems that accommodate all needs of providers and sites, and the ongoing challenge of raising awareness regarding the availability of federal funds to assist with implementation.

Unfortunately, progress in the implementation of EHR systems has been slower than the implementation of new technologies in other technology-dependent industries, such as aeronautics. The ability to access patient information at all sites at all times remains elusive. Accessible universal health records will most likely be developed and refined in the next decade. With new systems, access to patient care will become safer and more streamlined.

Medication Administration and Safety Technology

Medication administration today is safer than in the past because of barcoding technology that allows for scanning medications and the patient's identification bracelet with unique barcode to ensure compatibility. If there is incompatibility between medications, the barcode system signals that the scanned medication is unsafe for administration.

The uniformity of the physical setup of a medication administration environment and a consistent process for the ordering, processing, and delivering medication are equally important emerging technologies. The implementation of bar coding for administration of medication can result in a significant savings in the amount of time used to administer medications. The safety of bar coding in terms of decreasing errors, however, is more difficult to prove. Since most nurses are hesitant to report near-miss drug errors, the only reported errors prior to bar coding were those reported in incident reports. Incident reports have usually been considered to be punitive; thus underreporting of potential or actual errors in medication administration occurs.

The critical piece of tracking adverse events is the process, which includes multiple providers and settings. Just tracking one simple order for acetaminophen for a child with a fever may involve the following:

1. Provider places order in computer physician order entry (CPOE) and gets error message if dose is inappropriate

2. Pharmacy dispenses the medication and double-checks with other pharmacist to ensure correct medication, dose, and route

3. Medication is transported to floor

4. Nurse gathers medication from delivery area and checks the "rights" of dose, patient, route, drug, and time. Nurse then administers medication to the patient.

Talking with the patient and family each time a medication is given also helps to decrease the likelihood of error. The family can help with identification of allergies, appropriate medications, and whether the patient has received the medication before.

Systems must also be set up to recognize common characters and letters that can be read two ways and cause mistakes. Included in the program for bar coding is the *Do Not Use* list of abbreviations, such as using "mL" instead of "cc" (The Joint Commission, 2004). The goal is to limit any risk for misinterpretation (ISMP, 2004). Another new safety check is the use of Tall Man names for similar drugs such as PredniSONE versus PrednisoLONE. The Institute for Safe Medication Practices (ISMP) is committed to making medication administration as safe as possible (ISMP, 2011).

To improve the safety of medication administration, all nurses must move beyond negative feelings about error reporting. The National Association of Children's Hospitals and Related Institutions (NACRI) works to ensure benchmarking and productivity for safety. This group meets to discuss approaches to medication reconciliation, that is, making sure medications are administered in the safest manner possible. NACRI is a national organization, but more locally, nursing quality councils within individual hospitals focus on process improvement, continually reviewing incidents that need to be addressed to make the hospital safer.

Telehealth

Many terms used in the discussion of technology need clear definitions. Technology use in the medical context includes a range of human interaction with phones, computers, and diagnostic instruments, and is often referred to as informatics. The terms "telehealth" and "telemedicine" are often used synonymously. However, there are differences (see Box 9-1). The Office for Advancement of Telehealth (OAT) identifies telehealth as using electronic information and telecommunications to support long-distance clinical healthcare treatment plans and interventions, patient and professional health-related education, and public health and health administration (Amer, 2006). Telehealth is a broad interprofessional approach to the use of information systems. By contrast, telemedicine is more focused on specific diagnostics, such as phone interpretation of heart sounds to diagnose heart murmurs, and thus is defined as the use of electronic

BOX 9-1 FREQUENTLY CONFUSED TECHNOLOGY TERMS

Electronic health record (EHR): Digital version of patient data found in traditional paper record

Electronic medical record (EMR): Legal record of a single encounter or visit

Personal health record (PHR): Lifelong tool for patients to use to manage health information

Telehealth: Use of technology to assist with health assessment, diagnosis, treatment, and promotion of health to patients at other locations

Telemedicine: Branch of telehealth that uses technology to deliver medical care and services to patients at other locations

communication and information technologies to provide or support clinical care at a distance.

Using telehealth, healthcare providers can assess patients in locations anywhere in the world. For example, with a video-conference connection guided by a surgeon, a provider not trained as a surgeon can help a person in a remote location who needs emergency surgery. Other examples may be less dramatic but nevertheless are important. Nurses in rural health locations can transmit heart sounds and ear exams via stethoscopes and otoscopes that have computer connections to other providers. Cardiac tracings can be transmitted to cardiologists who can determine the best treatment for arrhythmias.

The potential range of emerging telehealth and information systems abilities can be broad and futuristic. Nurses and physicians should be prepared to design and use innovative systems to accomplish their work in the future, including the ability for treatments to be globally accessible through telehealth. The diagnosis and treatment of illness will be only a small part of the range of health provision that can be provided. Standard care scenarios can be constructed to help guide rural or other remote practitioners. Such scenarios delivered by video conference or web conference can help patients in all nations.

Future Directions in Technology

Future nursing care will include small handheld or wearable devices that can track patient progress and telemetry; provide laboratory and radiology data; allow the patient, family, or staff to call the nurse; and provide safety alerts for patients and the environment. Such devices are being used now in select nursing units. There is great potential in using smart phones or personal digital assistant (PDA) devices for managing nursing care. However, as with any technology, the human factor must be included. Nurses need to continue to have human-to-human contact with patients. Nurses must assess patients thoroughly and provide human touch along with the technology that can assist with safe care. Another emerging technology, HPS (high fidelity patient simulation), uses computer patient models in the nursing education setting. This soon to be standard education tool will be discussed in more detail later in this chapter. Figure 9-1 delineates how technology can be used and its outcomes for healthcare providers and patients.

Robots

Many high-level technological breakthroughs were not imaginable as recently as 2000. One example is the use of robotics for a variety of tasks, from precision surgery to prosthesis work. Robots pull supplies, stock supplies, and enter data into hospital computers. Some new robots are similar in appearance and demeanor to humans and are used to simulate patient care situations for nursing education. Robots will never replace nurses; however, their use can help to streamline nursing tasks and increase productivity and efficiency.

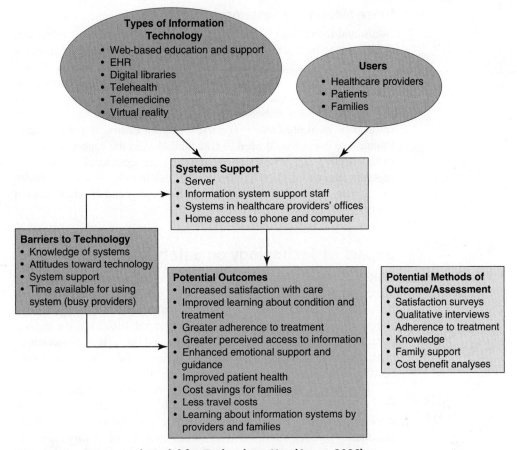

Figure 9-1   Conceptual Model for Technology Use (Amer, 2006)

This model depicts how technology can transform the healthcare system.

Amer, K. S. (2006). Innovations in pediatric health care technology: A multidisciplinary conceptual framework for using and evaluating information systems. *Children's Health Care 35*(1), 5–10.

Global Positioning Systems

Global positioning systems (GPSs) are another new technology that has become accessible to most people. In past years, GPS units were large and cumbersome, often the size of a large coffee cup. Now these systems are included in most smart phones and can be added to other useful patient care devices. GPS can be especially useful with patients who may wander away from safety, for example, patients with Alzheimer's disease or patients who have psychiatric disorders. The GPS can alleviate anxiety by easily tracking patients if they wander outside of their homes or hospital rooms. The devices can be worn as a bracelet that looks like a watch, or they can be added to shoes. These devices are only a few of the new technologies that keep people safe and have the ability to influence health outcomes.

Nurse Monitoring Systems

Additional technology of the future can only be imagined at this point. One idea is to have a monitoring system for nurses that triggers an alarm when a nurse falls asleep or has symptoms of stress and fatigue. Nurses are notorious for working long shifts with no breaks. A high-risk time for errors occurs during the final hours of a 12-hour shift. A watch or necklace that could monitor body temperature, heart rate, and blood pressure could be a great predictor of a nurse's risk for errors. When the alarm sounds, the nurse would need to take a break, and the supervisor would automatically come to cover. Although this may seem idealistic, the concept may come to fruition like many ideas that initially seemed unobtainable. Nurses need to continue to think about unique and different ways to ensure safety and quality care.

Impact of Technology on Safety and Quality

EHRs and other technologies can dramatically affect health outcomes. More needs to be done to elevate the status of EHR systems to the level of safety tracking used in aeronautics. Health care, of course, is more complex than maintaining aircrafts and tracking destinations. But the use of simulation training for safety assurance and the design of models to track outcomes in the aeronautics field can be helpful in designing future healthcare systems focused on safety and quality.

The impact of technology on quality is much more abstract and complex than its impact on safety. Quality is a way to arrive at safe care through consistent patient-centered care. Quality care is not just patient satisfaction; while patient satisfaction can be a part of quality care, it is much more than that. Quality care is a process that includes a commitment to continually improving practice through safety reports, making changes to improve care, and being open to change. Ultimately, technology can play a part in the process, although there is no replacement for basic human judgment and decision making.

Nurses need to be involved in creating technological systems that are safe and flow well within their practice settings. For example, crash carts for sudden cardiac arrests should be set up according to the logical need for the drugs, a critical factor for ease of use and encouraging thorough documentation. Someone outside the healthcare field may want to organize the crash cart differently, perhaps alphabetically, but those who use the cart know that the best way to organize it is via the logical use of emergency drugs. Scrambling for emergency drugs can be just as frustrating during a code as endless scrolling through pages of computer screens to find the needed documentation screen.

In order to participate in technological solutions that will work for them, nurses need to master EHR systems and new technology as it emerges. But technology should not displace teaching basic nursing concepts. The basic caring concepts—hygiene, environment, and prioritization of care—remain the cornerstone of nursing education. The primary consideration for different units and other settings is how the workflow is structured, and only those who participate in the workflow can offer firsthand knowledge of it.

Consistency is key for safe care through workflow analysis. Errors are not solely caused by erratic individuals or bad technology; it is the lack of a systemic, predictable organizational factors that usually increases risk of error, a fact that is critical for all healthcare workers to grasp (Woods, Patterson, & Cook, 2007).

Meaningful Use

When investing in technology, a healthcare organization should focus on its suitability as well as its ease of use. The highest level of technology is not always needed for effective healthcare management. "Meaningful use" is a phrase that has been adopted to signify the appropriate design and proper application of information systems to those who will be using them. The American Academy of Nursing (AAN) developed a matrix and set of definitions and criteria for meaningful use, which is available at www.aannet.org.

User Perceived Need

In community and hospital settings, many healthcare professionals and even patients and families may be accessing the same system for patient information. For all users to benefit from technology, their needs must be considered when determining what specific technology to use and how it should be configured. Nursing involvement is essential in this

Evidence for Best Practices: Preparing for EHR

What is the best way to get ready for the implementation of EHR systems in a healthcare setting? Creating realistic scenarios in undergraduate nursing education is essential so that newly graduated nurses can master electronic systems prior to beginning their new jobs (Meyer, Sternberger, and Toscos, 2011). Textbooks with data mock ups prepare students for the electronic world of documentation and data management. The American Academy of Nursing (AAN), taking a future-oriented view of EHRs and meaningful use, recommends that EHRs should focus on healthy patients outside of hospitals in community-based settings. Providers should be delivering care that is documented as impacting the quality and outcomes of care. Electronic data systems must include patient-centered documentation elements from all disciplines so that nurses and other clinicians can explore data that is linked to better interventions, better outcomes, and more efficient and cost effective care. Documentation will be important in future technology systems (AAN, 2010), and newly graduated nurses who have been trained on the use of EHRs will be prepared to use it effectively.

process. Because of the inclusive nature of the nursing process, nurses have a more holistic view of patients than other interprofessional team members. However, other team members, such as ancillary staff, pharmacists, dietitians, physical therapists, and social workers, should also be included in assessing the needs for specific technology (AAN, 2010). Their feedback is necessary for consideration of the benefits and also potential risks of technology.

User Competence and Confidence

Much of the perceived need regarding technology is guided by the user's level of competence and confidence. If users are not confident in their ability to master information systems, their competency levels will never advance to fully master the technology. Positive reinforcement and good support during the transition to using new technology is of utmost importance. For example, an elderly patient with a new blood glucose monitor may not feel confident in his ability to master the new device. If proper demonstrations are done for the patient and the patient practices monitoring his glucose during the demonstration, there is a much greater chance the patient will use the device at home. If the patient is simply handed a box with the new device, the new technology may overwhelm him. Confidence guides competence with any technology.

Stages of Deployment and Technical Support

When new information systems are deployed, an organization must plan the launch with precision and technology support. With the implementation of EHR systems, staff and providers must be well oriented to the purpose and use of the system, and the orientation to it must be undertaken at a comfortable pace. The phase-in period must be done with support people on site initially and then available by phone. With good planning and technology support, users will be comfortable and positive at the end of the deployment. Conversely, if the proper introductory time period is not provided, or if there is poor technology support, the deployment can fail, and the users may never view the system in a positive light.

EHR and Upgrading Health System Access to Client Information

EHR systems can be an efficient resource if used appropriately. As stated previously, "meaningful use" is the term used to encourage providers to use medical record data for the benefit of the patient, help track trends in disease, or follow specific outcome measures.

Phasing in EHR or medication administration systems requires a well-executed implementation plan. During the initial phases of implementation of a computerized medication administration system, there is a high potential for mistakes. For example, if one physician orders a STAT medication by paper chart and another physician orders the same medication electronically, a system to catch the duplicate orders may not yet

CASE STUDY: *Stanley*

Stanley was doing his initial assessment of surgery patients at 7 p.m. at the beginning of a 12-hour shift. Ms. Meyer, a 90-year-old patient who had undergone gall bladder surgery, was his first assessment. She complained of discomfort in her left antecubital area, and Stanley noticed a reddened area where the intravenous (IV) catheter was inserted. He documented the variance in the PDA program and reviewed the previous hourly check by the day shift nurse. He stopped the IV antibiotic that was running immediately and called the hospitalist. The IV site was more edematous when the hospitalist arrived, and she told Stanley that he probably saved Ms. Meyer's forearm from a severe skin infiltration. Early identification of infiltrates can prevent severe burns and scarring. Checking intravenous sites regularly can be automatically programmed into the EHR system.

1. How might an EHR system have prevented the IV site from becoming edematous?

2. Which of Stanley's actions were important to identification of the problem?

be in place. To ensure safe care, the system designer and support people must be available to edit and change the system in the early phase. If a product fails to provide continual service, it may be time to change vendors and try a new system. An example of outcome tracking in EHR is described in the case study about Stanley.

Rates of documented infiltration prior to EHR implementation were three times less than the rates after the documentation was done on the electronic record in a Transforming Care at the Bedside (TCAB) hospital, Children's Memorial Hospital in Chicago, described in chapter 8. This appears to be a case of underreporting. The goal is not to be punitive, but to begin to identify trends and risks that can be addressed to decrease the likelihood of future infiltration events. Electronic documentation is key to tracking the measured standard, such as infiltration rates.

Tracking Outcomes Focused on Quality

The EHR and medication delivery systems in current use have limited ability to retrieve aggregate data on long-term outcomes. The focus on population health, as outlined by the ONC and HITECH, requires the development of technological systems that can pull out data from categories of patients and analyze the health of populations. The focus on population health, or looking at broad aggregate data on a large geographical cohort of people who have a similar health issue, is a feature of the early development of the ONC. Frameworks for technology to report population health are being designed, revised, and implemented with the support of many agencies and organizations.

The Agency for Healthcare Research and Quality (AHRQ) has many ongoing research projects that support exploring long-term quality outcome measures. One example is the Template of Measure Attributes, the primary tool used to develop National Quality Measures Clearinghouse

(NQMC) measure summaries (AHRQ, 2011), a listing of the measures, grouped by domain, that can be tracked. The goal is to develop quality common measures that can be universal. There are many domains of potential measures of quality. In the population health domain, health quality measures include structure, process, access, experiences, health state, cost, health knowledge, social determinates of health, and environment. Such measures are excellent in theory; however, designing universal measures to integrate into all EHRs becomes a labor-intensive task. Ultimately, a well-designed EHR system will incorporate critical tracking of such outcomes, and the data will be easy to access. This will allow all healthcare providers and government regulators to assess progress toward safe and quality health care in the United States.

Home Health-Focused Technology in Community Care

Nurses need to focus on all aspects of patient health when it comes to technology in and out of healthcare institutions. The hospital setting is the most common place to provide care; however, the home care environment is becoming important in consumer health and information technology.

Many factors determine how well a patient does after discharge from the hospital. If nurses and physicians neglect to assess a patient's home and community context, the outcomes are worse (Olson, 2010). For example, the patient may be at risk for falling or poor adherence to her medication regimen. The National Academy of Science published a guide for human factors design consideration that focuses on the best use of information technology in the home (see Figure 9-2). The model incorporates multiple factors, including the person, equipment, tasks, and environment. The technology, however, is only as good as the user's ability. Patients have a wide variety of technological aptitude influenced by factors such as age, education, gender, ethnicity, health status, knowledge and skills, healthcare beliefs, technological competence, and healthcare readiness (Olson, 2010). A complex interaction needs to be structured to take into account the patient's context, equipment complexity (e.g., blood glucose monitors versus home ventilators), and the collaboration required to accomplish the tasks. Coordination of care processes can be done to ensure the mastery of technology so that the best care and outcomes are achieved.

Consumer-Based Health Information and Wikis

The AHRQ is in the final phase of evaluating the feasibility of using wikis, that is, web pages that can be accessed and edited by all users. If approved, the wiki could be used for reviewing draft reports of evidence-based outcomes and for development of peer reports. Potentially, it could also be used as a platform for report publication, updating, and disseminating. This is just one way that the AHRQ is working toward making outcomes more easily reported and reviewed (Erinoff, 2011). The benefit of using wikis is the ability for all users to add content. This accessibility

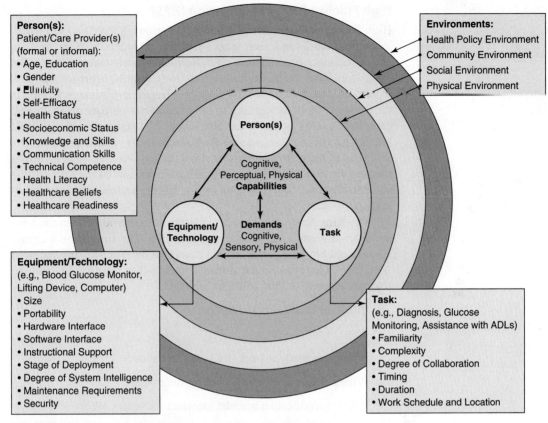

Person(s):
Patient/Care Provider(s)
(formal or informal):
• Age, Education
• Gender
• Ethnicity
• Self-Efficacy
• Health Status
• Socioeconomic Status
• Knowledge and Skills
• Communication Skills
• Technical Competence
• Health Literacy
• Healthcare Beliefs
• Healthcare Readiness

Environments:
Health Policy Environment
Community Environment
Social Environment
Physical Environment

Person(s)

Cognitive,
Perceptual, Physical
Capabilities

**Equipment/
Technology**

Demands
Cognitive,
Sensory, Physical

Task

Equipment/Technology:
(e.g., Blood Glucose Monitor,
Lifting Device, Computer)
• Size
• Portability
• Hardware Interface
• Software Interface
• Instructional Support
• Stage of Deployment
• Degree of System Intelligence
• Maintenance Requirements
• Security

Task:
(e.g., Diagnosis, Glucose
Monitoring, Assistance with ADLs)
• Familiarity
• Complexity
• Degree of Collaboration
• Timing
• Duration
• Work Schedule and Location

Figure 9-2 Model of Human Factors in Health Care in the Home
Key elements of health at home involve the person, the task, and the equipment or technology.
Consumer health information technology in the home: A guide for human factors design considerations
Copyright © 2011 National Academy of Sciences. All rights reserved.

can also be a problem when inappropriate or inaccurate information is posted. The future of this technology in the context of health care is yet to be determined.

Informatics and Nursing Education

Educational programs that offer nursing informatics graduate degrees focus on the design and use of healthcare records, medication administration systems, Internet-based health information, and online storage and use of healthcare information (Meyer, Sternberger & Toscos, 2011). A future focus of informatics should be on the knowledge needed for nurses to design specific health information systems that ensure safe care, provide guidance about health promotion and disease management, and give patients and providers access to all health records. Many companies are already designing such systems, and nurses need to be part of the development teams.

High Fidelity Patient Simulation (HPS)

High fidelity patient simulation (HPS) is a growing technological teach-ing tool for nurses and many other healthcare providers. HPS involves the use of computer-programmed manikins that simulate real situations. The simulators have the ability to generate lung sounds, heart sounds, gas-trointestinal problems, and much more. The primary strength of HPS is the bridge from book learning to direct contact with patients in clinical care. During HPS, students can take charge of a serious health situation, making decisions and observing the consequences of their decisions in a safe setting. Instructors can assess strengths and weaknesses in groups of students instead of assessing clinical care behaviors in the hospital one student at a time. Students perceive the HPS experience as overwhelm-ingly positive.

Dr. Kim Amer developed a simulation scenario presentation for an HPS simulation conference in April 2010. The simulation was of a 10-year-old boy with acute asthma exacerbation. The scenario included 10 safety violations that the students were told to identify. Most of the students succeeded. The violations included:

- Lifesaver candy at back of throat

- (Fake) vomit on floor

- Suspicious mark on back (rule out child abuse)

- Wrong albuterol dose for nebulizer treatment

- Patient identification bracelet incorrect

- Unsafe materials left in bed (used syringes)

- Side rail left down after treatment

- Oxygen not connected correctly

- Adult visitor not related to patient

- Hand hygiene noncompliance

Each scenario done in nursing programs can stage multiple safety breaches, ensuring that all students know to identify the safety issues so that the behavior routine is established.

CHAPTER HIGHLIGHTS

- EHRs are being implemented in healthcare settings to improve access to patient information and enhance quality care outcomes.

- The U.S. government has passed legislation such as HITECH and the Patient Care and Affordability Act that provide funding and support for technological innovations that track patient information and patient outcomes to improve overall safety in health care.

- Patients will benefit from new innovations in technology such as global positioning systems technology to monitor patients with Alzheimer's disease.
- Emerging healthcare innovations such as simulations of patient care safety situations will assist with nursing education that is focused on improving quality patient care.

Pearson Nursing Student Resources

Find additional review materials at
nursing.pearsonhighered.com
Prepare for success with additional NCLEX®-style practice questions, interactive assignments and activities, web links, animations and videos, and more!

REFERENCES

Amer, K. S. (2006). Innovations in pediatric health care technology: A multidisciplinary conceptual framework for using and evaluating information systems. *Children's Health Care 35*(1), 5–10.

AHRQ (2011). Template of Measure Attributes retrieved from http://www.qualitymeasures.ahrq.gov/about/template-of-attributes.aspx

American Academy of Nursing (AAN). (2010). *To meet the needs of patients, the American academy of nursing says we need to go beyond meaningful use.* Retrieved from http://www.aannet.org/i4a/headlines/headlinedetails.

Erinoff, E. G. (2011). Feasibility study of a wiki collaboration platform for systematic reviews. *Agency for Healthcare Research and Quality.* Retrieved from http://www.AHRQ.gov/.

Gartee, R., & Beal, S. (2012). *Electronic health records and nursing.* Upper Saddle River, NJ: Prentice Hall.

Health Information Technology for Economic and Clinical Health. (2009). *American Recovery and Reinvestment Act of 2009,* Title XIII.

Institute of Medicine (IOM). (1999). *To err is human: Building a safer health system.* Retrieved from http://www.iom.edu/Reports/1999/To-Err-is-Human-Building-A-Safer-Health-System.aspx.

Institute for Safe Medication Practices. (2004). *ISMP's list of error-prone abbreviations, symbols, and dose designations.* Retrieved from www.ismp.org/tools/errorproneabbreviations.pdf.

The Joint Commission. (2004). *Official do not use list.* Retrieved from http://www.jointcommission.org/nurses.aspx

Meyer, L., Sternberger, C., & Toscos, T. (2011). How to implement the electronic health record in undergraduate nursing education. *American Nurse Today, 6*(5), 40–44.

Olson, S. (2010). *The Role of Human Factors in Home Health Care: Workshop Summary* (National Academies Press) by Committee on the Role of Human Factors in Home Healthcare, National Research Council.

Woods, D. D., Patterson, E. S., & Cook, R. I. (2007). Behind human error: Taming complexity to improve patient safety. In P. Carayon (Ed.), *Handbook of human factors and ergonomics in health care and patient safety* (pp. 459–476). Mahwah, NJ: Lawrence Erlbaum Associates.

PERSON-CENTERED CARE

Mario Ortiz

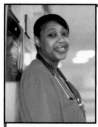

Blend Images /
Shutterstock.com

Betty is beginning her shift by admitting a new patient to the hematology oncology unit. She has worked on the unit since she graduated from nursing school eight years ago. Her patient, Pete, is a 57-year-old mechanic who has worked for 35 years at the same garage. For two months, he had pain in his right hip and his stomach. He was diagnosed with late-stage stomach cancer with bone metastasis. He has had extensive consultation with hematologist oncologist Dr. Levitsky and Pete has decided he does not want chemotherapy or radiation. He simply wants to work until he gets sick, and then he wishes to die at home. Maria, his wife, is very angry, and at consultations she tries to convince Pete to do everything possible to help him live. She wants him to be treated with chemotherapy and radiation, and she wants him to quit his job to get treated. Betty recognizes that much of her day will be focused on organizing a team approach to help the family make decisions about Pete's care.

CORE COMPETENCY

Communicate the impact of person- and family-focused care on quality and safe care.

LEARNING OUTCOMES

1. Describe person- and family-centered care in the context of planning nursing interventions.
2. Explore the links between person-focused care and safety and quality outcomes.
3. Demonstrate the ability to integrate person-centered care in clinical situations.
4. Demonstrate an understanding of the importance of cultural differences on how patients and families behave and respond during hospitalization.

Nurses must maintain a delicate balance while coordinating patient and family care. They must be aware of the disparate approaches to care decisions between patient and family members so that adjustments can be made to the treatment plan. The long-term care resources and approach will determine the quality of care for the whole family.

The purpose of this chapter is to outline the importance of person- and family-centered care. Person-centered care is defined as nursing practice that recognizes the beneficial relationships between all healthcare providers, patients, family, and other caregivers. It differs from patient-centered care in its holistic approach and in its recognition of humanistic values for all persons engaged in healthcare practice. Mutual respect, understanding, and the individual right to self-determination are the foundation of person-centered care (McCormack, Dewing, & McCance, 2011). Consequently, person-centered care will be used throughout this chapter.

Importance of Person-Centered Care

Care that is centered on each person as a unique individual has become more important than ever in the delivery of safe, quality health care. Often referred to as patient-centered care, person-centered care is a perspective that explicitly views the experiences, values, and beliefs of individuals as important and central to the way health is lived, and to any healthcare plan or regimen. Every healthcare plan or regime must be developed in a manner that includes the person experiencing a health situation as an integral component (Ponte et al., 2003). This personal experience contains many "answers" or what really matters within interactions with healthcare team members and the healthcare system. Gerteis, Edgeman-Levitan, Daley, and Delbanco, (2002) described seven important dimensions of person-centered care. When these were renamed, the Picker Institute added an eighth dimension to the principles:

1. Respect for patients' values, preferences, and expressed needs

2. Coordination and integration of care

3. Information, communication, and education

4. Physical comfort

5. Emotional support and alleviation of fear and anxiety

6. Involvement of family and friends

7. Transition and community

8. Access to care

Respect for Patients' Values, Preferences, and Expressed Needs

Persons have a right to care that recognizes them as unique. The ways in which life is lived by each person is shown in the values that every person brings to any healthcare situation. It is important to recognize personal values and to treat each person with dignity and respect. It is also important to focus on certain aspects of a person's uniqueness to consistently support autonomy. These aspects are *quality of life, involvement in decision making, dignity,* and *needs and autonomy* (Gerteis et al., 2002).

Quality of life is whatever a person says it is. This means that quality of life is "the incarnation of lived experiences" (Parse, 1998, p. 31). Quality of life is lived moment-to-moment and is lived as health. Because of this living of health and quality of life, it is important to understand what a person values and prefers. It is also important to gain insight into a person's needs, as these needs may be expressed in ways that are different from what a healthcare team member may expect or what the healthcare system may see as normal. Questions should be asked to understand more about a person's quality of life (Gerteis et al., 2002, p. 6):

- What impact does the illness or treatment have on the patient's quality of life or subjective sense of well-being?

- How is this mediated by life-style, cultural values, or religious beliefs?

- How can health care help patients achieve their short-term and long-term goals?

- What are the limitations of the treatment?

Involvement in decision making is another aspect of respecting a person's values, preferences, and expression of needs. Involvement is a way for persons to take action within their health and healthcare plan in a manner that is consistent with what they believe and hold as important. The involvement of a person is not always constant, however. Involvement shifts moment-to-moment, day-to-day, or week-to-week. These shifts arise out of each person's changing view of health, values, priorities, goals, and hopes. The daily living of life colors the ways in which a person may see what was important, what is important, and what may be important. For example, a person may initially choose an aggressive treatment plan for a health-related issue. However, as time passes and experiences are lived, the person may decide to alter or cease the treatment plan, despite explanations of positive progress, milestones, or negative consequences. Therefore, some initial and ongoing important questions to ask may be (Gerteis et al., 2002, p. 6):

- What level of involvement do patients want in decision making?

- How does this vary over time, or with the degree of illness?

- How much, and to whom (clinician, family, friends), would patients prefer to defer?

Dignity is central to valuing the ways in which a person chooses to live health. The ways in which dignity symbolizes the importance nurses convey to those they care for is important because it connects what nurses do and say to how they respect those they care for within practice situations. These connections provide a means for persons receiving care not only to feel respected but to retain dignity in all care settings and interactions. Important questions to focus on when practicing are (Gerteis et al., 2002, p. 6):

- Are patients' physical and emotional needs for privacy and individual expression respected?

- Are they treated with dignity, respect, and sensitivity to their cultural values?

- Do staff treat patients kindly and respectfully?

The *needs and autonomy* of all persons serves as a central aspect of their experience of respect and dignified care. The needs and autonomy of persons must be supported and enhanced so that those receiving care are not left feeling helpless or without a sense of control (Shaller, 2007). Within most healthcare systems, the rules, regulations, policies, and procedures are structured in a manner that places persons receiving care into a passive, and sometimes submissive, role. So, the needs of persons receiving care must be understood by nurses and other healthcare providers to ensure the autonomy of persons remains intact, supported, and the driving force of care. Some important questions to ask when initiating a dialogue about the needs and autonomy of patients are (Gerteis et al., 2002, p. 6):

- What do patients need, want, or expect from their encounter with a healthcare provider or system?

- How do these needs and expectations differ from those perceived by providers?

- How much can patients do on their own, and how much do they want to do?

- How does this mesh with the provider's expectations?

Coordination and Integration of Care

There are many facets to the experiences persons have when they are receiving care. The complexity of the coordination of services affects the care processes and healthcare experience of persons and their loved ones. Patients report feeling vulnerable and powerless in the face of illness. Proper coordination of care can ease those feelings (NRC Picker, 2011). The experiences of persons receiving care are shaped by three factors: *coordination and integration of clinical care, coordination and integration of ancillary and support services,* and *coordination and integration of frontline patient care.*

Coordinating Clinical Care

A care coordinator or case manager provides a bridge or link between health care, supportive services, and the person or family receiving care. Questions that may arise within the coordination of a person's or family's care are:

- Who is in charge of the patient's care?

- Is that person recognized by the patient, as well as by the members of the clinical team?

- How are clinical services coordinated so that members of the team communicate effectively with each other and deliver a consistent set of messages to the patient and family?

The coordination and integration of ancillary and support services should be done with one professional acting as point person. Case managers or care coordinators are now sometimes called nurse navigators or health advocates. These professionals are responsible for coordinating and integrating frontline patient care from admission to discharge and health maintenance at home.

Information, Communication, and Education

Patients and families have the right to know all information about their care, and they should be involved in the plan of care. White boards in patients' rooms have helped to communicate to the patient and family the scheduling for the day and to update them about visits with various providers. The healthcare provider should clearly articulate the person's prognosis to all people involved in the person's care, based on the person's wishes.

Education should include a clear presentation of all options that are available, and the patient and family should be able to demonstrate knowledge of the education and understanding of the plan of care. In the vignette that opened this chapter, the patient did not wish to receive care after he was diagnosed with cancer. He and his family needed to know what comfort care would be available when he grew sicker and when referrals to hospice should be made.

Physical Care

All care situations involve patients with their unique values and beliefs. Eliciting the perspective of the patient and family is one of the nurse's most important functions. The combination of person, family, and other contextual factors such as cultural meaning of illness form the whole experience of the person.

Pain Management

Pain experiences are a good example of how person, family, and other contextual variables affect the individual's experience. Now defined as the fifth vital sign, pain is what the person reports. No other individual

CASE STUDY: *Edward*

Edward, a middle-aged male who was recently discharged from the hospital after cardiac bypass surgery, had several prescriptions to fill at the pharmacy. He sorted through the prescriptions and sent his wife to get all but one of them. Edward decided that the pain medication was not needed. Twelve hours following discharge, his wife, Nancy, called the nursing station in a panic because her husband could not move and was breathing fast, and his heart rate seemed high. His lack of pain control had affected all systems. Two weeks later at his outpatient follow-up visit, the nurse explored Edward's decision to not get pain medication. Edward said he thought he had a high enough pain threshold to "gut it out." He also said that in his culture, pain and suffering were viewed as "good in the eyes of the Lord." In exploring the patient's perceptions, the nurse was able to understand the context of Edward's experiences and the broader cultural and spiritual perspectives.

1. What is a proper response by the nurse to the wife and patient?

2. Why is it important to have the patient and family express their concerns and hopes for treatment?

can express or define a person's pain experience. Because of this individual experience, the nurse must be flexible and willing to explore the patient's perspectives in depth. There are many perspectives that must be assessed, including the person's previous experiences with pain, family response to illness and pain, and the cultural or spiritual meaning associated with pain. Without a comprehensive assessment of an individual's pain experience, pain management will likely not be fully effective.

Activities of Daily Living

While a patient is still in the hospital, the nurse should explore with the patient and family what aspects of the home environment and day-to-day activities might be a challenge to navigate. If a person has work and home environments that will not allow basic daily functions to be achieved, the nurse must ensure that a solution is created. If a person leaves the hospital with limited ambulatory function, the home and work environments must be assessed to make sure that the patient will be safe and able to perform all activities of daily living (ADLs). If nurses do not assess and intervene appropriately, the safety of the patient is compromised due to negligent care planning. The nurse's primary focus should be on the patient and the patient's lived experience of day-to-day life, not just the disease or recovery from surgery or treatments.

Care Environment

Whether the person is having a simple surgical procedure or heart surgery, the assessment of the individual's perceptions of the hospital experience, past experiences with treatments or medications, and cultural understanding of the hospitalization should be considered. The environment must be constructed to align with the person and family's best interest and input regarding the light, sound, and other aspects of the hospital room, such as shutting doors and turning off lights. All senses should be accommodated, including sound, temperature, visual perceptions, and sense of smell.

Emotional Support and Alleviation of Fear and Anxiety

The most effective approach to preventing anxiety is providing information and assessing the patient and family's emotional status. Making sure that their issues are addressed is the key focus. Questions need to be framed with a target in mind. "What are your concerns?" or "What questions do you have?" are good examples of person-focused queries. Also, if the nurse shares with the patient and family common concerns from other patients or other experiences, the patient may be more likely to express his or her own anxiety and fear.

Involvement of Family and Friends

As recently as 1990, patients could have visits only from immediate family, meaning parents, children, siblings, and spouses. The definition of family was narrowly defined. Currently, a broader, more enlightened view of family is defined as those persons who are the closest people in the patient's life, as articulated by the patient. This definition includes a broader cast of partners, good friends, and community members. The primary issue is being able to develop a good rapport with patients and their loved ones, so that there is an open dialogue about their wishes.

Accommodation of Family and Friends

Allowing family and friends to visit patients and integrating these important people into the patient's care are integral to comprehensive patient care, in both inpatient and outpatient settings. When family and friends are involved, the patient can be supported with care that is coordinated by the patient and facilitated by those around him or her. When the patient is the focus, the care is not just physical but holistic, including psychological, social, and community concerns.

Involving Family in Decision Making

When the patient is on good terms with family, they can ask for help with decision making. Ultimately everyone surrounding the patient should honor the patient's wishes first and foremost. Exceptions do occur when patients have altered mental status or psychological impairment. The family's involvement can make all persons feel better throughout the care process.

Supporting the Family as Caregiver

Another rather recently developed concept in person-centered care is recognizing the family as patient and the stressors of family caregiving. *Caregiver burden* is the perception of stress and alteration of daily life when faced with caring for a dependent family member. The range of caregiver burden is wide. The degree of burden does not always correlate with the intensity of the care needed. For example, a child who is ventilator dependent and is being cared for at home by parents may be perceived as producing minimal caregiver burden in contrast to an elderly parent who has mild diabetes and heart disease and who is living with adult children. The main issue is how the caregiving is perceived.

Recognizing the Needs of the Family

Since nurses cannot generalize or assume what the needs of any particular family will be, nurses must ask both patients and families about the specific day-to-day resources that may be needed to care for their loved one. Needs may be as simple as getting bus passes to ensure that the patient returns to the clinic for follow-up visits or as complex as setting up a hospital bed with intravenous infusions in the family home. The most important aspect of person-centered care is focusing on the individual's unique needs and the associated family needs.

Allowing for Cultural Considerations

Cultural competency is an increasingly important aspect of person-centered care. The demographic characteristics of the United States are rapidly changing as the nation becomes more culturally, racially, and ethnically diverse. According to a recent study of the U.S. population, it is estimated that by the year 2050, 14.6% of those living in the United States will be African American, 8% will be Asian American, and 29% will be Latino (Passel & Cohen, 2008). With increasing minority populations, health disparities become more of a challenge. Part of the disparity may be related to the inability to communicate with and understand cultures that differ from the provider's.

The Institute of Medicine (IOM, 2002) and the Sullivan Commission (2004) reported that cultural competence is key to improving quality of care and eliminating racial and ethnic disparities in health care. The goal of cultural competence is to create a healthcare system and workforce that can deliver the highest quality care to every patient regardless of race, ethnicity, culture, or language proficiency. Leininger (1995) emphasized that to be culturally competent, healthcare providers need to understand their own world-view and those of their patients, while avoiding stereotyping and misapplying scientific knowledge. They also need to be knowledgeable, respectful, and responsive to the issues surrounding cultural diversity so that positive outcomes are more likely to occur.

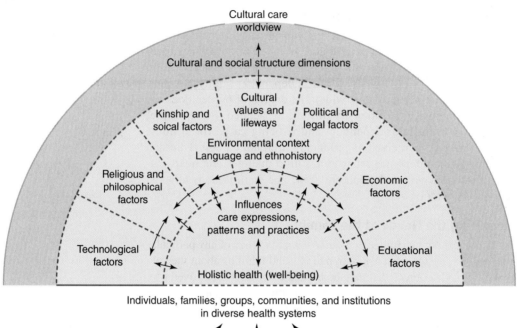

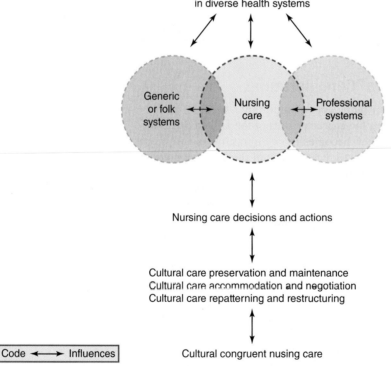

Figure 10-1 Leiningers' Sunrise Model (Wheel of Culture)

Source: Lippincott Williams & Wilkins Instructor's Resource CD-ROM to Accompany Psychiatric Nursing: Contemporary Practice, Third Edition, by Mary Ann Boyd and Diane Schweisguth. (2005)

Conceptual Framework

Leininger's Transcultural Nursing Theory (Leininger, 1995) provides the foundation for understanding the importance of cultural competence in health care. The legitimacy of transcultural nursing comes from the right and expectation of all people to have their cultural values, beliefs, and needs met by nurses.

In transcultural nursing, culture is viewed as an integral and essential aspect of the person, and cultural care must recognize the need for respect and acknowledgement of the wholeness of human beings, regardless of culture, race, ethnicity, heritage, or religion (Leininger, 1995). Cultural care values that patients are greatly influenced by kinship, language, and environment. Nurses must try to fully understand and accept differences in cultural care values to provide culturally competent nursing care that reasonably fits with the patient's cultural needs, values, and worldview (Leininger, 1995). This type of nursing practice contributes to the well-being of individuals and family members within their environmental context.

Providing culturally competent nursing care not only contributes to better health outcomes but helps facilitate communication and develop a strong patient-nurse relationship. According to Leininger (1995), culturally congruent and competent nursing care is a practice by which nurses become responsive and sensitive to the practices, beliefs, emotions, values, and problems faced by patients belonging to a different culture, as Figure 10-1 depicts. Without cultural competence, patients may exhibit signs of stress, cultural conflict, noncompliance, and misunderstanding between themselves and healthcare providers.

Culturally competent care is frequently defined as behaviors, attitudes, and policies that support a negotiated process of appropriately caring for people across languages and cultures (Cross, Bazron, Dennis, & Isaacs, 1989). This does not mean healthcare providers must have significant knowledge of all cultural groups, but they must be willing to listen to and learn from members of diverse cultures and to provide services based on knowledge of their patients' culture and language (Won, Krajicek, & Lee, 2004). Because perspectives may differ by race and ethnicity, culturally competent care should be based on patients' perspectives, not on some set criteria. Nurses have an important role in delivering culturally appropriate care, especially in acute care settings where intense bedside care is sometimes provided for days. Recognizing and understanding the issues surrounding culturally incompetent care related to health disparities and poor health outcomes in minority populations can have a significant impact on safety and care quality.

The following case study describes a specific example of a failure to focus on the person and family, and the resulting damage. The purpose of this family-focused case analysis is to provide a comprehensive overview of the effect of cultural competence on minority health outcomes by examining the case of a young, female Korean American immigrant admitted to an acute care setting and to make recommendations for safe nursing care by incorporating cultural care.

CASE STUDY: *A Family's Story*

By Young-Me Lee PhD, RN and Hyemin Lee BSN, RN

J. L. was the daughter of a Korean immigrant family. Her parents immigrated to Chicago in 1982. They had two daughters who were born in the United States. J. L. was the first daughter, and when her illness occurred, she was attending college and close to graduation. Previously, J. L. was diagnosed with a brain tumor when she was 11 years old. J. L. underwent brain surgery and received radiation and chemotherapy afterward. The surgery and other treatments were successful, and the cancer was eradicated. But the treatment left her with brain damage and pituitary dysfunction, including diabetes insipidus. She was prescribed desmopressin (DDAVP) and was advised to drink adequate amounts of water daily to control the hypernatremia. J. L. had a good recovery, adjusting well to school and managing her medical condition. Over time, she regained her health and performed well in school.

During the years after surgery, J. L. was also diagnosed with diabetes mellitus and hypothyroidism. Four years after her surgery, she changed her primary doctor to a Korean doctor who specialized in endocrinology. During her teens, J. L. maintained her health with her parents' help. She was majoring in special education and hoping to become a teacher. Her parents owned a dry cleaning business, which they had for more than 20 years. The business was a good source of income, and J. L.'s family was financially stable. J. L.'s sister had just entered college in Boston with a four-year scholarship. J. L.'s family was happy until J. L.'s health crisis happened.

J. L. went to the hospital with severe vomiting and diarrhea. Her parents took her to the nearest emergency department (ED) as her condition was worsening. Since J. L.'s parents knew that dehydration could lead to a critical problem for her, they tried to tell the ED nurse that she was a high-risk patient, but the nurse's response was that J. L. had to wait her turn. The nurse did not look up J. L.'s record. Finally, after four hours of waiting, J. L. was seen by the doctor. She received intravenous (IV) fluid administration, and lab work was done. Her parents were relieved. J. L.'s heart rate was a little low, so she was admitted to a telemetry floor to be closely monitored. Her primary doctor was notified, and she was admitted under his care.

On the telemetry unit, J. L.'s sodium level was closely monitored, and she continued to receive IV fluids. The next morning, her parents saw an improvement in her condition. The doctor thought that food poisoning was the cause of the crisis. Her sodium level was down to her baseline, and she slowly tolerated a clear liquid diet. They restarted her medications, including DDAVP. After seeing the improvement in J. L., her parents left for work. J. L. was transferred to a general medical floor, as her condition was stable and she no longer required telemetry monitoring.

J. L.'s parents went to see her after they finished work around 7 p.m. J. L. said she had been eating well and felt like she was ready to go home. But around 11 p.m., she started having some lower abdominal pain. Her parents noticed her abdomen was distended and called the primary nurse to assess her. The nurse assessed J. L. and seemed perplexed. J. L.'s father asked the nurse to call the doctor, but the nurse left the room and did not return for an hour. J. L.'s parents started to get worried and called the nurse again. The nurse told them that she had paged the doctor, but the doctor was not responding to the page.

J. L.'s dad started to get frustrated and insisted that the nurse call the doctor again. The nurse appeared to be getting annoyed with him. He returned to J. L.'s room and waited for an order from the doctor. Her parents suspected that J. L. was probably overloaded with fluids this time. Finally, the nurse returned after talking with the doctor. The doctor told the nurse to monitor J. L.'s condition and said that he would see J. L. early in the morning. The parents were frustrated with the doctor's actions. They tried to explain that

J. L. needed something done immediately to fix her sodium imbalance. The nurse replied that she could not do anything without a doctor's order. It was hard for J. L.'s parents to fully express their concerns and thoughts in English. They tried hard to convince the nurses to do something but were unable to do so. They were frustrated and felt powerless that they could not do anything for their daughter.

Toward dawn, J. L.'s parents noticed a change in her mental status. She seemed lethargic and less responsive. They called the nurse to come immediately. The nurse assessed her patient's vital signs and said they were stable, so she decided to continue to monitor. J. L.'s father could not understand why they were not taking any action to help his daughter. He tried to argue with the nursing staff, but the nurse did not seem to understand or be concerned about J. L. He did not want to deal with the nurses anymore. Their responses were all the same, blaming the doctors for not taking any action. J. L.'s father insisted that the nurse call the doctor right away. The nurses said that they had called the doctor, but again there was no response or action. There was nothing J. L.'s parents could do except wait for the doctor. They felt powerless, hopeless, and very angry about the senseless response of the medical staff.

The primary doctor showed up around 7 a.m. J. L.'s parents were glad that he was there. First, the doctor shook J. L. hard and called out her name. J. L. moaned in response. The doctor told her parents that she was conscious and they did not need to worry so much. They were relieved, even though they were angry about what had happened overnight. The doctor left orders to place a urinary catheter, stop the IV fluids, hold the DDAVP, and obtain a nephrology service consultation. Later that morning, J. L.'s parents found out that her blood sodium level was extremely low. They were very concerned since J. L. had never had a low sodium level before. Her father requested that the nurses perform blood sodium levels more frequently, but the nurse said that they could not do that due to the floor policy. The parents did not understand how the floor could have a policy that prohibited addressing patient care needs. As ordered, the IV fluid infusion was stopped and the urinary catheter was inserted. When the catheter was inserted, over a liter of urine was removed. J. L.'s father went to work after watching the orders being carried out, while J. L.'s mother remained at the hospital. Slowly, J. L.'s condition began to improve. She became more alert and awake. Her father stopped by the hospital after work and saw that she had improved. He then went home to sleep.

Around 10 p.m., J. L. started became more irritable. She complained about the urinary catheter, saying that it was uncomfortable and felt like it was leaking. Her mother assured her that it was not leaking and her skin was dry. But J. L. was becoming more agitated and stated that she wanted the catheter taken out. Her mother called the nurse and asked if the catheter could be removed. At first, the nurse convinced J. L. to keep the catheter in until the morning. But later, J. L. stated that she still wanted it taken out, and the nurse responded in a cold voice that if the catheter came out, J. L. would have to walk to the bathroom on her own and she would not help J. L. with the bedpan. J. L. answered that she would walk to the bathroom if she could have the catheter removed. The nurse returned to the room to remove the catheter after about an hour. J. L.'s mother thought that the nurse had to phone the doctor before removing the catheter. The catheter was finally removed, but unfortunately doing so did not relieve J. L.'s discomfort. She still complained about feeling uncomfortable. J. L.'s mother kept reassuring her and tried to calm her down. The nurse offered a pain medication to J. L., and she received morphine intravenously. She fell asleep after a morphine injection around 2 a.m.

At 4 a.m., J. L.'s father came to the hospital. He noticed that J. L. was lethargic again and barely arousable. He immediately called the nurse for help. J. L.'s father told the nurse that J. L. needed DDAVP. He thought that her sodium was going up this time. The nurse said that lab draws would be done soon, so he should wait. He yelled, "I cannot wait anymore! Call the doctor. I'll talk to him." He could not let the same thing happen to J. L. again. The nurses finally paged the doctor for him. J. L.'s father went back to the room to assess her, but she still looked lethargic and was not responding to his voice and shaking. Thirty minutes passed before the doctor returned the page. J. L.'s father was getting aggravated by the slow callbacks from the doctor, so he went back out to the nursing station and called the nurse again. This time, the nurse told him to wait in the room without even listening to him. The time was almost 6 a.m.,

CASE STUDY: *A Family's Story* *(continued)*

and J. L.'s father still had not received a call back from the doctor. J. L.'s parents were desperately waiting for the doctor, who usually made rounds early in the morning. But that day, the doctor was not coming in early. It was almost 7 a.m. J. L.'s father could not stand waiting anymore and asked for the head nurse to come assess his daughter. The head nurse went to see J. L. and seemed to sense that something was wrong with J. L.'s condition. She paged the house doctor to come see J. L. The house doctor responded in 10 minutes. He assessed J. L. and reviewed her chart. Meanwhile, J. L.'s primary doctor showed up and took over her care. J. L.'s father begged the primary doctor to do something so that his daughter could get better. The doctor said he would take care of it and left the room. Until 8 a.m., there were no interventions other than the blood draw at 7 a.m. J. L.'s parents called the nurse again to ask what the doctor had ordered for J. L. The nurse said that the doctor just ordered levothyroxine medication for her hypothyroidism. J. L.'s parents felt hopeless at that point. They were devastated and did not know where to turn for help.

At 8 a.m., J. L. was found to be unresponsive and not breathing. The rapid response team (RRT) was activated. She was intubated and transferred to the intensive care unit (ICU). J. L.'s parents were asked to stand aside when the emergency teams were in the room. Her parents were shocked, and her mother almost fainted. They were speechless and felt helpless. All they could do was follow J. L. to the ICU.

In the ICU, J. L.'s parents had no idea how bad her condition was because nobody was there to explain what was going on. They just wanted the medical team to bring their daughter back to normal. The team was busy oxygenating her and giving her medications. After the situation became more settled, the ICU nurses told J. L.'s parents that she needed to be monitored more closely. Soon after, they found out from the lab results that her sodium level was too high, which was exactly what J. L.'s father had thought was the problem. He could not that believe his daughter's condition had become critical. The sodium level was closely monitored in ICU and was slowly decreasing. J. L.'s father tracked the sodium level as it decreased. J. L.'s parents thought that she would be back to normal once the sodium level got corrected, but when that happened, she still did not wake up.

After two days in the ICU, the doctors told J. L.'s parents that she needed a tracheostomy and tube feeding placement, which they hoped would be temporary. J. L.'s father stayed with her in the ICU. He thought that the staff disliked him for staying there. He slept on a chair in the small ICU room to watch his daughter. He could not leave her alone there because he felt that he could not trust anyone in the hospital. J. L. stayed in the ICU for three weeks.

One day, the primary doctor asked J. L.'s parents to come to a family meeting. They were scared about what the doctors were going to say. They called their other family members to come with them to the meeting for support. At the meeting, they were told that J. L.'s condition was in a chronic state. The neurologist said that J. L. had severe brain damage from the imbalanced sodium level. They diagnosed her with cerebral myelinolysis. They told the family that they had done everything that they could do, but they could not save her. J. L.'s family was in shock; her parents had still been somewhat hopeful. It was the first time they had heard from the doctors that her condition was irreversible. J. L. was transferred back to the general medical floor and was discharged home. J. L.'s parents could not send J. L. to the suggested skilled nursing facility because they felt it looked unclean and unsafe, so they decided to care for her at home. Her father learned everything he had to know to care for J. L. and became her 24-hour caregiver since she was still in a vegetative state. A year later, the family was engaged in a lawsuit with the hospital due to the poor care they feel J. L. received.

1. What factors contributed to the poor outcome in J. L.'s case?

2. What can nurses do to help to prevent an event like J. L.'s from happening?

Cultural Conflicts between Family and Healthcare Teams

In the preceding case study, J. L. and her family's experience in a different culture presented the healthcare team with the challenge of identifying cultural barriers. When the cultural barriers were not recognized and addressed in the acute care setting, poor outcomes resulted. J. L. and her parents did not have much experience with the healthcare system, other than when J. L. was hospitalized for a brain tumor during her childhood. Therefore, they were lacking the information they needed about the current hospital system. First, they did not understand the different care levels of each department within the hospital and had only a general idea relating to the severity of conditions. For example, J. L.'s parent sensed that J. L.'s condition was improving and that was why she was being transferred to a different department, but they thought the same kind of care would be continued. Their expectations of care were the same on the general medical unit as the telemetry unit. When the parents' request for frequent sodium blood levels were denied by the nurse on the general medical unit, they did not understand why the nurses could not draw blood as requested and felt frustrated because they felt it was important for J. L. Second, J. L.'s parents were lacking information about resources available to them, such as family support services that hospitals have for any kind of issues or concerns that the family may face in the hospital. They could have utilized services such as having a patient representation or a social worker to help resolve their issues with the hospital care. Third, they did not know that a translation service was available for them. Since J. L. was fluent in English, communication was not a problem in the beginning of the hospitalization. But as her condition declined, the language translation service was essential for appropriate communication with her parents.

Language Barriers

A nursing intervention early in J. L.'s hospitalization could have solved the language barrier issue. A translator or a family advocate from their cultural group could have ensured that all the medical information was communicated and that the family was satisfied with the care. The language barrier was one of the leading causes of stress and frustration for J. L.'s parents while J. L. was in the hospital. Her parents had difficulty delivering the message that they were trying to tell the nurses in English, especially when J. L.'s condition was acutely changing. They were sensitive to changes related to her sodium level and alerted the nurses immediately whenever an acute change was noted. Since they had dealt with J. L.'s hypernatremia for a long time, they quickly knew when changes were occurring. They knew that J. L.'s sodium level was abnormal. The message that J. L.'s father was trying to tell the nurse was not delivered effectively because of the language barrier. If J. L.'s father had been fluent in English, he could have convinced the nurses of his knowledge of his daughter's condition, and perhaps the nurse could have taken action immediately. The nurses did not correlate J. L.'s condition with the sodium level as her parents did. A translation service was essential for J. L.'s parents to understand what was happening.

Lack of Communication Skills

The communication between J. L.'s parents and the medical staff was ineffective, but not only because of language barriers. J. L.'s parents did not receive prompt responses from the nurses and doctors. There was a long period of time spent waiting for the each response from the medical team. The nursing staff did not obtain translators or assure the family that they were going to resolve the issues. Clear communication between J. L.'s parents and nurses did not exist. In the end, J. L.'s parents felt hopeless and powerless. This situation also led to anger and mistrust directed toward the nursing staff.

Cultural assessment, including the ability of patient and family to communicate with healthcare providers, is a priority in care planning. The nurses should have more comprehensively assessed the situation.

Lack of Assurance and Advocacy

While a nurse should advocate for patients and families, J. L.'s parents felt isolated while J. L. was in the hospital. They felt powerless about not being able to do anything while they watched their daughter's condition decline. They reported that the nurses did not carefully listen to their opinions and concerns. After J. L. ended up in the ICU, her parents' anger and blame toward the insensitive and inconsiderate nurses grew, and they felt they could not trust any of the nurses. J. L.'s parents expressed great anger toward the nurses who were not carefully handling their daughter.

Cultural Insensitivity

The nurses and doctors from this case study displayed cultural insensitivity. J. L. and her family's values and cultural beliefs were not appropriately assessed and therefore, their needs were not fulfilled. Providing a translation service should have been a basic part of providing culturally competent care, but it was not provided for J. L.'s parents. The hospital staff did not acknowledge the hardships or difficulties that an immigrant minority family could have when they come to the hospital. The nurses should have sensed that J. L.'s parents needed assurance when they were anxious about her condition. As J. L.'s parents were very involved with J. L.'s care, the nurses could have involved them in her care instead of telling them to step out of the room. The nurses were task oriented instead of caring for the needs of the family. The relationship between the nurses and J. L.'s parents was not positive as opposed to the trusting relationship that should have developed.

As Yang (2002, 2008) notes, the main characteristic of "Koreanness" can be described as familism, which is a unique social characteristic that highly emphasizes family cohesion, interdependence, and kinship. Koreans are expected to sacrifice their individual needs for the sake of family interests (Jung & You, 2001). If the family had been assessed in depth, the nurses would have discovered how much the parents were involved in J. L.'s life. These tight family relationships, or familism, of Korean culture were not well understood by the nurses. J. L.'s parents may have appeared overly sensitive or too involved with their child's care to the nurses. In a culturally competent setting, familial beliefs and practices would have been valued and not dismissed.

Culturally incompetent health care can change the life of not just the person but also the entire family. It is important for all healthcare providers to realize the issues underlying culturally competent health care and come together as a team to achieve the goal of cultural competence.

Transition and Community

Encounters with healthcare providers during illness or hospitalization can dramatically change the lives of patients and families. Once patients are discharged, they may face significant barriers to maintaining their health. The new functioning level of patients may limit their ability to get groceries or obtain medications from the pharmacy. Even the functioning of others in the home may be affected. The following case study about Penny and Chris exemplifies a situation in which the person and family had a distinct need that would lead to poor health in the family if not addressed.

Coordination and Planning

Several European countries have postnatal visits for new families that focus on the maternal-child bond and the multiple factors that assist with normal growth and development. Proper nutrition and stimulation of the infant are key to long-term health. The reciprocal interaction between parents

CASE STUDY: *Penny and Chris*

Penny and her partner, Chris, were ready to go home with their three-day-old newborn. When Chris came to pick up Penny and the baby with their four-year-old son, Cody, Penny began to cry uncontrollably. Chris was distraught and asked Penny why she was so sad. They always wanted two children, a girl and a boy, and now their little baby Ruby had been born healthy and everything was coming together. Their dreams were coming true. Chris told Penny to get dressed and that they would all grab a milkshake on the way home. Chris said, "We'll all feel better after a chocolate milkshake, right?"

The nurse came to discharge Penny and Ruby, and asked if everything was okay. Chris said, "We are all really happy. No problems." And the nurse gave Penny her books and new mother diaper bag. They left the hospital for home with no follow-up appointment and no material about how Penny could take care of herself or her sadness.

1. What family-centered care strategy could help Penny and her sadness?

2. Did the nurse intervene appropriately?

3. What could be the cause of Penny's crying, and what diagnosis would need intervention?

Evidence for Best Practice: Person-Centered Care and Safety

How does person-centered care affect safety or perceived quality of care? When persons are involved in their care, safety improves. For example, before administering a medication, the nurse should show the medication to the patient and ask whether the patient has taken the medication in the past. If family members are present and wish to be involved in routine care, they should be included in discussions and teaching. Nurses should take the opportunity to find out about the home and community that the person will be returning to and any health concerns or safety issues there. The need for visiting nurses or other care in the home should also be assessed (DiGioia, 2010).

Wolf, Lehman, Quilin, and Zullo (2008) conducted a clinical randomized study (posttest design) and examined whether patient-centered care (PCC) impacted patient satisfaction, perception of nursing care, and quality of care. Differences were seen in two of three subscales within the Baker and Taylor Measurement Scale. The PCC group rated satisfaction and quality of services higher than controls. PCC may impact patients' perception of the level of satisfaction and quality of care received. A well-educated patient provides a strong defense against errors (Hunter, 2011). For example, educating patients on the barcode system for medications as well as the armband barcode can only decrease the safety risk.

and infant is pivotal in the health promotion and long-term development of the child. The parent-child bond needs to be nurtured to make sure that the whole family is functioning at the optimal level. If postpartum depression is ignored and not treated, the family unit can become less functional and ultimately very unhealthy. In the preceding case study, an awareness of postpartum depression signs and the benefit of early treatment of such depression should have been stressed. Follow-up with primary care providers who are aware of signs of depression would have helped to ensure optimal health.

When a patient with a complex condition is being cared for in a hospital, the coordination or discharge may take many days or weeks. For example, a patient in cardiac rehabilitation will need to work up slowly to exercise again, and dietary and medication changes may need to be taught and mastered before discharge. When there are multiple stressors or cultural or family complexities, coordinating and planning for home care become much more challenging. The primary goal for coordination of care is an individualized plan for the patient and family.

Importance of Family-Centered Care

Family-centered care (FCC) is relatively new (Shields, 2008). The Institute for Family-Centered Care (2012) defines it as:

> An approach to the planning, delivery, and evaluation of health care that is grounded in mutually beneficial partnerships among health care providers, patients, and families. . . . Patient- and family-centered practitioners recognize the vital role that families play in ensuring the health and well-being of infants, children, adolescents, and family members of all ages.

Kyler (2008) outlined FCC as a ". . . purposeful inclusion of multiple stakeholders in the decision-making process and is often fraught with concern and controversy. When to include and who to include in the decision-making process is not clear" (p. 101).

Shields (2008) outlined the elements of FCC as proposed by the Institute for Family-Centered Care:

- Recognizing the family as a constant in the child's or patient's life
- Facilitating parent-professional collaboration at all levels of health care
- Honoring the racial, ethnic, cultural, and socioeconomic diversity of families
- Recognizing family strengths and individuality, and respecting different methods of coping
- Sharing complete and unbiased information with families on a continuous basis
- Encouraging and facilitating family-to-family support and networking
- Responding to child and family developmental needs as part of healthcare practices
- Adopting policies and practices that provide families with emotional and financial support
- Designing health care that is flexible, culturally competent, and responsive to family needs

All elements of FCC need to be part of nursing care philosophy and should be integrated with every person and family encounter. When such integration is present, outcomes will most likely improve.

CHAPTER HIGHLIGHTS

- Person- and family-centered care should be integrated into every nursing assessment and intervention.
- Culture is a key component of person- and family-centered care.
- Nurses who integrate the culture and family into patient care will be more likely to provide safe and effective nursing care.

Pearson Nursing Student Resources

Find additional review materials at
nursing.pearsonhighered.com
Prepare for success with additional NCLEX®-style practice
questions, interactive assignments and activities, web links,
animations and videos, and more!

REFERENCES

Cross, T. L., Bazron, B. J., Dennis, K.W., & Isaacs, M. R. (1989). *Towards a culturally competent system of care: A monograph on effective services for minority children who are severely emotionally disturbed.* Washington, DC: CASSP Technical Assistance Center, Georgetown University Child Development Center.

DiGioia, A. (2010). A patient-centered model to improve metrics without cost increase: Viewing all care through the eyes of patients and families. *Journal of Nursing Administration, 40*(12), 540.

Gerteis, M., Edgeman-Levitan, S., Daley, J., & Delbanco, T. (Eds.). (2002). *Through the patient's eyes: Understanding and promoting patient-centered care.* San Francisco: Jossey-Bass.

Hunter, K. (2011). Implementation of an electronic medication administration record and bedside verification system. *Online Journal of Nursing Informatics (OJNI) 15*(2). Retrieved from http://ojni.org/issues/?p=672.

Institute for Family-Centered Care. (2012). *Patient- and family-centered care.* Retrieved from http://www.ipfcc.org/pdf/CoreConcepts.pdf

Institute of Medicine (IOM). (2002). *Unequal treatment: Understanding racial and ethnic disparities in health care.* Washington, DC: National Academies Press.

Jung, H., & You, K. (2001). *Ga-jock-gwan-gay (family relations).* Seoul, Korea: Hack-gee-sa.

Kyler, P. L. (2008). Patient-centered and family-centered care: Refinement of the concepts. *Occupational Therapy in Mental Health 24*(2), 100–120.

Leininger, M. M. (1995). *Transcultural nursing: Concepts, theories and practices.* New York: McGraw-Hill.

Leininger, M. M., & McFarland, M. R. (2002). *Transcultural nursing: Concepts, theories and practices.* New York: McGraw-Hill.

McCormack, B., Dewing. J., & McCance, T., (2011). Developing person-centred care: Addressing contextual challenges through practice development. *The Online Journal of Issues in Nursing*, (16)2, Manuscript 3. doi: 10.3912/OJIN.Vol16No02Man03

NRC Picker. (2011). *Eight dimensions of PCC.* Retrieved from http://www.nrcpicker.com/member-services/eight-dimensions-of-pcc/

Parse, R. R. (1998). *The human becoming school of thought: A perspective for nurses and other health professionals.* Thousand Oaks, CA: Sage.

Passel, J. S., & Cohn, D. (2008). US population projections: 2005–2050. Washington, DC: Pew Research Center.

Picker Institute. (2012). *Principles of patient-centered care.* Retrieved from http://pickerinstitute.org/about/picker-principles/

Ponte, P. R., Reid, P., Conlin, G., Conway, J. B., Grant, S., Medeiros, C., et al. (2003). Making patient-centered care come alive: Achieving full integration of the patient's perspective. *Journal of Nursing Administration, 33*(2), 82–90.

Shaller, D. (2007). *Patient-centered care: What does it take?* Picker Institute. Retrieved from www.pickerinstitute.org.

Shields, L. (2008). Questioning family-centered care. *Journal of Clinical Nursing 19*, 2629–2638.

Sullivan Commission. (2004). *Missing persons: Minorities in the health professions: A report of the Sullivan Commission on diversity in the healthcare workforce.* Retrieved from www.sullivancommission.org.

Wolf, D., Lehman, L., Quinlin, R., & Zullo, T. (2008). Effect of patient-centered care on patient satisfaction and quality of care. *Journal of Nursing Care Quality 23*(4), 316–321.

Won, J., Krajicek, M., & Lee, H. (2004). Culturally and linguistically competent care of a Korean-American child with autism. *Illness, Crisis & Loss, 12*(2), 139–154.

Yang, S. (2002). *Korean-American mothers' meanings of academic success and their experiences with children in American schools.* Unpublished doctoral dissertation, University of Minnesota.

Yang, S. (2008). A mixed methods study on the needs of Korean families in the intensive care Unit. *Australian Journal of Advanced Nursing 25*(4), 79–86.

QUALITY HEALTH CARE, POLICY, AND ETHICS

Kim Siarkowski Amer

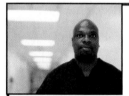

Blend Images /
Shutterstock.com

Kevin was on the night shift on the postsurgical unit with two new graduates and Nancy, his supervisor. Kevin was assigned two patients who had returned from surgery earlier in the day. Orders for morphine administered intravenously every four hours if needed had been prescribed for both patients. Every four hours, Kevin went through the procedure of drawing up the doses of morphine from the vial, while Nancy checked the medication and dosage. Each time, Nancy insisted that Kevin give her the vial with the remaining morphine. At first, Kevin did not think anything was unusual. Then Kevin noticed that every time they had remaining morphine, Nancy went into the bathroom after placing the vial in her tunic pocket. He was struck with a sick feeling in his stomach. Was his supervisor saving up the morphine? Or even worse, was she using it while she was at work? Kevin felt a panic because he had never learned about this possibility in nursing school. What would happen if Kevin reported Nancy? What were his rights—and Nancy's?

CORE COMPETENCY

Apply ethical and legal frameworks to nursing's role in quality improvement in health care.

LEARNING OUTCOMES

1. Describe policy examples that have emerged to make quality improvement more attainable.
2. Provide examples of legislation passed to improve the safety of patient care.

3. Examine ethical dilemmas that nurses face when observing unsafe care practices.

A culture of safety in health care needs structure founded on research and consistent policy. The culture must value ethical practices and open communication focused on the best patient outcomes. Recently, the profession of nursing has focused attention on increasing awareness of safety concerns in health care. Many new healthcare-focused safety programs, laws, policies, and initiatives have been designed and implemented. The process of putting policies and laws into action in a timely manner can be challenging. Changes proposed by policy and ethics committees can take months to years before the changes are implemented within the institution. This chapter will describe some of the ethical, legal, and policy issues that continue to challenge patient safety and the overall healthcare system. Even though many initiatives are presently in place, there is much more to do to ensure that they are used and monitored. Efforts are also needed to track outcomes and evaluate efficacy.

This chapter focuses on select political policy, legal action, and technological advancements motivated by injustices, stressors, and safety. Ethical issues will be addressed, from public policy suggestions to practical steps for establishing quality and safety in the healthcare setting. While this book has outlined many safety risks, models of change, transitions to practice, empowerment issues, and patient-centered care models, all initiatives and issues are undergirded by the notion that there must be major structural, philosophical, and behavioral changes made to address these challenges.

While nurses across the globe face different career challenges, this chapter will present issues most pressing to nurses in the United States today. Due to the ever-evolving nature of health care, nursing will see new challenges in the future. The steps needed for nurses are awareness of issues, acting on policy need, and disseminating knowledge about the healthcare improvement. Patients should be able to count on receiving care that is safe, meets their needs, and meets standards that apply across the United States.

Current Events in Quality and Ethics

One example of nursing awareness and action is related to collective bargaining and the right to strike. The largest strike in nursing history to date took place in Minnesota in June, 2010, with 12,000 nurses picketing for an environment of safety. The nurses were seeking patient-to-nurse ratios that safely put patient care first (Gomstyb, 2010). The Minnesota Nurses Association is one of many nursing unions in the United States, the largest of which is in the state of California. In many states, union-represented healthcare systems require that each nurse be a union member. Nursing unions remain controversial, and as in any profession, union membership presents both benefits and disadvantages. However, in terms of quality, nursing unions can mandate workers' pay, safe staffing ratios, and level of education needed for nursing practice. In December 2009 the National Nurses United became the largest registered nursing union and professional association in an attempt to create a single nursing standard nationwide. Nursing standards may be implemented with the help of a union; however, unions alone will not be able keep nurses politically aware or act in their place to design policy.

Quality and safety are also being redefined in other areas of health care. Awareness of high rates of central line infections motivated Peter Pronovost, an intensive care specialist at Johns Hopkins Hospital in Baltimore, Maryland, to design a checklist of five simple tasks that are credited for saving 1,500 lives and $100 million in the state of Michigan over an 18-month test period in 2010. Pronovost's checklist protocol before central venous catheter insertion includes the following simple steps:

1. Washing hands with soap before inserting a central line

2. Cleaning the patient's skin

3. Using sterile drapes

4. Utilizing sterile kits

5. Inserting in the direction away from the groin area, which is harder to clean

These simple steps or standard protocols are often overlooked by medical professionals, who tend to dislike being monitored or micromanaged, skip steps to save time, or do not give adequate importance to such simple steps (Provonost, 2010).

These protocols are not novel or ingenious ideas. Adequate staffing, cleanliness, and a place to set materials are foundations of safe nursing practice. Implementing these key concepts with each patient can make the difference between life or death. Another simple yet crucial aspect of quality and safety, as illustrated in the opening scenario, is reporting wrongdoing within the healthcare setting. Whistleblowing, that is, reporting a colleague for disciplinary action, is an important issue facing nurses today and is addressed later in this chapter.

The Ideal Practice Environment: High Reliability Organizations

The best safety practices in all organizations, not just in health care, can be found in high reliability organizations (HROs). These organizations have a sustained safety record in the face of complex and challenging environments. Henriksen, Dayton, Keyes, Corayon, and Hughes (2008) describe the characteristics that workers should have when working in HROs such as health care, aviation, and nuclear power plants. These workers should have mindfulness that includes a set of cognitive processes that allows the worker to be aware of the potential for mistakes and the ability to prevent such mistakes. Workers in HROs are qualitatively different than workers who are not part of HROs because they are mindful of different things than workers in less reliable organizations.

Evidence for Best Practices: Do Rapid Response Teams Really Help?

Failure to rescue is the clinician's inability to save a patient who has had complications of hospitalization or surgery. Often the event can be traced back to a clinician who is not experienced enough to recognize serious signs of demise. When rapid response teams (RRTs) are in place in clinical sites, outcomes are much different. Nurses who were hesitant to call codes for fear of upsetting the physician are now encouraged to call the RRT to evaluate the situation. Failure to rescue is not intended to be a negligence accusation; rather, it is intended to draw attention to the potential for prevention of death in future similar circumstances (Garretson, Rauzi, Mesiter, & Schuster, 2006). Thomas, VanOven Force, Rasmussen, Dodd, and Whildin (2007) identified that 91% of all nurses who observe a patient's status changing for the worse felt that calling the RRT helped prevent a cardiac arrest. There was also a trend toward better interdisciplinary communication and collaboration. RRTs have reduced the incidence of cardiac arrest outside the intensive care unit (ICU) by 50% (Buist et al., 2002). Thus RRTs offer many benefits, including better patient outcomes as well as better staff communication and positive attitudes.

There are five mindfulness processes that help nurses and other workers in HROs prevent errors (Henriksen et al., 2008):

1. Preoccupation with failure, or always being aware of the risks
2. Reluctance to simplify interpretations, or always seeking out more information and following hunches or intuition if there is a sense that something is not correct
3. Sensitivity to operations, or seeing the big picture of the whole patient and procedure
4. Commitment to resilience, or responding to errors that include easy solutions such as putting emergency equipment closer to the patient
5. Deference to expertise, or utilizing a frontline person who can assist when unexpected events occur

An example of the last process is the use of rapid response teams to prevent failure to rescue situations. (See Evidence for Best Practices box.)

The best quality care can be accomplished when nurses design their own best practice situations. The safety components of nursing integrate select elements that will help nurses focus on designing, implementing, and following up on quality outcomes. The goals of nurses should include these safety components:

- Safe staffing
- Safe work environments that include 15-minute off-unit breaks every two to four hours and at least one 30-minute off-unit break during the shift
- Shared governance models of leadership that include all nurses in decision making

- Care provision that always follows the standard of care with evidence-based interventions

- Technology innovation that increases the time nurses spend with patients

Some technology innovations that increase the time nurses spend with patients and decrease non–nursing task time include:

- Bar coding for safer medication administration

- Robotic technology to help with non-nurse duties

- Electronic health records (EHRs) for easily accessible patient data

- Personal digital assistant (PDA) devices, pagers, or cell phones that allow nurses to access resources and information more quickly

Even in an ideal environment, there will never be zero mistakes. The human factor will be present, providing both benefits to patients and potential risks. Human factors research is described in the Agency for Healthcare Research and Quality (AHRQ) publication by Henrickson and colleagues (2008). This research applies "knowledge about human strengths and limitations to the design of interactive systems of people, equipment, and their environment to ensure their effectiveness, safety, and ease of use" (Henrickson et al., 2008, p. 51). In other words, the tasks that nurses perform, the technology they use, the work environment in which they function, and the organizational policies that shape their activities may or may not be a good fit for the nurse's individual strengths and limitations. When these system factors and the sensory, behavioral, and cognitive characteristics of care providers are poorly matched, substandard outcomes frequently occur. Areas that may be affected include effort expended, quality of care, job satisfaction, and perhaps most importantly, the safety of patients. Fortunately, if a position is not a good fit for a nurse, other options exist. There are many healthcare institutions with a variety of roles for nursing professionals. Schools, churches, community centers, health clubs, and clinics are just a few of the multitude of career environments from which a nurse can choose.

Whistleblowing

Although nursing is rated the "most ethical" profession according to the Gallup Poll News Service, whistleblowing is still necessary in today's healthcare environment. Whistleblowing is an attempt by a member or former member of an organization to issue a warning about a serious wrongdoing or danger (Martin, 1999). There are many situations in which whistleblowing occurs, but at its core, the practice involves advocacy for those who have been or may be harmed. Nurses are responsible for advocating for their patients, and healthcare policy should protect them when they do (Lachman, 2008).

Perspectives on Whistleblowing

There are many arguments for whistleblowing. It is ethical, responsible, and part of the nurse's inherent role. It enhances patient care and encourages responsibility. Whistleblowing can include such practices as submitting incident reports and reporting verbally to managers when something happens in a healthcare setting that endangers a patient. Examples of whistleblowing occurences include reporting unethical colleagues, healthcare fraud, or failure to adhere to policy. Reporting misconduct is morally required in nursing in particular and the healthcare field in general, where nurses are trained in accountability, ethics, and virtue theory. Human nature defines right and wrong within individual preferences and socially accepted norms. Virtue theory requires each individual to exemplify integrity and courage based on their own definitions. Nurses, by nature of their training, demonstrate loyalty and courage in providing relief to suffering patients. Ignoring practices that go against that goal would be a violation of the nursing Code of Ethics (Lachman, 2008).

Arguments against reporting misconduct claim that it encourages dissension in the workplace, threatens patient confidentiality, raises healthcare costs, or is unnecessary. Some see whistleblowing as a "form of dissent resulting in public disclosure of perceived wrongdoing by members of one's own organization" (Martin, 1999, p.17). It may inhibit trust and loyalty among employees of healthcare institutions and cause everyone to "look over their shoulder."

Because nurses are already required by law to report abuse, some think that additional whistleblowing laws are unnecessary. Statute and common law require, for example, nurses to report any suspected child abuse or a patient's intent to harm others. Because reporting these abuses is mandatory by law, protection and support for nurses reporting other issues, like understaffing, is sometimes viewed as a lesser concern.

Legislation currently varies from state to state regarding whistleblower protection. In New Jersey, for example, nurses are protected when reporting any action defined as a "common act of misconduct," such as diversion of drugs, providing medical care under the influence of alcohol, or stealing personal property. Yet nurses in some states (e.g., Minnesota) have no legal protection when they report these occurrences. Because of variation in the state legislation, nurses should be aware of policy changes and must stay up to date and educated on the laws in the state in which they work. Although 20 states in the United States currently have whistleblower protection, many nurses still fear termination and discrimination in the workplace.

Nurses should hold one another accountable for ethical behavior that follows standards of care and hospital policy. Such conduct is inherent in the nurse's role as caregiver but should be protected nationwide. There is a need for consistency and standard protocol, and the federal government must enact legislation to ensure whistleblowing is allowed. Federal law must change to define misconduct worth reporting and lay out protocols for both reporting misconduct and protecting whistleblowers. These protocols should include mechanisms for handling complaints, procedures for disclosure, guarantee of anonymity, guarantee of prompt investigation of any report, and protection for employees making the report. In addition to federal law protecting whistleblowers, effective internal structures within healthcare settings are necessary to minimize the need for whistleblowing. When nurses have protocols regarding how and when to voice a concern, they are more comfortable reporting misconduct. But they must have job security so that fear does not interfere with safety. Once a nurse draws attention to a concern, there must be a protocol for the way the concern is addressed and investigated. Nurses should have a supportive work environment so that issues can be solved from the inside instead of going outside the organization through legal action or media attention (Lachman, 2008). Knowing the precise course of action that will be taken, and that it will occur every time, will encourage nurses to report wrongdoing when necessary.

Motivating Factors for Ethical Policy Implementation

Nurses have a unique vantagepoint within the healthcare community because they help patients navigate complex systems with many providers. By nature of their training and responsibilities, nurses witness interactions between staff, patients, and doctors; coordinate care; and advocate for families. This perspective makes them ideal monitors of the healthcare field. They must be able to report their experiences with a system in place that hears and protects them. Guidelines such as those in New Jersey are necessary nationwide so that nurses can in fact know what actions are reportable and how to address them.

Many recommendations have emerged from this exploration of whistleblowing. Nurses should continue to be educated in ethics and encouraged by their preceptors and institutions to act morally. Nurses who are involved in whistleblowing should have the right to be protected from discrimination and victimization (Martin, 1999). Federal guidelines should be put in place to establish protocols for whistleblowing practice and requirements such as paperwork, verbal report procedure, time constraints, and consistent hospital response across the nation.

Reciprocity and Nursing Practice Policy

At this writing, a nurse's ability to practice in multiple states is limited. Varying requirements can make it challenging for an individual to obtain licensure in multiple states even though the testing to become a registered nurse (RN) is the same for everyone. Legislation to standardize the licensure of RNs in the United States would eliminate this problem. The movement of RNs from state to state is a quality and safety issue because discipline and standard of care can be compromised when nurses are held to many differing standards. Thus, reciprocity across states remains an issue of safety in need of attention.

The Nurse Licensure Compact (NLC) is a first step toward a nationwide nursing standard. It authorizes a nurse licensed and residing in a compact state (home state) to practice in other compact (remote) states without obtaining additional licensure. The NLC facilitates nursing practice among the compact states by requiring the nurse to maintain active licensure in only the nurse's "primary state of residence," and granting "multi-state privilege" to practice in other compact states. This privilege requires that the nurse practice according to the laws and regulations of the state in which he or she is practicing.

Nancy Spector of the National Council of State Boards of Nursing spoke about the importance of the NLC at the fifty-eighth annual National Student Nurses Association conference in April 2010. She identified it as a key issue for nurses today related to their licensure and the current NLC. The benefits of NLC encompass the growing need for nursing practice to occur across state lines, the growth of the settings and/or technologies nationwide that create a need to work across state lines, consumers' growing need to have access to nurses across state lines, the need for efficient and expedient authorization to practice, and the ability to incorporate more uniformity in laws across practice modalities in the nursing discipline.

Although standardized nursing licensure nationwide is a sound and practical ideal, the reality is that nurses in the United States are not currently practicing in this matter. The states outside the NLC maintain their own standards for nursing licensure. To keep nursing quality consistent and to hold nurses accountable to one standard of education and safety, a nationwide licensure program must exist. Nursing reciprocity will be effective only when nurses can easily move from state to state and be fully licensed as RNs, regardless of location.

Nursing Roles and Quality

An increasing population of nurses are advanced practice registered nurses. As these nursing professionals practice in a broader scope and with greater autonomy, they increase patients' access to cost-effective, comprehensive, and high quality care in a patient- and community-centered environment. In addition, patient-centered, community-centered care coordination models that include nurse practitioner provider options have proven to be a cost-effective and efficient means of improving health outcomes. Nurse practitioners should be fully recognized and utilized as healthcare providers in leading coordinated care models.

Ethical board membership is another relatively new role for nursing, one in which it is essential for nurses to be involved. Ethical boards are structured for the benefit of patients and families and to ensure interdisciplinary communication. The role of the ethics board is to discuss all aspects of complex genetics cases or cases where the treatment decsions are complicated. For example, if a baby needs a risky experimental heart surgery and the parents disagree on the treatment plan, the ethics board could meet and make a recommendation to help diffuse the situation. Every ethics board should have a least one nurse included along with the social workers, ethicists, physicians, hospital administrators, lay community representatives, and select family members when applicable. Ethical dilemas are present every day in patient care situations, and nurses need to examine their own ethical framework and focus on the best responses for both the patient and the healthcare team.

Awareness of Patients' Rights

Both the Patient Care Partnership adopted by the American Hospital Association (AHA) (www.aha.org), and the Declaration of Human Rights (www.un.org/ed/documents/udhr) are excellent examples of legal and ethical standards for treatment of all patients. The Patient Care Partnership, which replaced the Patients' Bill of Rights in 2006, focuses on the close relationship of patients and healthcare providers, and the patient's rights to a high quality hospital care environment, involvement in the patient's own care, protection of the patient's privacy, help when leaving the hospital, and help with billing issues. The United Nations' Universal Declaration of Human Rights is published in hundreds of languages and is more global in scope than the Patient Care Partnership. The declaration is a reminder that respect and dignity should be afforded to everyone, including prisoners, illegal citizens, and those who are poor or without health insurance. The rights include the right to have a name; be free of torture; receive fair treatment under the law regardless of race, color, sex, language, social, or national origin; and pursue life, liberty, and security of person. Nurses need to be aware of this document to ensure that it is honored.

The most powerful instrument nurses can use to ensure ethical behavior and respectful care delivery is their own practice. The nurse should model care that is dignified and holistic with a clear desire for excellent quality outcomes. This practice, when observed, influences all nurses from supervisors to students and can also influence other healthcare providers. To develop such nurses, we must foster excellent clinical instructors and ensure the best clinical and classroom experiences to develop ethical nurses.

Agency for Healthcare Research and Quality (AHRQ): Policy and Ethics in Action

In 2008, the federal AHRQ published a comprehensive 1,300-page volume entitled *Patient Safety and Quality: An Evidence-Based Handbook for Nurses*. One of its most influential chapters provides a conceptual framework for using evidence-based practices in nursing. This framework integrates dissemination of knowledge generated by AHRQ to generate and encourage activities that include knowledge transfer in clinical settings and nursing schools, social marketing, behavior change, and social innovation to help keep patients safe. The primary focus areas, as mentioned earlier in this book, are person-focused care and interdisciplinary collaboration. The volume is currently available online and is an invaluable source of administrative and clinical strategies for safe and effective healthcare delivery.

Nurses at all levels need to be more involved in policy and ethical research, with a clinical focus on safety, wellness, and health promotion strategies. This will yield significant improvements in healthcare outcomes nationwide and produce long-term cost savings that can be reinvested into achieving a healthier population. Transparent reporting of clinical measures and health outcomes by all providers gives the public important information upon which to evaluate the safety, quality, and cost of healthcare services and helps build an evidence base to inform processes of care and identify opportunities for improvement.

Challenging Times for Nurses Today

Nursing is a career that offers hard-working, creative, and critical thinkers an opportunity to better the lives of patients in healthcare settings. As patient advocates and professionals, nurses serve through compassionate, genuine care; patience; and curiosity. Research, new techniques, and technology make nursing a desirable career that must not lose its personal element and commitment to quality and safety. An integral part of nursing is the responsibility to remain educated on current issues and events that shape the nursing world. By voicing concerns, practicing safely, and working in an ethical manner, nurses have the opportunity to advance a dynamic and unique field of care and advocacy.

Nurses are the largest group of healthcare providers and the profession that society trusts the most. The moral and ethical frameworks that nurses practice from are rooted in doing the best for the patient and family, and honoring patients' autonomy. The most important part of patient care is mutual respect among all healthcare providers. To ensure safety and continued improvement of safe care delivery, nurses need to also embrace veracity, or the obligation to tell the truth when a mistake is made. If mistakes are addressed immediately, the likelihood of a better outcome is higher and the threat of litigation against a nurse or healthcare institution decreases (Kelly, 2007). With increased numbers of nurses holding advanced degrees, including the doctorate of nursing practice (DNP), more policy and ethics positions should be created in healthcare settings along with more nursing faculty positions. The higher profile of nurse scholars should help shape policy and law.

CHAPTER HIGHLIGHTS

- The ethical legal issues facing nurses today are complex and require competencies in safety, quality, and a strong ethical framework for practice.

- Whistleblowing is a challenging issue for nurses since they are faced with exposing colleagues' wrongdoing.

- Nurses have many opportunities for career growth and development; however, the lack of reciprocity between states can impede nurses from relocation and expanding practice options.

- Ideal practice sites are rich in resources for nurses, and encourage independent thought and mindful practice.

Pearson Nursing Student Resources

Find additional review materials at
nursing.pearsonhighered.com

Prepare for success with additional NCLEX®-style practice questions, interactive assignments and activities, web links, animations and videos, and more!

REFERENCES

American Hospital Association. (2012). The patient care partnership: Understanding expectations, rights and responsibilities. Retrieved from http://www.aha.org/advocacy-issues/communicatingpts/pt-care-partnership.shtml

Buist, M. D., Moore, G. M., Bernard, S. A., Waxman, B. P., Anderson, J. A., Nguyen, T. V. (2002). Effects of a medical emergency team on reduction of incidence of and mortality from unexpected cardiac arrests in hospital: Preliminary study. <http://www.bmj.com/content/324/7334/387.short> BMJ 2002; 324 doi: 10.1136/bmj.324.7334.387 (Published 16 February 2002)

Gomstyb, A. (2010). Thousands of nurses strike in Minnesota. ABC News Unit. Retrieved from http://abcnews.go.com.

Garretson, S., Rauzi, M., Mesiter, J., & Schuster, J. (2006). Rapid response teams: a proactive strategy for improving patient care. *Nursing Standard* 21(9), 35–40.

Henriksen, K., Dayton, E., Keyes, M. A., Carayon, P., & Hughes, R. (2008). Understanding adverse events: a human factors framework. In *Patient safety and quality: An evidence-based handbook for nurses*. Rockville, MD: Agency for Healthcare Reaseach and Quality. *volume 1*, p. 5.1–5.19.

Kelly, P. (2007). *Nursing leadership and management* (3rd ed.). Clifton Park, NY:Delmar Cengage Learning.

Lachman, V. D. (2008). Whistle-blowers: troublemakers or virtuous nurses? when is a Whisleblower morally required to tell? *Dermatology Nursing* 20(5), 390–393.

Martin, B. (1999). Whistleblowing and nonviolence. *Peace and Change, 24*(3), 15–28.

Provonost, P. (2010) Checklists alone won't change healthcare.

Huffpost. Retrieved from www.huffingtonpost.com/peter_provonost.

Thomas, K., VanOven Force, M., Rasmussen, D., Dodd, D., &

United Nations. *The universal declaration of human rights*. Drafted in 1948. Retrieved from http://www.un.org/en/documents/udhr/.

FUTURE-FOCUSED QUALITY NURSING

Bernadette Curry

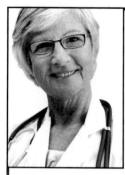

Source: Yuri Arcurs /
Shutterstock.com

Jennifer is an experienced nurse executive, responsible for the operation of the nursing division of a large urban hospital. She holds quality as a priority over financial cost and is concerned about patient outcomes and professional performance. She routinely attends leadership conferences and has developed a network of peers. Though outcomes and performance rank high at her hospital according to recognized standards, she looks beyond current day processes and strives for continual improvement. To that end, she engages a quality care consultant and initiates an institutional assessment that involves all personnel. The assessment purpose emphasizes the ongoing journey for quality to achieve improved patient outcomes and increased professional performance and satisfaction.

Since all personnel are involved, a team mentality evolves, and new and varied perspectives are brought forth in practical strategies. The focus is placed on the future and innovation. The motto is "How can we do this better?" Education plays a paramount role.

Recent studies are acknowledged, and Jennifer seeks additional funding from foundations to increase the number of nurses who the hospital subsidizes for baccalaureate and advanced degrees. In addition, alliances with academic institutions are formed to enhance educational opportunities. Employees are sent to conferences, especially those that feature research and development. The premise is that advanced education will breed advanced ideas and processes, and precipitate vision for the future.

Emerging technologies are assessed and incorporated to enhance point of care situations as well as communication and administrative processes. Leadership retreats are held for key personnel, as are management seminars to develop specific skill sets among clinical nurses promoted to managerial positions. An interdisciplinary view is adopted to embrace, respect, and implement valuable concepts. A formal mentoring program is designed and implemented to have a future focus. Nurses are selected to sit on marketing and planning committees to present a more accurate image of the nurse's role to the community at large.

The concern of one nurse executive is responsible for the domino effect of ideas and actions regarding quality and facing the challenges of the future with preparation, innovation, and commitment.

CORE COMPETENCY

Develop quality-focused insight into the profession of nursing guided by evidence-based research to function effectively in the evolving healthcare environments.

LEARNING OUTCOMES

1. Explore attributes of leaders who promote change and motivate colleagues to advance vision and expertise.

2. Describe the need for nurses to participate in change and the benefits from interprofessional and technological endeavors.

3. Describe possible professional career goals that exhibit advancement in expertise and position.

4. Describe the importance of engaging in professional activities, organizations, and scholarly efforts to increase the body of knowledge and address policy via research, publication, and presentation.

The future is now, the vision for tomorrow begins today, and quality is the byword. The nursing profession today is involved in a quest for quality, and there is no substitute for excellence when one is involved in the well-being of an individual. These tenets are vital and emphasize the necessity of forethought regarding a wide scope of knowledge and competencies, accompanied by a global perspective.

Characteristics of the future-focused nurse center around scholarship, dedication, and autonomy. The future-focused mindset promotes inquiry, diligence, motivation, and commitment. Nursing must go far beyond competence. Practice must reflect expertise, the full extent of passion for the profession, and commitment to quality.

The quest for quality in health care is a profound priority. The profession of nursing has been evolving at an increasingly rapid pace, and quality has been an integral aspect of the evolution. It is imperative to bear in mind that nurses are responsible for the vast majority of direct care. They are truly on the front line of the provision of care and arc heavily invested in quality. With continual advances, the road to quality has become more complex. Technological developments and the information explosion have created a synergistic effect, and a plethora of information can be available at the touch of a computer key. The increasing focus on quality will intensify as technological and biomedical advances evolve. The challenge for nurses is to analyze and synthesize information effectively in order to use it to its full potential in the context of quality.

Communication: Messages for the Future

Communication is the conduit for concepts, thoughts, and the expression of emotions. It is the "exchange of messages and the creation of meaning" (Andrews & Boyle, 2008, p. 20). It is the pathway for directives, an essential element in society and an imperative in healthcare. Effective communication propels the delivery of quality care and infuses compassion into the process. Effective communication is holistic and addresses all aspects of care for the patient, and it encompasses the varied disciplines of health care. The importance of communication cannot be overestimated. The quality of communication feeds directly into the quality of care. Communication has always been at the core of nursing. It remains in that vital place, yet there are additional considerations now and for the future.

Communication has been enhanced and advanced by technological developments. This has created both a blessing and a challenge for nursing. New computerized systems and devices require orientation and time for assimilation. Once healthcare providers have mastered the technology, communication can be more rapid, widespread, and permanent. However, there are two cautions: (1) Technology depends on accurate data entry and programming, and (2) technology will continue to change and advance. Ongoing education becomes essential to quality care. In addition, the healthcare team is expanding; it incorporates more disciplines and individuals involved with the patient and increases the sphere of communication.

It is important to remember that the patient is at the heart of the communication complex. In spite of the most recent technological devices, it is quality patient–nurse interaction that leads to quality care. As technology advances and assists members of the healthcare team, the nurse–patient interaction becomes imperative. Though the interaction may be occurring via technical devices, the basic principles of communication must apply. Communication is a reciprocal activity in which a sender and receiver are involved. Each must be clear about the message in order to be effective.

The art of listening should not be underestimated. Although attention often focuses on the speaker and minimizes the role of the listener, listening is a talent that must be cultivated and plays a formidable role. Nurses must be attentive and insightful listeners to accurately assess and address patient situations and to be active, valuable participants of the healthcare team. It is in the moments of listening that one can learn; learn from peers, learn from patients. The information explosion coupled with steadily advancing technology calls for nurses to be diligent listeners and learners. The growing plethora of technological systems and devices applicable to health care can facilitate the speed and documentation of information; however, at times, it can eliminate or minimize visual interaction with the patient. That visual image, in person or electronically, provides a wealth of information to the nurse. Likewise, audible interaction relays not only content of the exchange but demonstrates affective components as well. Nonverbal and paraverbal aspects can add significantly to communication and confirm or question congruence of the verbal message. When information is delivered electronically in a visual word-based format, it is important to

be "listening with your eyes." Electronic devices have been found to assist in conveying thoughts; however, the emotional component of the communication does not transfer readily (Dickerson, Stone, Pachura, & Usiak
2007). The nurse must be attentive to the tone of the written message and
draw on strong assessment skills and a formidable base of knowledge.

Globalization and Health Care

Globalization has influenced healthcare delivery and will continue to affect communication in health care. Increasing numbers of cultures are
entering the healthcare system as patients and as professionals. It is incumbent for healthcare providers to be prepared to address health needs
with an understanding of and a respect for culture. Cross-cultural communication calls for more than mere translation of words. It goes far beyond
the ability to speak the language. It requires understanding of the values
and the nuances of the culture, and the context of the communication.
Effective interaction demonstrates an awareness of the varied perspectives, including those related to formality, gender, eye contact, touch, and
silence. Silence is an interesting aspect of communication that spans a
broad range of meanings across cultures.

Cross-cultural interactions may fail to convey a patient's true sense of
trust. Kosoko-Lasoki, Cook, and O'Brien (2009) note that patients are more
trusting of those with whom they share race, ethnicity, and gender. Trust is
also an essential ingredient in cross-cultural professional interactions. That
trust is built when the nurse exhibits a sensitivity to the patient's cultural
background and beliefs with an emphasis equal to the nurse's scientific
knowledge of the patient's disease and diagnostic data. The nursing profession in the United States comprises approximately 80% Caucasian men and
women and 20% Hispanic, African American, Native American, Pacific Is-
lander, Asian, and other ethnicities (American Association of Colleges of
Nursing, 2011). Yet as a profession, nurses are expected to care for all patients with cultural competence and understanding. Incorporation of varied
cultures into the profession will expand perspectives of all the professionals
on the healthcare team and position communication to be effective and contribute to quality care.

Technology and Health Care

Peer professional communication is a core element of effective health
care. For centuries, spoken and handwritten words have transported
thoughts that have alleviated pain, consoled, motivated, and promoted
quality care that contributed to quality of life. Today, similar words, both
spoken and written, often are conveyed via an electronic mode. The contemporary nurse must be adept with current and evolving communication technology. Many changes have occurred since the time when nurses
wrote notes with printed letters, and the only cursive writing was used
for a signature. The current mode of documentation is often via computer
keyboard, and many providers use dictation and translation programs
for documentation. The keyboard may be a component of a variety of

CASE STUDY: *PDA Use*

A study funded in part by Transforming Care at the Bedside (TCAB) was initiated in 2004 at Molloy College in Rockville, New York, to examine the use of personal digital assistants (PDAs) by graduate and undergraduate nursing students. The purpose of the project was to explore lines of communication and access to and use of valid resources. Twenty-eight students participated over a six-week period. Four faculty, who supervised the students in their respective clinical areas, also participated. Students were provided with a PDA that contained several applications appropriate to their respective academic level, graduate or undergraduate. Throughout the study, each student entered into a journal information regarding date, nature of inquiry, and perceived value of site accessed. Students were encouraged to explore sites and databases to access new and varied information. Emphasis was placed on determining the validity and value of the sites.

Students were enthusiastic during the project. Three students, two graduate and one undergraduate, reported a slight degree of anxiety related to lack of familiarity with electronic devices. Students were assessed by a self-reporting survey for technology competency and associated level of confidence. At the conclusion of the six-week period, feedback was positive, surveys and journals were analyzed, and students met in groups (graduate and undergraduate) with the principal investigator. Several students asked to continue using the PDA through the remainder of the semester. Students reported that the preloaded applications were helpful and assisted in both clinical and theory aspects of courses. Several students reported that in the clinical setting, personnel asked them to search for information and viewed them as a reliable resource. Faculty reported similar instances and reported the PDA to be beneficial for communication. Students stated the PDA was a valuable resource and should be required of all students. Seven stated they would buy one even if not required. Students reported frequent sharing of sites and related information among one another. Results indicated PDA use was beneficial to access and expansion of information as reported by the participating students. The process facilitated the acquisition, utilization, and dissemination of information.

computerized systems including laptops and handheld devices. In addition to acute care settings, electronic devices assist peer communication and patient care documentation in the many venues of continuing care such as home care, clinics, and assisted living environments. Healthcare situations where the patient is not in direct and constant proximity to the provider have benefitted from implementation of electronic communication. Nurses must be open to change and innovation, and prepared for the continuing evolution of technology.

Sharing Information

Nurses will need to continue to address change and evolution of the profession in the many nursing journals. Sharing developments with other nurses advances the profession and contributes to quality outcomes. There is a distinct need for nurses to publish in journals for the public at large in addition to scholarly journals. All too often, the scholarly endeavors of nurses are not seen by the public. It is important to disseminate information throughout the profession; however, nursing should not "preach only to the choir."

Nurses must have an awareness of, and appreciation for, the public media as well as the professional media. Health is a popular and bona fide topic of concern, and nurses can contribute their knowledge and expertise to journalistic operations. Likewise, there is opportunity to represent the profession as consultants to films, television, and other media in order to convey an accurate image to the public. Members of the profession should be future-focused and proactive, seeking out opportunities to communicate the expertise and value of nursing.

There are numerous occasions when nurses are called on to interact spontaneously with public or professional media. Contemporary nurses must be prepared to respond skillfully and accurately. The context of a formidable response can be lost in a brief "sound bite" on the six o'clock news. These situations call for forethought and interprofessional communication to be prepared for such situations. These principles apply today, and they must be integrated into the evolution of health care.

Healthcare communication operates on a platform of accuracy, importance, and urgency. The interactions, whether in person or electronically, must convey the essential elements of the message. The exchange must be conducted with exacting professional terminology and demeanor to address the situation with the deserved dignity and importance. This mode of communication can be contrary to current social electronic communication, which often is casual and rife with symbols and abbreviations that can lead to confusion and miscommunication. There is no room for miscommunication in health care. The contemporary nurse must be attuned to the varied forms of communication, open to both human and electronic nuances, and act as guardian of the accuracy of the message to ensure safety.

Collaboration: Working Together Into the Future

Communication serves as a vehicle for collaboration and is the conduit for team activities. Collaboration builds on communication. It places value on all participants and recognizes the unique perspective each person brings to the team. There is no hierarchy in true collaboration. However, the diverse talents and expertise of the members allow for individuals to take the lead at various points in evolving situations. Members frequently negotiate for roles and responsibilities. The dynamics of collaboration foster creativity and motivation, and bring a sense of energy to the project. There is a synergistic effect that can be construed as $1 + 1 = 3$. This synergy means that two people thinking together may be more effective than two people working in isolation ($1 + 1 = 2$ in isolation versus $1 + 1 = 3$ when working together). Participants encourage, support, and challenge one another as they formulate and work toward a common goal.

Boxer and Goldfarb (2011) emphasize the importance of involving others and note benefits such as enhanced perspectives and investment in the work. However, collaboration can also introduce the challenge of competition, as Rossen, Bartlett, and Herrick (2008, p. 390) note when they state, "American norms value competition rather than consensus." It is that challenge that can propel the activities of the team.

The nature of the work of nursing has already created teams within the profession that are categorized according to specialty areas (e.g., maternal-child, pediatrics, critical care). These intrainstitutional teams, however, do not necessarily focus on collaboration. Their focus is instead on communication of treatment plans, scheduling of patients, or covering patient care. The logistics are centered on team building or ongoing education.

When the concept of collaboration is introduced as the focus, group dynamics can be accelerated and elevated. Finkelman (2012) notes how collaboration can bring about an increase in interaction and a coordination of team efforts and potential outcomes. Collaboration can also promote job satisfaction and a sense of professional growth for the healthcare provider. In addition, institutions may benefit from providing the structure for interprofessional collaboration, as that type of environment promotes creativity and coordination (D'Amour & Oandasan, 2006). Collaboration is a significant opportunity for nurses to bring their strengths and creativity to the table. Nurses who are concerned about high-quality health care in the future need to initiate same-specialty teams comprised of members from varied institutions. Formation of these teams can expand networking and result in an exchange of best nursing practices and research potential, which are essential elements to the formation of future health care. The huddles described in Chapter 8 and developed through the TCAB project are an example of collaborative teams that can have a significant impact.

When nurses take part in interprofessional endeavors, exchanges with the varied personnel of healthcare teams promote a holistic approach to quality and safety, and broaden the perspective of all involved. This team approach can generate a new point of view, a different level of understanding, and respect for individuals. A collaborative team has the potential to support a comprehensive perspective that allows it to address healthcare quality and patient safety through the broadest possible lens. Interprofessional collaboration, along with effective communication, is cited by Ierardi as being "crucial to patient safety" (2010, p. 33). In 2002, an Institute of Medicine (IOM) report noted the importance of the disciplines' ability to interact collaboratively for patient benefit. The American Nurses Association (American Nurses Association, 2012) cites collaboration as a standard for the profession.

Collaboration is not limited to an institution, community, organization, region, or country. All spheres of health care operate in a global community and must interface with the challenges and assets of the world. Pearson notes that "nations and cultures are more alike than they are different. . . . Collaboration increases the scale of a research exercise, shares the work across nations and professions, and accelerates the production of knowledge" (Pearson, 2007, p.69). Interaction with colleagues in other countries can contribute significantly to the growing body of knowledge and processes, and increase perspectives that pave the way for future endeavors.

Triple Aim Health Care Goals

The Institute for Healthcare Improvement (IHI) has developed three goals, called the Triple Aim, for healthcare institutions that are partnering with them to target. Since 2007, more than 50 organizations and institutions have participated in the program with reported success. The goals of the Triple Aim are to improve the experience of receiving health care through a broader view of aiming to improve population health and reducing the per capita cost of health care. The three parts of the Triple Aim are (Berwick, Nolan, & Whittington, 2008):

1. Improve the care experience.

2. Improve the health of populations.

3. Decrease the per capita cost of health care.

These goals can be accomplished only if there is universal access to care and organizational willingness to accomplish them. The best way to achieve them is to have a philosophy that values partnering with patients and families, provides accessible preventative health care for all persons, and employs educated healthcare providers who know about population health and can manage the broader health system policy and cost issues. The structure of the Triple Aim focus can be used in all countries.

Collaboration During Education

The ideal time for instituting the process of thinking and functioning collaboratively should not be after a nurse is hired but before, during basic nursing education (Benner, Sutphen, Leonard, & Day, 2010). To date, nursing education has isolated students into compartments with little or no interaction with other members of the healthcare team. This void was emphasized by Pamela Thompson, CEO of the American Organization of Nurse Executives, in an address at a nursing leadership conference of the North Shore–Long Island Jewish Health System (Thompson & Stanowski, 2009). She noted the extremely low numbers of new nurses who had experienced a conversation with a physician as a student. Elements of collaboration need to be part of nursing education with ample opportunity for cognitive and practical experience for students. Brown, White, and Leibbrandt (2006) refer to collaborative activities between educational and clinical sectors of nursing as the "cornerstone of successful clinical experience for nursing students" (p. 170).

The shared vision and diverse expertise of the collaborative team can forge a strong bond and an informed determination to address issues at hand. These same characteristics can forecast future implications and encourage teamwork on a proactive basis. The group dynamics can serve as an impetus for both current and future action, and be instrumental in laying the groundwork for policy. The collaborative team can also be a mechanism to acquire funding for various projects. Varied backgrounds and networks can increase the sphere of inquiry and access, and possibilities for success. Criteria for funding opportunities often require that more than one discipline be involved in the endeavor. The value of collaboration is recognized as an effective method to optimize potential. It is an essential element of the professional nurse's mindset.

Continuous Quality Improvement: Methods for Today and Tomorrow

High-quality health care should be available at all times, for all patients, in all institutions and agencies. Quality is an evolving concept. It is not a finite goal but rather an ongoing process that is subject to the changing needs of society and the knowledge, expertise, and creativity of the healthcare team and the scientific community. In theory, quality is expected to improve continuously and requires vigilant efforts by many. The importance of continuity is demonstrated in the Continuous Quality Improvement (CQI) process, also referred to as Total Quality Management (TQM), first instituted in the business field by W. Edward Deming. It is a philosophy that asserts increasing quality, proactivity, employee empowerment, and continuous improvement. The process "trusts the employees to be knowledgeable, accountable, responsible, and provides education and training for all employees at all levels" (Marquis & Huston, 2009, p. 548). Though the CQI/TQM concept began as a business model for industry, it has been applied in a variety of venues, and Deming's 14 management principles have been the hallmark for quality processes and success for decades.

The approach Deming designed has been used in conjunction with the CQI philosophy in healthcare organizations and has effected the desired transformation. Known as PDCA (plan, do, check, and act), its primary themes include embracing a philosophy and purpose to improve a product continuously (in the case of nursing and health care, the product is safe nursing care) and provide a reward or a gain for improvement of care as illustrated in Figure 12-1. Once a process resulting in safe nursing care is established, it should continue to be reevaluated and reassessed. Teamwork and investment in the team members' individual goals also need to be integrated into the process (Deming, 1986).

The PDCA approach to CQI combines seemingly simplistic principles with practical applications that can guide multiple situations. The efficacy of PDCA in an acute care setting, specifically nephrology, was cited by Williams and Fallone (2008) to demonstrate how CQI can influence the practice environment. CQI provides a format for improvement applicable to all aspects of health care. Baker and Newland (2008) recounted the

FOCUS–PDCA

Find a process to improve, such as medication administration.

Organize a team that knows the process, such as an interdisciplinary team of nurses, pharmacists, physicians, and social workers.

Clarify current procedures and how to do the process.

Understand causes of process changes that affect safety.

Select the safety and quality process improvement.

Plan – Do – Check – Act

Source: Adapted from Yoder-Wise, P. S., & Kowolski, K. (2006). *Beyond leading and managing: Nursing administration for the future.* St. Louis, MO: Mosby/Elsevier.

Figure 12-1 FOCUS–PDCA

benefits of CQI implementation related to cardiopulmonary bypass, and the role of electronic data collection and statistical control charts.

The CQI process is geared toward achieving quality and then analyzing, evaluating, and modifying. There can be efforts to reduce variation and achieve error-free performance. Robbins (2005) notes that a 99.9% error-free performance may seem extremely successful. However, he points out, that level of functioning by the U.S. Postal Service would bring about a loss of 2,000 pieces of mail per hour. The goals of the CQI process are usually high, and when projects focus on patients, the importance and motivation of the endeavor increase significantly. McLaughlin and Kaluzny (2004) refer to CQI as a "structured organizational process for involving personnel in planning and executing a continuous flow of improvements to provide quality healthcare that meets or exceeds expectations" (p. 3).

In the delivery of daily care, nurses routinely assess the outcomes of treatment regimens and are in an ideal position to implement CQI. They should enter clinical practice with knowledge of and exposure to CQI philosophy and strategies. Nursing education can use CQI to introduce students to the CQI process. Doing so can demonstrate CQI in action, emphasizing the importance of utilizing information and processes from other disciplines and the value of interdisciplinary interaction. Kyrkjebo (2006) designed and conducted a program to teach CQI in nursing schools in which she emphasized the need to connect theoretical and experiential learning as well as the importance of faculty and students participating in ongoing improvement activities. Incorporation of CQI into a community health nursing course at a Massachusetts college resulted in improved nursing curricula and improved collaboration between the academic institution and community agencies (Teeley et al., 2006). Integration of CQI

Evidence for Best Practices: Nursing and Financial Knowledge

Do nurses really need to have financial knowledge and skills? Nurses need to have an understanding of many levels of healthcare structure, function, and cost. Nurses are the largest group of healthcare providers. In most cases, they are paid based on hospital budgets and suffer cuts when budgets need to be decreased. Such models for nursing salaries can decrease the safety and quality of nursing care. Every nurse should recognize the link between staffing, care delivery, revenue, and costs (Sanford, 2011). Nurses should be able to track their patient outcomes and determine how to balance a unit budget. Most hospitals collect data that includes finance, information technology, utilization management, quality, medical records, and human resource records. Nurses should be able to use these resources to examine data being collected that influences patient outcomes, nurse staffing, and nursing salaries (Sanford, 2011; Nosek, Androwich, & Amer, 2011).

into undergraduate nursing education can prepare nurses to be acutely aware of the pursuit of quality, and to function proactively to initiate policies and practices as emerging needs occur.

Nurses must be ready, armed with knowledge and experience about the varied and effective processes in play, to be active participants on the healthcare team and to achieve quality care. Professional education is a life-long process and requires graduate nurses to engage in dialogue, literature, seminars, and conferences to convey and expand their perspectives. Contemporary nurses must be attuned to evolving plans and methods, and current and potential roles to address quality.

Healthcare Economics: The Price of Quality

The pursuit and achievement of quality health care costs time, effort, and money. Nurses must understand the economic status of health care and have an awareness of the economic macro environment. The economies of health care are colored by the events and demographics of society. Life occurs in a global community, and the economic well-being of a nation is often meshed with that of others. The health economy comprises a large part of the gross domestic product. Over 17% of the gross domestic product in the United States goes to the health sector (Folland, Goodman, & Stano, 2012). It is important for nurses to recognize the major influences on health care in order to be an advocate for quality.

In varied ways, nurses interface with fiscal issues and processes on a daily basis. Nurse leaders who have ultimate responsibility for an institution or a system rely on nurses at all levels to report and/or manage financial issues. Though the individual patient is a nurse's prime focus, that patient is accompanied by personal financial issues, institutional fiscal policies, and procedures related to care that must be considered.

Nursing has always promoted a holistic approach to patient care. Current economics may bring more intense focus on the financial aspect of care for both the patient and the institution. The nurse is positioned to provide input regarding the promotion and maintenance of quality care. Contemporary nurses must acquire a familiarity with fiscal terminology to develop insight into economic issues. As nurses advance on the career ladder and functions expand, budgetary responsibility is often included. Knowledge of the principles and language of fiscal planning and budgeting processes is essential for nurses. However, this knowledge is not innate, and steps must be taken to acquire the information and practical methods of applying it. Many schools of nursing are including basic information on healthcare economics in the curriculum, providing a foundation for those who choose to advance in that area.

Healthcare finance is not simply a matter of providing for the latest and greatest in equipment. It also requires knowledge of the most current and effective products and, most important, an understanding that for safe and quality patient care to occur, the most effective numbers of nurses with the most appropriate expertise should be allocated for a specific unit on a given day. Quality is the driving force in budget allocation. A budget is essentially a plan that forecasts expenditures and revenues. In health care, that plan is devised to support the needs of the patient and personnel. It all reverts to quality care for the patient.

In some institutions, nurses may be called on to serve on a budget committee, and it is important to recognize the opportunity for input that this provides. The committee may be composed of nurses only or include representation from all disciplines of an institution or system. To be active and contributing members, nurses should have a clear understanding of the financial processes. This type of membership can allow for creative planning for the future and the expression of vision and advocacy for quality. Committees often lead to networking and can include interaction with managerial personnel in the financial offices and on occasion the chief financial officer (CFO). This provides an opportunity for nurses to gain a balanced, nonclinical perspective, learn benchmark data related to operational performance, and interpret financial data and cost estimates (Thompson & Stanowski, 2009).

The chief nurse executive (CNE) of an institution, agency, or system often holds a master's degree in business administration (MBA), which prepares the nurse with financial and administrative knowledge and experience. The combination of clinical and administrative skills can lead to formidable insights and effective outcomes. These insights can help to foresee potential projects that increase quality of care and address patient safety. The CNE is often on an administrative level with the CFO, and the two usually interact on a regular basis. Much of the CNE's responsibility is related to the economic well-being of the entity. Current economic downturns have brought additional pressures to healthcare institutions. Nurse leaders are faced with increasingly difficult decisions and are challenged to be more creative than ever to address quality of care for patients and to provide a positive and supportive work environment for personnel. Collaborative and entrepreneurial activities are requisite (Henderson & Hassmiller, 2007), and nurse leaders must be willing and able to engage and to role model for all of nursing. Constituting a significant portion of the healthcare workforce, nursing should be energized as a profession to participate in activities to advance the quality of care in financially creative ways.

The importance of the financial aspects of nursing is confirmed by the existence of a journal entitled *Nursing Economics.* It—along with the *Wall Street Journal,* the *New York Times,* and the business pages of regional or local newspapers—should be required reading for nurses. As professionals, it is incumbent upon nurses to keep current on the economic status of the country and world, and the implications for health care. Health care may be considered a service industry; however, humanity is at the center, and quality is essential.

Leadership: Vision and Influence for the Future

Leadership in its simplest form is the the power to influence a person or group to achieve shared goals. Leadership is needed, sought after, and valued. Leaders are people who are focused on success of the endeavor at hand with the mindset of addressing and accomplishing the mission. It is about the "absence of ego, not its presence" (Porter-O'Grady & Malloch, 2007, p. 168). The leader shows concern for the work, rather than the self, and demonstrates a genuine sense of concern for the quality of the process and the quality of the outcome.

Variations in leadership function and characteristics abound. There are formal leaders who are in the role of holding a title, authority, and credentials. In any large organization, there are levels of leadership and skillful leaders who are responsible for operations and personnel. They are people of vision and talent, and are recognized in the role. However, informal leaders, that is, those who do not hold the formal title or authority of a leader, also have the ability to influence others and to contribute to a successful operation. Styles of leadership—autocratic, democratic, or laissez-faire—are practiced in accord with the nature and philosophy of the business. Most leaders will use a combination of approaches, depending on the situation. Naturally, each leader brings his or her own nuances to the situation.

Leadership Qualities and Characteristics

Leadership characteristics can be expanded to include a compendium of qualities and behaviors as illustrated in Table 12-1. They present a relatively complete picture of a leader and depict a person of action, with mind, body, and spirit in focused motion. Despite changing times and situations, many of the same qualities and behaviors required in the past surface as successful means to the desired end today. Traits such as self-motivation, creativity, self-confidence, and persistence may be the driving elements that propel an individual in the role of

TABLE 12-1 ■ Leadership Abilities for Success

Personal and Personality Strengths	Behaviors	Characteristics	Overall Descriptors
• Positive view • Perseverance • Ability to see other points of view • Ability to cope with stress of change and innovation • Team player with self-knowledge	• Strong critical-thinking and problem-solving skills • Creativity • Respect for individual differences • Clear communication • Good listening skills • Persistence • Focus on goals and outcomes • Ability to be flexible and change course	• High intelligence and skill level • Ability to accept criticism • High self-motivation; takes initiative • Willing to take risks • Self-confidence and assertiveness	• Fair-minded and wise • Brave and willing to explore options with all viewpoints considered • Poised and articulate • Loyal and dedicated • Insight into self and others • Well rounded

Adapted from: Catalano, J. T. (2003). *Nursing now! Today's issues, tomorrow's trends* (3rd ed.). Philadelphia: F. A. Davis.

leader (Catalano, 2003). However, some people have these traits but are not leaders.

Most discussions of leadership include the topic of vision. It can be described as an intangible of significant value. As Jonathan Swift wrote, "Vision is the ability to see things invisible." Vision brings foresight and sets the stage for proactivity. The leader with vision is acutely aware of the present and what needs to be done to address future needs. It is more than accommodation; it is seeing the possibilities and methods for advancement. In the rapidly changing world of health care, it is essential for nurses to develop and perfect their gift of vision to advance quality delivery of care. A leader's vision can chart a course that others may not see. It is that ability to project that sets the leader apart from others.

Passion, another attribute often connected with leaders, brings intensity to a project that can be palpable and infuse others with enthusiasm and motivation. "Attitude can be contagious," according to Yoder-Wise and Kowalski (2006, p. 132), and the leader can set the positive tone and expectations for success. Passion can ignite courage, the element that often brings a leader to the forefront of challenges. Crigger and Godfrey (2011) have identified courage as a fundamental virtue for nursing. Courage has many avenues, some more visible than others. Yet it is a constant thread in the fabric of effective leadership.

Courage can be manifested when a leader:

■ Operationalizes vision into reality

■ Takes reasonable risks

■ Is willing to be the lone voice

■ Serves as a staunch advocate for quality

Leadership is not simply having the courage to finish, but rather the courage to start. Follow-through is extremely important, but the intellectual and emotional strength to initiate paves the way for the opportunity to finish. A likely metaphor would be the marathon. The runner must have the vision, the passion, and the courage to stand at the start.

Specific attention to leadership in nursing is presented in a summary of chief nursing officer (CNO) leadership characteristics:

- Character
- Commitment
- Connectedness
- Compassion
- Confidence

Character is emphasized as a pivotal element, but all of these characteristics are integral to leadership. Nursing leaders such as Porter-O'Grady and Malloch (2003) speak to the importance of character.

Specific leadership behaviors of nurse leaders flow from a combination of the characteristics and the functions of the leadership role, as depicted in Table 12-2. These behaviors exhibit the many facets of the nurse leader role and the enormity of the responsibility. One important aspect is bringing out the best in people. This involves role modeling, mentoring, and empowerment. A good leader works to recognize and appoint leaders at varied levels, and to create a team of enthusiastic and competent people dedicated to the mission of the organization. That team capitalizes on the varied talents and experiences of its members. A prime example of that occurred when nurse leaders at select institutions formed and led teams in the TCAB project described in Chapter 8. The project brought thought, talent, and leaders to the surface and fostered a high-level exchange of ideas, innovation, and networking. As the project progressed, the team of chief nursing officers, directors of nursing, unit managers, and staff returned to their respective institutions as a cadre of newly empowered nurse leaders armed with enthusiasm and an extremely positive, proactive attitude toward quality. Their titles were varied, but their commitment and concern for quality care were similar.

Supporting staff to achieve their potential is important to the individual, the leader, and the institution. Wiseman and McKeown (2010) write about the benefits to all involved when leaders encourage and support employees, and accompanying methods. They also note how some leaders can stifle the creativity and talents of a team, potentially rendering the team useless and bringing stasis to the organization. Contrasting behaviors of leaders are presented as "multipliers" and "diminishers" and depict how a leader can potentiate or minimize a worker's ability and effectiveness. (See Table 12-3.)

TABLE 12-2 ■ A Summary of the Chief Nursing Officer's Leadership Behaviors

Behavior	Description	Example
Visioning	A guiding purpose or an overarching, compelling vision, in which the necessary people are enrolled	Wants the facility to become a Magnet hospital; talks among the directors and staff enthusiastically, pulling them into the vision of a Magnet hospital
Building trust	Being accountable, predictable, reliable, persistent, and an expert	Accepts ownership of results; demonstrates consistent and known behaviors; can be relied on to keep promises; does not give in when obstacles appear; demonstrates a set of skills
Empowering people	Bringing out the best; encouraging and promoting a positive mindset	Is publicly appreciative for specific efforts of the senior leadership group in solving some of the problems related to acquiring Magnet status
Coaching	Asking questions and leading the coached through a process of delivery	Establishes specific times for coaching and supports the coached in personal and professional growth
Getting results	Focusing on the outcomes	Focuses on determining the cause of falls and builds interventions to reduce falls
Acknowledging	Staff are acknowledged for who they are and what they do by making the acknowledgement person-to-person, specific, from the heart, appropriately timed, and public when possible	Comes to the unit (even with the chief executive officer [CEO]), brings treats or rewards, speaks to each staff nurse individually, and thanks him or her for the work done on the plan to decrease falls; knows at least one specific thing that each person did; speaks to each staff nurse as soon as the results are known, and does it publicly

Source: Yoder-Wise, P. S., & Kowolski, K. (2006). *Beyond leading and managing: Nursing administration for the future.* St. Louis: Mosby/Elsevier.

TABLE 12-3 ■ The Five Types of Multipliers and Diminishers in Leadership Style

Diminishers (Focus on Self or Ego)	Multipliers (Focus on Workers)
The Empire Builder	*The Talent Magnet*
Hoards resources and underutilizes talent	Attracts talented people and uses them to their highest potential
The Tyrant	*The Liberator*
Creates a tense environment that suppresses people's thinking and capabilities	Creates an intense environment that requires people's best thinking and work
The Know-It-All	*The Challenger*
Gives directives that demonstrate how much he or she knows	Defines an opportunity that causes people to stretch their thinking and behaviors
The Decision Maker	*The Debate Maker*
Makes centralized, abrupt decisions that confuse the organization	Drives sound decisions by cultivating rigorous debate among team members
The Micromanager	*The Investor*
Drives results through his or her personal involvement	Gives other people ownership of results and invests in their success

Source: Wiseman, L., & McKeown, G. (2010). Bringing out the best in your people. *Harvard Business Review,* May, 117–121.

Leadership and Change

Change is a constant challenge that leaders face. Though it may be uncomfortable for some, it is a natural and expected part of health care that has brought about many developments to alleviate pain, erase disease, and improve the quality of care. Nurses should be aware that they are the sources of new innovation, and since changes do not ask for permission, the opportunity never waits for readiness. They need to be ready to innovate at all times (Porter-O'Grady & Malloch, 2007).

Anticipating change is proactive as opposed to reactive. It can be extremely helpful to view change as an opportunity rather than an enemy. A positive mindset about change can color the discussions and actions related to the project and the attitudes of those involved. Leaders must be prepared to listen for the sounds of change (Porter-O'Grady & Malloch, 2007). Ideally, the leader will anticipate and be attuned to themes, messages, and undercurrents suggestive of change. Listening skills are vital to the flow and connotation of quality communication in a culture of safety in the midst of change. Developing a sense of the "temperature in the room" can incorporate previously unspoken thoughts and ideas and generate efforts in a productive direction.

The subject of change is closely aligned with the role of leader and research. At times, the need for change brings about research, and at other times, research demonstrates a need for change. In either scenario, the leader is involved and may be the driving force. An effective nurse leader is current with research related to heath care and aware of potential collaborations to execute studies. Leaders network with a variety of colleagues to lay foundations for funding of research projects, making the entrepreneurial skills of a leader a distinct advantage. Additionally advantageous is the direct participation of the leader in the research study. It brings a special level of expertise that combines clinical and administrative insights and offers a valuable perspective on the specific needs for research and how it may be implemented to influence the type and timing of the research.

Research often leads to policy development, and policy provides a direct link to quality care. Nurse leaders at all levels need to know, abide by, and revise the policies of an institution, which must be in accord with the professional policies as well as state and federal laws. In this time of healthcare reform in the United States, nurses have the opportunity for input into the developing policies. Though policy may be crafted upon a foundation of research, it is the active participation of professional nurses and nurse leaders that will enact policy. Mason, Leavitt, and Chaffe (2007) emphasize that nurse leaders are people of influence and are capable of and positioned for policy creation and change.

Though some people may be considered natural-born leaders, usually the mindset and skills of leadership are developed and nurtured over time. Nursing curricula have increased the emphasis on leadership and management, but there must be a formidable base of knowledge accompanied by experiential opportunities for it fully to take root. Leadership cannot be relegated to a course in the last semester of a program nor considered on-the-job training. Jones and Sackett (2009) propose a three-course approach initiated in the third year of a nursing undergraduate program to facilitate development of leadership behaviors and to promote assimilation of concepts and the acquisition of skills. New graduates can enter the workforce with more solid grounding in, and an appreciation for, the functions that address patient safety and quality care.

Successful leaders never stop learning (Maxwell, 2007). They are eager to learn, and even more eager to use the knowledge in pursuit of quality. Nursing education is an ongoing process that is recognized by effective leaders because they routinely engage in self-development and are responsible for supporting the professional development of others. It is not personal aggrandizement but rather developing the talents of the team and achieving the goal that is the focus of the leader. This premise of leadership has been succinctly stated and has served as a guidepost for leaders for more than a century. In 1859, Florence Nightingale wrote, "Let whoever is in charge keep this simple question in her head (not how can I always do this right thing myself, but) how can I provide for this right thing to always be done?" (p. 24).

Quality is a global goal in constant evolution, an ever-increasing standard that can be elusive. Society, nursing, and health care are in transition and in pursuit of quality of life and quality delivery of care. Contemporary society is besieged by challenges and advancements. Socioeconomic events have challenged both patients and the healthcare system. Even the most positive advancements bring change and the need for education and adaptation. Future-focused nurses must be mindful of the successes and complications of today to address the issue of quality as complexity increases. The signposts for the challenges of tomorrow already exist.

Future Trends

Ten trends that will impact the future of nursing have been cited and explored for solutions (Heller, Oros, & Durney-Crowley, 2007). Each of these trends holds significant implications for quality care, nursing practice, and nursing education. The trends have begun to influence quality of life and quality of care. (See Box 12-1.)

Nurses must be proactive to address the trends and not become silent but disgruntled victims of change. There are many positive aspects among the trends, and nurses must use their assessment and evaluation skills to gain insight and create advantages specific to their area of practice. These trends are not to be feared, but embraced. Addressing them will take time and effort. Porter-O'Grady and Malloch (2010) note that in this "age of innovation" it is not sufficient to be an innovator, but rather necessary to nurture and expand the innovation dynamic. This requires specific skills and is akin to being "keeper of the flame." Nurses should interact with other disciplines to increase and share perspectives, to gain the benefits of a team pursuing a common goal, and to increase the likelihood of success. It is important for nursing as a unified body to be a significant player in the changes and a continual advocate for patient safety and quality care.

| BOX 12-1 | FUTURE TRENDS WITH NURSING IMPLICATIONS |

1. Interacting with an educated consumer about traditional and alternative care

2. Changing demographics with more cultural and racial diversity

3. Global economy and society with accessibility to healthcare for all

4. Increasing focus on care of populations

5. Keeping updated on healthcare policy and regulation

6. Awareness of the cost of health care and ethics of access to health care

7. Innovations that need nursing expertise

8. Understanding and using interprofessional education and collaborative practice

9. Opportunities for lifelong learning and workforce development

10. Opportunities for and awareness of advances in nursing science and research

Source: Adapted from Heller, B. R., Oros, M. T., & Durney-Crowley, J. (2007). The future of nursing education: ten trends to watch. *NLN: National League for Nursing Newsletter*. Retrieved from www.nln.org/nlnjournal/infotrends.htm.

Nurses can be active participants in each of the trends and bring the nursing mindset and the quality imperative to these new endeavors. Polifko (2010) emphasizes the importance of analyzing the traditional role of the nurse and nursing education and devising a new model that will incorporate contemporary advances and meet the increasingly complex health issues of society. Nursing education must be transformed to position nurses to meet the challenges of contemporary nursing and to anticipate those of the future. The nurse of every era should be prepared with cutting edge knowledge and carry a firm commitment to the patient and quality. As Sulmasy wrote, "Competence remains the first act of compassion" (p. 50).

CHAPTER HIGHLIGHTS

- Future nurses will need to be excellent communicators, collaborators, and masters of outcome data in order to provide quality care.
- New methods for monitoring continual quality improvement are emerging, and nurses need to be aware of the methods and engaged in developing new technology.
- Healthcare economics needs to be included in the curriculum of all nursing programs.
- The type of leadership in a healthcare organization will have a strong influence on staff attitude and motivation.

Pearson Nursing Student Resources

Find additional review materials at
nursing.pearsonhighered.com

Prepare for success with additional NCLEX®-style practice
questions, interactive assignments and activities, web links,
animations and videos, and more!

REFERENCES

American Association of Colleges of Nursing. (2011). Enhancing diversity in the workforce. Retrieved from http://www.aacn.nche.edu/media-relations/fact-sheets/enhancing-diversity

American Nurses Association. (2012). ANA participates in partnership to determine national quality measures. Retrieved from http://nursingworld.org/MainMenuCategories/ThePracticeofProfessionalNursing/PatientSafetyQuality/Collaborative-Activity/ANA-Partnership-National-Quality-Measures.html

Andrews, M. M., & Boyle, J. (2008). *Transcultural concepts in nursing care*. Philadelphia: Wolters Kluwer.

Baker, R. A., & Newland, R. F. (2008). Continuous quality improvement of perfusion practice: The role of electronic data collection and statistical control charts. *Perfusion 23*, 7–16.

Benner, P., Sutphen, M., Leonard, V., & Day, L. (2010). *Educating nurses: A call for radical transformation*. San Francisco: Jossey-Bass.

Berwick, D.M., Nolan, T.W., & Whittington, J. (2008). The triple aim: Care, health, and cost. *Health Affairs 27*(3), 759–769. doi: 10.1377/hlthaff.27.3.759

Boxer, B. A., & Goldfarb, E. M. B. (2011). *Creative solutions to enhance nursing quality*. Sudbury, MA: Jones & Bartlett.

Brown, D., White, J., & Liebbrandt, L. (2006). Collaborative partnerships for nursing faculties and health service providers: What can nursing learn from business literature? *Journal of Nursing Management 14*, 170–179.

Catalano, J. T. (2003). *Nursing now! Today's issues, tomorrow's trends* (3rd ed.). Philadelphia: F. A. Davis.

Crigger, N., & Godfrey, N. (2011). *The making of nurse professionals: A transformational ethical approach*. Sudbury, MA: Jones & Bartlett.

D'Amour, D., & Oandasan, I. (2006). *Interprofessional education for collaborative patient-centered practice: An evolving framework*. Montreal, Canada: University of Montreal.

Deming, W. E. (1986). *Out of crisis*. Cambridge, MA: MIT Press.

Dickerson, S., Stone, V., Pachura, C., & Usiak, D. (2007). The meaning of communication: Experiences with augmentative communication devices. *Rehabilitation Nursing 27*, 215–230.

Finkelman, A. W. (2012). *Leadership and management in nursing*. Upper Saddle River, NJ: Pearson/Prentice Hall.

Folland, S., Goodman, A., & Stano, M. (2012). *The economics of health and health care*, Seventh Edition. Upper Saddle River, NJ: Pearson/Prentice Hall.

Heller, B. R., Oros, M. T., & Durney-Crowley, J. (2007). The future of nursing education: Ten trends to watch. *NLN: National League for Nursing Newsletter*. Retrieved from http://www.nln.org/nlnjournal/infotrends.htm.

Henderson, T., & Hassmiller, S. (2007). Hospitals and philanthropy as partners in funding nursing education. *Nursing Economics 25*(2), 95–100.

Ierardi, J. (2010). Back in the day. *Nursing 2010 40*(4), 32–33.

Institute of Medicine (IOM). (2002). *Crossing the quality chasm: A new health system for the 21st century.* Washington, DC: National Academies Press.

Jones, J., & Sackett, K. (2009). Integrating leadership and management content across the curriculum. *Nurse Educator 34*(5), 204–208.

Kosoko-Lasaki, S., Cook, C., & O'Brien, R. (2009). *Cultural proficiency in addressing health disparities.* Sudbury, MA: Jones & Bartlett.

Kyrkjebo, J. M. (2006). Teaching quality improvement in the classroom and clinic: Getting it wrong and getting it right. *Journal of Nursing Education 43*(2), 109–116.

Marquis, B. L., & Huston, C. J. (2009). *Leadership roles and management functions in nursing: Theory and application* (6th ed.). Philadelphia: Wolters Kluwer.

Mason, D. J., Leavitt, J. K., & Chaffee, M. W. (2007). *Policy and politics and healthcare* (5th ed.). St. Louis: Saunders / Elsevier.

Maxwell, J. (2007). *The 21 irrefutable laws of leadership.* Nashville, TN: Thomas Nelson Incorporated.

McLaughlin, C. P., & Kaluzny, A. D. (2004). *Continuous quality improvement in healthcare: Theory, implementation, and applications.* Sudbury, MA: Jones & Bartlett.

Nightingale, F. (1859). *Notes on nursing.* Facsimile of first edition reproduced 1946. Philadelphia: J. B. Lippincott.

Nosek, L. J., Androwich, I. M., & Amer, K. (2011). *Basic clinical health care economics.* In Kelly, P. (2011). (Ed.), *Nursing leadership and management* (3rd ed.). Clifton Park, NY: Delmar Cengage Learning.

Pearson, A. (2007). Exploiting the potential of international collaboration in nursing. *International Journal of Nursing Practice 13* (p. 269).

Polifko, K. (2010). *The practice environment of nursing: Issues and trends.* Clifton Park, NY: Delmar Cengage Learning.

Porter-O'Grady, T., & Malloch, K. (2003). *Quantum leadership: A textbook of new leadership.* Boston: Jones & Bartlett.

Porter-O'Grady, T., & Malloch, K. (2007). *Quantum leadership: A resource for health care innovation* (2nd ed.). Sudbury, MA: Jones & Bartlett.

Porter-O'Grady, T., & Malloch, K. (2010). *Innovation leadership: Creating the landscape of health care.* Boston: Jones & Bartlett.

Robbins, S. (2005). *Organizational behaviors.* Upper Saddle River, NJ: Pearson/Prentice Hall.

Rossen, E., Bartlett, R., & Herrick, C. (2008). Interdisciplinary collaboration: The need

to revisit. *Issues in Mental Health Nursing 29,* 387–396.

Sanford, K. (2011). Making the business case for quality and nursing. *Nurse Leader 9*(1). 28–31.

Sulmasy, D. P. (1997). *The healer's calling: A spirituality for physicians and healthcare professionals.* Mahwah, NJ; Paulist Press.

Teeley, K., Lowe, J., Beal, J., & Knapp, M. (2006). Incorporating quality improvement concepts and practice into a community health course. *Journal of Nursing Education 45*(2), 86–90.

Thompson, P., & Stanowski, A. (2009). Maximizing nursing productivity: The benefits of improved collaboration between nursing and support services. *Healthcare Financial Management,* January, 76–85.

Williams, H., & Fallone, S. (2008). CQI in the acute care setting: An opportunity to influence acute care practice. *Nephrology Nursing Journal 35*(5), 515–522.

Wiseman, L., & McKeown, G. (2010). Bringing out the best in your people. *Harvard Business Review,* May, 117–121.

Yoder-Wise, P. S., & Kowolski, K. (2006). *Beyond leading and managing: Nursing administration for the future.* St. Louis: Mosby/Elsevier.

Appendix

QUALITY AND SAFETY ELEMENTS: BASIC PRACTICE ELEMENTS IN THE NCLEX®-RN BLUEPRINT, THE COPA MODEL, AND THE QSEN COMPETENCIES

NCLEX®-RN Blueprint (Client Need)			
Safe Effective Care Environment	**Health Promotion and Maintenance**	**Psychosocial Integrity**	**Physiological Integrity**
• **Management of Care** Providing and directing nursing care that enhances the care delivery setting to protect clients, family/significant others and health care personnel. • **Safety and Infection Control** Protecting clients, family/significant others and healthcare personnel from health and environmental hazards. **Example**: Proper hand washing and infection control for isolation	The nurse provides and directs nursing care of the client and family/significant others that incorporates the knowledge of expected growth and development principles, prevention and/or early detection of health problems, and strategies to achieve optimal health. **Example**: Home safety assessment prior to discharge from the hospital	The nurse provides and directs care that promotes and supports the emotional, mental and social well-being of the client and family. **Example**: Person-centered care in assigned care plans in clinical experiences	The nurse promotes physical health and wellness by providing care and comfort, reducing client risk potential, and managing health alterations. • **Basic Care and Comfort** Providing comfort and assistance in the performance of activities of daily living. • **Pharmacological and Parenteral Therapies** Providing care related to the administration of medications and parenteral therapies. • **Reduction of Risk Potential** Reducing the likelihood that clients will develop complications or health problems related to existing conditions, treatments, or procedures. **Example**: Medication reconciliation and hypothetical root cause analysis worksheet for medication error

COPA Model

Assessment and Intervention Skills	Critical Thinking Skills	Teaching Skills	Human Caring and Relationship Skills	Teaching Strategies
• Safety and protection • Assessment and monitoring • Therapeutic treatments and procedures	• Evaluation; integrating pertinent data from multiple sources • Problem solving; diagnostic reasoning; creating alternatives • Decision making; prioritizing • Scientific inquiry; research process	• Individuals and groups; clients, coworkers, others • Health promotion; health restoration	• Morality, ethics, legality • Cultural respect; cooperative interpersonal relationships • Client advocacy	Teaching Strategies • High fidelity patient simulation (HPS) with 10 safety breaches

Leadership Skills	Knowledge Integration Skills	Management Skills		Teaching strategies
• Collaboration, assertiveness, risk taking • Creativity, vision to formulate alternatives • Planning, anticipating, supporting with evidence • Professional accountability, role behaviors, appearance	• Nursing, healthcare, and related disciplines • Liberal arts, natural and social sciences, and related disciplines	• Administration, organization, coordination • Planning, delegation, supervision of others • Human and material resource utilization • Accountability and responsibility; performance appraisals • Communication • Oral skills • Talking, listening with individuals • Interviewing; history taking • Group discussion, interacting • Telling, showing, reporting • Writing skills • Clinical reports, care plans, charting		• Professional role development course • Continual quality improvement project assessing unit policy and procedures and revising for best practices for safe care

QSEN Competencies

Patient-Centered Care	Teamwork and Collaboration	Safety and Informatics	Evidence-Based Practice	Quality Improvement	Teaching Strategies
K: Integrate understanding of multiple dimensions of patient-centered care: physical comfort and emotional support. **S:** Elicit patient values, preferences, and expressed needs as part of clinical interview, implementation of care plan, and evaluation of care. **A:** Value seeing the healthcare situation through patients' eyes.	**K:** Describe scopes of practice and roles of healthcare team members. **S:** Function competently within own scope of practice as a member of the healthcare team. **A:** Value the perspectives and expertise of all healthcare team members.	**K:** Describe the benefits and limitations of selected safety- enhancing technologies (such as barcodes, computer provider order entry, medication pumps, and automatic alerts/alarms). **S:** Demonstrate effective use of strategies to reduce risk of harm to self or others. **A:** Value the contributions of standardization / reliability to safety. *Informatics* **K:** Identify essential information that must be available in a common database to support patient care. **S:** Navigate the electronic health record. Document and plan patient care in an electronic health record. **A:** Value technologies that support clinical decision making, error prevention, and care coordination.	**K:** Explain the role of evidence in determining best clinical practice. **S:** Participate in structuring the work environment to facilitate integration of new evidence into standards of practice. **A:** Value the need for continuous improvement in clinical practice based on new knowledge.	**K:** Recognize that nursing and other health professions and students are parts of systems of care and care processes that affect outcomes for patients and families. **S:** Participate in a root cause analysis of a sentinel event. **A:** Appreciate that continuous quality improvement is an essential part of the daily work of all health professionals.	• Integrated throughout curriculum • Clinical experiences, high fidelity patient simulations

K = Knowledge
S = Skills
A = Attitudes

Cronenwett, L., Sherwood, G., Barnsteiner, J., Disch, J., Johnson, J., Mitchell, PI, et al. (2007). Quality and safety education for nurses. *Nursing Outlook, 55*(3), 121-131.

Glossary

Quality and Safety for Transformational Nursing: Core Competencies

Glossary of Terms and Resources

A

Acute Care   Care for patients who need medical treatment for illnesses or injuries lasting less than 6 months or who are recovering from surgery.

Affordable Care Act (ACA)   Healthcare reform legislation aimed at increasing healthcare insurance coverage for the millions of people in the United States who are not insured or underinsured. Includes pay for performance components and incentives for primary care provision and nursing education tuition assistance to help bridge the faculty shortage gap. Signed into law March 2010. (http://www.healthcare.gov/law/full/index.html)

Adverse Drug Event (ADE)   A negative response to administration of a medication or treatment. Negative responses can range from mild side effects, such as gastrointestinal upset, to severe anaphylaxis (allergic reaction) and death.

Agency for Healthcare Research and Quality (AHRQ)   Government funded leader in research on healthcare quality, costs, outcomes, and patient safety. AHRQ is the health services division of the U.S. Department of Health and Human Services (HHS) and the sister agency of the National Institutes of Health (NIH). AHRQ has research centers that specialize in healthcare research, including clinical practice and technology assessment, healthcare organization and delivery systems, and primary care. AHRQ is a source of funding and technology innovations related to health services. (www.AHRQ.gov)

Aligning Forces for Quality (AF4Q)   Organization established to help improve health and health care in communities across the United States. The group focuses on prevention and early treatment of chronic conditions such as diabetes, asthma, depression, and heart disease. The philosophy of AF4Q is that no single person, group, or profession is able to influence the quality of care without the support and commons goals with others. AF4Q promotes quality improvement by aligning key forces, including healthcare providers (physicians/physician groups, nurses, clinics), healthcare purchasers (employers and insurers), and healthcare consumers (patients). (http://forces4quality.org)

American Association of the Colleges of Nursing (AACN)   One of the accreditation organizations for schools of nursing. The AACN has responded to the need for more quality and safety education in nursing schools by developing the Quality and Safety Education in Nursing (QSEN) group to provide support for nursing educators. (www.aacn.nche.edu)

America's Health Insurance Plans (AHIP)   The national association representing nearly 1,300 member companies that provide health insurance coverage to more than 200 million Americans. Member companies offer health insurance, long-term care insurance, disability-income insurance, dental insurance, supplemental insurance, stop-loss insurance, and reinsurance to consumers, employers, and public purchasers. AHIP's goal is to give consumers more information to make better decisions about their health, support innovations that facilitate patient-centered care, help patients stay on their treatment plans, promote patient safety, change incentives for health promotion, collaborate on quality improvement efforts, and address the disparities in health care. (www.ahip.org/Who-we-are)

American Health Quality Association (AHQA) A central hub for quality improvement organizations and professionals, sharing information about best practices with providers, hospitals, and nursing homes. Linking educational, governmental and nonprofit associations dedicated to promoting and facilitating fundamental change with the goal to improve the quality of health care in America. (www.ahqa.org)

American Hospital Association (AHA) An independent organization that represents and serves all types of hospitals, healthcare networks, and their patients and communities. The AHA is a resource for education for healthcare leaders and a source of information on healthcare issues and trends. AHA facilitates the members' perspectives and needs being heard and addressed in national health policy development, legislative and regulatory debates, and judicial matters. The group has active advocacy efforts including in Washington's legislative and executive branches as well as the legislative and regulatory arenas. Nearly 5,000 hospitals, healthcare systems, networks, other providers of care, and 37,000 individual members come together to form the AHA. (www.AHA.org)

American Nurses Association (ANA) The professional organization representing the nation's 3 million registered nurses (RNs) through its 54-constituent member associations. The ANA advances the nursing profession by fostering high standards of nursing practice, promoting the rights of nurses in the workplace, projecting a positive and realistic view of nursing, and lobbying Congress and regulatory agencies on healthcare issues affecting nurses and the public. (www.ana.org)

Attending nurse Suggested terminology used to provide a parallel status between the discipline of nursing and that of medicine. Patients will have a choice of nurses just as they choose physicians.

B

Benchmark (benchmarking) Benchmarking is used to establish goals in quality and safety efforts. It was used in the Transforming Care at the Bedside Project (TCAB) to analyze the effectiveness of tests of change and innovations in quality data to identify best practices of care and improve quality.

Best practices The most up-to-date patient care interventions that result in the best patient outcomes and minimize patient risk of death or complications (based on research). Evidence-based practice is the cornerstone of best practices.

C

Caregiver burden The perception of stress and alteration of daily life when faced with caring for a dependent family member.

Center for Health Care Strategies (CHCS) A nonprofit health policy resource center dedicated to improving the quality and cost effectiveness of healthcare services for low-income populations and people with chronic illnesses and disabilities. CHCS works directly with states and federal agencies, health plans, and providers to develop innovative programs that better serve people with complex and high-cost health care needs. (www.CHCS.org)

Center for Health Improvement (CHI) A national, independent, nonprofit health policy organization focused on improving population health and encouraging healthy behaviors. Started in 1995, CHI uses evidence-based research to help public, private, and nonprofit organizations strengthen their capacity to improve the quality and value of health care and enhance public health at the community level. (www.CHI .org)

Center for Studying Health Systems Change A nonpartisan policy research organization located in Washington DC. The center designs and conducts studies focused on the U.S. healthcare system that are used by policymakers in government and private industry. Additional efforts are focused on healthcare policy research that enables decision makers to understand change and the national and local market forces driving that change. (www.HSC.org)

Centers for Medicare & Medicaid Services (CMS) Seeks to provide effective, up-to-date healthcare coverage and to promote quality care for beneficiaries. Ultimately, CMS is working to transform and modernize the healthcare system. (www.cms.gov)

Chief financial officer (CFO) Person primarily responsible for managing the financial risks of the corporation through financial planning, record-keeping, and financial reporting to higher management.

Chief nursing executive (CNE) Nurse at the highest level of the organization who collaborates with the clinical and operational domains, translating clinical performance demands into operating strategies and tactics.

Chronic disease An illness that lasts more than 6 months or recurs. Examples include diabetes, asthma, heart disease, kidney disease, and chronic lung disease.

Clinical practice guidelines A set of systematically developed standards, based on scientific evidence, that guides providers in making decisions about appropriate health care for specific medical conditions. Clinical practice guidelines focus providers so that they can identify and evaluate the most current information about prevention, diagnosis,

prognosis, therapy, risk–benefit, and cost effectiveness.

Collaboration A complex phenomenon that brings together two or more individuals, often from different professional disciplines, who work to achieve shared aims and objectives.

Competence The ability to demonstrate an integration of the knowledge, attitudes, and skills necessary to function in a specific role and work setting.

Consumer An individual who uses, is affected by, or is entitled or compelled to use a health-related service (i.e., clients, families, or patients).

Consumer Assessment of Healthcare Providers and Systems (CAHPS) A group that develops and supports the use of standardized surveys to evaluate providers. Healthcare consumers and patients report on and evaluate their healthcare experiences. The surveys cover topics that have been identified as important to consumers such as communication skills of providers and accessibility of services. (www.CAHPS.org)

Consumer engagement Patients and families who take an active role in their own health care. The consumers, who are patients and families, put effort into understanding their own conditions and available treatments. They also seek out and make decisions in collaboration with providers based on information about treatment options and the past performance of healthcare providers.

Consumer-driven (or directed) care A form of more affordable health insurance that combines a high-deductible health plan with a tax-favored health savings account, flexible spending account, or health reimbursement account to cover out-of-pocket expenses. These accounts are "consumer driven" in that they give participants greater control over their own health care, allowing individuals to determine on a personal basis how they choose to spend their healthcare account funds.

Continuous quality improvement (CQI) process (also referred to as total quality management [TQM])   A process of constant awareness of the status of quality in organizations and the effort to always be increasing quality, proactivity, employee empowerment, and continual improvement.

Coordination of care   A central comprehensive plan for the best health care for each patient. All providers must have equal access to, and take into consideration, all required information about a patient's conditions and treatments to ensure that the patient receives appropriate healthcare services.

Core measures   Clinical measures that assess the quality of care provided in a given focus area, which may be disease specific, such as acute myocardial infarction (AMI).

Crew resource management (CRM)   Safety model derived from aviation safety operations that helps nurses communicate effectively to keep patients safe and improve care team vitality.

Culturally competent care   Behavior, attitudes, and policies that support a negotiated process of appropriately caring for people across languages and cultures.

D

Data collection   The acquisition of healthcare information or facts based on patient and consumer race, ethnicity, and language. Data collection gives healthcare providers the information needed to perform benchmarking measures on healthcare systems to determine areas where improvement is needed in providing care.

Declaration of Human Rights   A universal declaration of the United Nations General Assembly that declares the common standard of achievement for all peoples and all nations. It outlines the fundamental human rights to be universally protected. (www.un.org/en/documents/udhr)

Deliberate practice   Focused learning with an engaged learner that involves repetitive performance of psychomotor or cognitive skills coupled with rigorous assessment, informative feedback, and opportunity for reflection.

Department of Health and Human Services (HHS)   The U.S. government's principal agency for ensuring the health of all Americans. The agency funds research focused on quality health care.

Doctor–nurse game   A stereotypical pattern of interaction first described in the 1960s in which female nurses, deferring to the doctor's authority (in past scenarios, usually male), learn to show initiative and offer advice.

E

Effective care   Healthcare services with proven value and potentially positive outcomes, such as insulin for type 1 diabetes patients, that are backed by well-established research and strong evidence of efficacy, determined by clinical trials.

Electronic health record (EHR)   A digital version of patient data found in the traditional paper record.

Electronic medical record (EMR)   A legal record of a single encounter or visit.

Emancipatory theoretical frameworks   Structures that outline nursing practice and the commonly held notions of how health care is delivered, often suggesting possible routes to change.

Evidence-based practice   The use of the current, best available scientific research with proven effectiveness in daily practice. Evidence is critical for developing performance measures for select health conditions.

F

Family-centered care (FCC)   An approach to the planning, delivery, and evaluation of health care that is governed by mutually beneficial partnerships between healthcare providers, patients, and families. FCC applies to patients of all ages, and it may be practiced in any healthcare setting.

G

Goal-based evaluation A summative way to track how a program is performing in terms of meeting outcomes or meeting the established metrics.

Globalization The increased interconnectedness and interdependence of peoples and countries. Includes the opening of borders to increasingly fast flows of goods, services, finance, people, and ideas across international borders and the changes in institutional and policy regimes at the international and national levels that facilitate or promote such flows.

H

"Heads-up" or "hot topics" meetings Short conferences that focus on quality initiatives, interprofessional communication, and collaboration. The model for these meetings is built on the premise that members of healthcare teams can learn from one another. The collaborative process includes communication, compassionate caring, and conciliatory interactions to solve problems.

Health information technology (HIT) A global term that encompasses electronic health records and personal health records to indicate the use of computers, software, electronic devices, and the Internet to store, retrieve, update, and transmit information about patients' health.

Health Plan Employer Data and Information Set (HEDIS) A set of healthcare quality measures for informing employers or consumers about the performance of health plans regarding their compliance with accepted care standards for prevention and treatment. Formerly known as the Health Plan Employer Data Information Set.

Health Resources and Services Administration (HRSA) An agency of the U.S. Department of Health and Human Services that provides information and research to help improve access to healthcare services for people who are uninsured, isolated, or medically vulnerable.

High fidelity patient simulation (HPS) The use of computer-programmed manikins that simulate real situations. The manikins have internal computers that respond to student treatments.

High reliability organizations (HROs) Organizations with a sustained safety record due to the cognitive processes they maintain that allow workers to be aware of the potential for mistakes and the ability to prevent mistakes.

Hospital Consumer Assessment of Hospitals, Providers, and Systems (H-CAHPS) A standardized survey instrument for measuring patients' perspectives on hospital care. H-CAHPS provides core questions that can be combined with customized, hospital-specific questions to produce information that complements the data hospitals currently collect to support improvements in internal customer service and quality-related activities.

Hospital Quality Alliance (HQA) A public–private collaboration seeking to improve the quality of care provided by the nation's hospitals by measuring and publicly reporting on that care. (www.hospitalqualityalliance.org)

Huddles Daily scheduled rounds that can easily be built into the schedule of all providers for a patient.

Human factors research Applies knowledge about human strengths and limitations to the design of interactive systems of people, equipment, and their environment to ensure their effectiveness, safety, and ease of use.

I

Informatics The use of information systems technology in health care or nursing.

Institute for Healthcare Improvement (IHI) An independent nonprofit organization leading the effort to improve the safety and quality of health care throughout the world. Founded in 1991 and based in Cambridge,

Massachusetts, IHI works to improve health care by building the will for change, cultivating innovative concepts for improving patient care, and helping healthcare systems put those ideas into action. IHI was a co-founder of the Transforming Care at the Bedside (TCAB) project along with the Robert Wood Johnson Foundation (RWJF). (www.ihi.org)

Institute of Medicine (IOM)   A nonprofit organization with esteemed membership that works outside the framework of government to ensure scientifically informed analysis and independent guidance on matters of nursing, biomedical science, medicine, and health. The IOM provides unbiased, evidence-based, and authoritative information and advice concerning health and science policy for policy-makers, professionals, leaders in every sector of society, and the public at large. A critical leader in the safety and quality in healthcare publications, the IOM published a series of reports that focused on the notion that health care needs to reform and look toward other industries and use engineering improvement methods to aim for top quality, efficiency, and safety. (www.IOM.org)

International Council of Nurses (ICN)   Federation of more than 130 national nurses associations representing nurses worldwide. Founded in 1899, ICN is the world's first and widest reaching international organization for health professionals. ICN works to ensure quality nursing care for all, sound health policies globally, the advancement of nursing knowledge, and the presence worldwide of a respected nursing profession and a competent and satisfied nursing workforce. (www.icn.ch)

Interprofessional   A model of team communication and collaboration among many disciplines used in patient-focused care planning. Can be applied in education settings such as health professions colleges or used in health care settings.

Intersectionality   A framework for analyzing interlocking systems of power and domination in social and cultural relationships at the interpersonal, community, corporate, and national identity levels. Intersectionality posits that all intolerances and socially unjust systems, beliefs, rituals, habits, and behaviors are related to how persons experience prejudicial treatment and limited opportunity.

J

Joint Commission (JCAHO)   The Joint Commission (formerly Joint Commission on Accreditation of Healthcare Organizations [JCAHO]) is a private, nonprofit organization that evaluates and accredits hospitals and other healthcare organizations. The range of organizations extend from acute care hospitals to providing home care, behavioral health care, ambulatory care, and long-term care services.

K

KSA   An acronym for knowledge, skills, and attitudes, all of which are necessary for safe nursing practice with optimal patient outcomes.

L

Leadership   Influencing the actions of a person or group to attain desired objectives.

Lewin's force-field analysis   A model created by Kurt Lewin, a German-American psychologist and social science innovator, that is used to assess the impact of change on the status quo. The theory discusses forces that are opposing, like a tug of war, that change when one side is stronger than the other. As Lewin describes, driving forces equal to restraining forces produce equilibrium. Persons are most comfortable with equilibrium. Opposing forces that are strong may produce unplanned and negative change, whereas driving forces that are built on consensus become a positive change environment. The Lewin model frames change in relation to the culture in which one is working.

It includes resistance to change from workers and administrators, willingness to be open to change, and assessed need for change.

M

Magnet status　An award given by the American Nurses Credentialing Center, an affiliate of the American Nurses Association, to hospitals that satisfy a set of criteria designed to measure the strength and quality of their nursing. A Magnet hospital is one where nursing delivers excellent patient outcomes, where nurses have a high level of job satisfaction, and where there is a low staff nurse turnover rate and appropriate grievance resolution.

Manifesto　A web-based evaluation of nursing ideas that speaks to emancipatory nursing and activism. (www.nursemanifest.com)

Meaningful use　A term that has been adopted to signify the appropriate design and proper application of information systems to persons. The American Academy of Nursing developed a matrix and set of definitions and criteria for meaningful use.

Medical error　A mistake that harms a patient. Adverse drug events, hospital-acquired infections, and wrong-site surgeries are examples of preventable medical errors.

Metric　The process of measurement in general, or a specific set of quantifiable and measured criteria.

Models of care　A conceptual object or diagram that guides the provision of current and future clinical services.

Muda　A Japanese word that describes activities that absorb resources but are not productive and create no value.

Multidisciplinary (Interdisciplinary) teams　Healthcare teams composed of healthcare professionals as well as health educators or community leaders.

N

National Hospital Quality Measures (NHQM)　Database and Web site that tracks the most effective ways to assess quality health care. Public resource for evidence-based quality measures and measure sets. (www.qualitymeasures.ahrq.gov)

National Committee on Quality Assurance (NCQA)　A private, nonprofit organization dedicated to improving healthcare quality through measurement, transparency and accountability. NCQA has been a central figure in driving improvement throughout the healthcare system and elevating the issue of healthcare quality to the top of the national agenda. The organization has helped build consensus around important healthcare quality issues by working with large employers, policy-makers, doctors, patients, and health plans to decide what is important, how to measure it, and how to promote improvement.

National Council of State Boards of Nursing (NCSBN)　Founded in 1978, the NCSBN is the vehicle through which boards of nursing act and counsel one another on matters of common interest. These member boards are charged with the responsibility of providing regulatory excellence for public health, safety, and welfare. NCSBN is devoted to developing a psychometrically sound and legally defensible nurse licensure examination consistent with current nursing practice. (www.ncsbn.org)

National Database of Nursing Quality Indicators (NDNQI)　This database is a quality measurement program that allows for a unit-based collection of performance reports and the opportunity for comparison to national averages.

National Health Plan Collaborative (NHPC)　A project that brings together health insurance companies in partnership with organizations from the public and private sectors to identify ways to improve the quality of health care for racially and ethnically diverse populations.

National Institutes of Health (NIH)　A part of the U.S. Department of Health and Human Services, the primary federal agency that conducts and supports medical research. Helping to lead the way toward important medical discoveries that improve people's health and save lives, NIH scientists investigate ways to prevent disease as well as the causes, treatments, and cures for common and rare diseases.

National League for Nursing (NLN) Founded in 1893 as the American Society of Superintendents of Training Schools for Nurses, the National League for Nursing was the first nursing organization in the United States. It is a preferred membership organization for nurse faculty and leaders in nursing education. NLN members include nurse educators, education agencies, health care agencies, and interested members of the public. The NLN promotes excellence in nursing education to build a strong and diverse nursing workforce to advance the nation's health. (www.nln.org)

National Quality Forum (NQF) A nonprofit membership organization created to develop and implement a national strategy for healthcare quality measurement and reporting. Members are from all parts of the healthcare system, including national, state, regional, and local groups. Members can include consumers, public and private purchasers of health insurance plans, employers, healthcare professionals, provider organizations, accrediting bodies, labor unions, supporting industries, and organizations involved in healthcare research or quality improvement. Together, the organizational members of the NQF work to promote a common approach to measuring healthcare quality and fostering system-wide capacity for quality improvement. Quality improvement measures endorsed by the NQF are considered the gold standard. (www.NQF.org)

Near miss An adverse event that was caught just before the treatment was given and could have been harmful or fatal. For example, preparing to give a medication to which the patient is allergic but catching the error prior to administration.

Never-events Mistakes that should never occur under any circumstances. For example, giving one patient's medication to another patient with a similar name.

O

Orientation The process of introducing staff to the philosophy, goals, policies, procedures, role expectations, and other factors needed to function in a specific work setting. Orientation takes place both for new employees and when changes in nurses' roles, responsibilities, and practice settings occur.

Outcome The result of a process and includes output, effects, and impact. Outcomes should be measured in a consistent and robust manner using data that can be compared over time and to other settings.

Outcome-based evaluation An evaluation focused on learning-centered activities or factors that is used to identify the successful operation of a nursing unit. Ultimately, the outcome-based evaluation measures the change that was supposed to result from the program, while the process evaluation measures the intervention itself.

Outpatient care Medical or surgical care that does not include an overnight hospital stay.

Overcrowding A situation experienced by many emergency departments across the nation when there are too many patients for the number of providers available. Patients may spend excessive time waiting for care. The safety and quality of care may be compromised, resulting in unhappy patients.

P

Patient Care Partnership A document created by the American Hospital Association focusing on communication and the close partnership between patients and healthcare providers. It replaces the Patient Bill of Rights. (http://www.aha.org/advocacy-issues/communicatingpts/pt-care-partnership.shtml)

Patient experience Patient satisfaction and quality health care as perceived by the user or client. This can include research or administrative reports that assess quality from the perspective of patients by requesting observations and opinions about what happened during the encounters in healthcare delivery. Patient experiences can encompass many varied indicators of patient-centered care, including access, patient satisfaction, communication skills, customer service, helpfulness of office staff, and information resources.

Patient registry A patient database maintained by hospitals, providers, or health plans that allows providers to identify their patients according to disease, demographic characteristics, and other factors. Patient registries can facilitate coordinated care for patients, provide data on new treatments, and improve overall quality of care. Electronic health records can include patient registries.

Patient satisfaction A measurement of a patient's satisfaction with the environment, treatment, and overall experience obtained through reports or ratings from patients about services received from an organization, hospital, physician, or healthcare provider.

Person-centered care Often referred to as patient-centered care, person-centered care is a perspective that explicitly views the experiences, values, and beliefs of individuals as important and central to the way health is lived, and to any health plan or regime. Every health plan or regime must be developed in a manner that synthesizes the person experiencing a health situation as an integral component.

Pay-for-performance (P4P) A method for paying providers and based on their demonstrated outcomes and adherence to standards of care. Healthcare quality objectives should be met before the provider or institution is paid. The idea is to reward providers for the quality, not the quantity, of care they deliver.

Payers The person or health plan that pays for health care. Examples include uninsured patients, self-insured employers, health plans, and health maintenance organizations.

Performance measures Sets of outcomes with established standards against which healthcare performance is measured. Performance measures are accepted as a method for guiding informed decision making as a motivation for improvement.

Personal digital assistant (PDA) A handheld device with software that allows for data to be captured and divided into value-added, nonvalue-added, and necessary categories, based on the TCAB study to measure how clinical instructors and students spent their time in a clinical setting.

Personal health record (PHR) A lifelong tool for patients to use to manage health information.

Praxis Professional practice that is explicitly guided and performed from social justice values and intentionally conducted for the good of persons and society.

Preceptor A competent nurse who has received formal training for the preceptorship role.

Preceptorship A formal relationship between a qualified preceptor and a newly licensed nurse that facilitates active learning and transition into practice.

Preventive care Primary healthcare services that prevent disease or its consequences. It includes primary prevention to keep people from getting sick (immunizations), secondary prevention to detect early disease (glucose testing for diabetes), and tertiary prevention to keep ill people or those at high risk of disease from getting sicker (helping someone with lung disease to quit smoking).

Price transparency Available listing of real costs of hospital care to ensure that consumers know what it will cost to receive a given healthcare service at a variety of outlets.

Primary care Care by providers who focus on general health care. They may be prepared as nursing practitioners, family practice, pediatrics, internal medicine, or gynecology.

Process improvement Quality management techniques, strategies, and steps implemented to solve healthcare problems. The process can occur in all outpatient and hospital settings, as well as in other health-system environment.

Provider incentives Motivators for efficient or positive outcome-focused health care. Examples include monetary rewards for providers who meet specific benchmark standards for their patient care.

Provider A healthcare professional engaged in the delivery of health services, including nurses, physicians, dentists, podiatrists, optometrists, clinical psychologists, and so on. Hospitals and long-term care facilities are also providers.

Q

Quality (of care) A measure of the ability of a provider for individuals and populations that increase the likelihood of desired health outcomes and are consistent with current professional knowledge. The quality of health care can best be carried out by doing the right thing, at the right time, in the right way, for the right person, and getting the best possible results. According to the mantra for the quality improvement movement, care should be safe, effective, patient-centered, timely, efficient, and equitable.

Quality (of life) The amount of happiness and balance in an individual's life measured by several research instruments such as Carol Farrans' quality-of-life assessment tool. Attention to good health will create a better quality of life.

Quality improvement (QI) In the healthcare context, the goal of quality improvement strategies is for patients to receive the appropriate care at the appropriate time and place with the appropriate mix of information and supporting resources. Healthcare systems should be designed in such a way so as not to be overwhelming to patients and families. Quality improvement tools can make recommendations or leave decision making largely in the hands of individual providers. Quality improvement efforts should be rooted in evidence-based procedures and integrate data collected about the various processes and outcomes.

Quality indicator An agreed-upon outcome measure that is used to determine whether the goal of quality care was achieved.

Quality measures Mechanisms used to measure the quality of care by comparing to a criterion.

Quality and Safety Education for Nursing (QSEN) Instruction on integrating quality and safety principles and strategies into all nursing programs. QSEN has an extensive Web site full of resources for all levels of nurse educators. (www.QSEN.org)

R

Rapid-cycle change Used in the Transforming Care at the Bedside (TCAB) project, a quality-improvement method that identifies, implements, and measures changes made to improve a process or a system. Teams identify issues that can be causing poor safety and quality outcomes and develop a PDSA (plan, do, study, act) cycle. The group begins by piloting several changes with small patient groups, measuring whether the desired effects of changes were met, then acting based on the data. When positive outcomes are identified, the change becomes a permanent part of the care. The fundamental concept of rapid-cycle improvement is that healthcare processes once defined, in place, and in effect should be continually improved upon by instituting a constant cycle of innovations or improvements.

Report card Objective assessment of the quality of care delivered by providers, hospitals, or health plans. Report cards can be published by states, private health organizations, consumer groups, or health plans.

Return on investment (ROI) The amount of expected improvement in care brought about by a certain investment versus the actual improvement. ROI can also refer to the theory that if you invest in healthcare quality now, the quality of care for patients will improve in the future.

Role socialization Becoming adjusted and competent in a new position both socially and professionally. New nurses must have a good understanding of their scope of practice as well as that of others on the healthcare team.

Root cause analysis The backtracking of events surrounding a medication error. Coexisting factors that lead to a mistake.

S

Safety   Little or no risk for harm.

SBAR   An acronym for situation, background, assessment, and recommendations. This tool is a situational briefing model developed to bridge differences in individual communication styles and rank (perceived authority or power gradient) of the people involved. It is used for reporting at change of shift or during changes in patient status.

Sentinel event   A serious and unexpected consequence culminating in an event in a healthcare setting that causes death or serious injury to a patient. Usually traced back to a provider not following the standard of care.

Stakeholder   Someone who has a stake, or concern, about a particular process or organization; someone who can affect, or be affected by, the nursing care provided.

Standard of care   The expected level and type of care provided by the average caregiver under a given set of circumstances that are supported through findings from expert consensus and based on specific research evidence.

Strategies and Tools to Enhance Performance and Patient Safety (STEPPS)   Program that provides structure to improve safety in an organization. Improving communication and conflict resolution within the healthcare teams and identifying threats to safety make up the first part of the process.

Synergy   A concept that posits that two minds working in collaboration may be more effective than two minds working independently of one another.

System work-arounds   Short-cuts that allow the nurse to get work done in spite of poor work processes.

T

Transforming Care at the Bedside (TCAB)   A national collaborative that took on the challenge of creating the ideal patient-care environment for the nurse and developing educational strategies to teach new nurses quality improvement methods necessary to keep patients safe and contribute to a workplace that can be vital and joyful. The funding for TCAB was provided by the Robert Wood Johnson Foundation (RWJF) and the Institute for Healthcare Improvement (IMI). A primary goal of TCAB was to highlight and improve medical–surgical nursing as a career destination for the nurse and a place where every patient received the right care, at the right time, in the right way, every time.

Telehealth   The use of technology to assist with health assessment, diagnosis, treatment, and promotion of health to patients at other locations.

Telemedicine   The branch of telehealth that uses technology to deliver medical care and services to clients at other locations.

Throughput   The ability of a medical facility, such as an emergency department, to complete a patient input and output cycle focused on improving quality.

Tikun olam   A Hebrew phrase that represents the Jewish value of repairing the world.

Transcultural nursing   A formal area of study and practice in nursing focused on comparative holistic cultural care, health, and illness patterns of individuals and groups with respect to differences and similarities in cultural values, beliefs, and practices with the goal to provide culturally congruent, sensitive, and competent nursing care to people of diverse cultures.

Transition to practice   A formal program of active learning, implemented across all settings, for all newly licensed nurses (registered nurses and licensed practical/vocational nurses) designed to support their progression from education to practice.

Transparency   Transparency is the process of collecting and reporting healthcare cost, performance, and quality data in a format that can be accessed by the public and is intended to improve the delivery of services and ultimately improve the healthcare system as a whole.

Triple Aim healthcare goals   Goals developed by the Institute for Heathcare Improvement (IHI) to improve the experience of receiving health care through improving population health and reducing the per capita cost of health care.

Tzdekah   A Hebrew phrase representing the Jewish value of giving to others.

V

Variation   An instance of change or deviation; unwarranted variation in the practice of medicine and the use of medical resources in the United States. For example, the underuse of effective care such as the use of beta blockers for people who have myocardial infarction and screening of people with diabetes for early signs of retinal disease.

W

Whistleblowing   An attempt by a member or former member of an organization to issue a warning about a serious wrongdoing or danger.

Work flow   A repeatable pattern of activity focused on efficiency and quality and dependent on the organization for resources, defined roles, and information into a process that can be documented and learned.

Index

A

AACN. *See* American Association of Colleges of Nursing (AACN)
Activities of daily living (ADL), 201
Acuity-adaptable pulmonary unit pilot, 176–177
Addams, Jane, 80
ADE. *See* Adverse drug events (ADE)
Admission process, 24
Adverse drug events (ADE), 7, 25
Advisory Board Company, 65–66
Agency for Healthcare Research and Quality (AHRQ), 37, 107, 191, 192, 220, 224–225
  Patient Safety Indicators, 144
AHRQ. *See* Agency for Healthcare Research and Quality (AHRQ)
Aiken, L. H., 25, 78–80
All the Women Are White, All the Blacks Are Men: But Some of Us Are Brave (Hull, Scott, & Smith), 89
Always a Sister (Daniel), 80
Amer Hybrid Model of Change, 36
American Academy of Nursing (AAN), 189
American Association of Colleges of Nursing (AACN), 12, 19, 45, 99, 105–106, 137
American Health Care Association, 54
American Hospital Association, 6, 76
American Nurses Association (ANA), 6, 99, 234
American Nurses Credentialing Center (ANCC), 20, 154
American Organization of Nurse Executives (AONE), 6, 37, 174
Americans with Disabilities Act (ADA), 201
ANA. *See* American Nurses Association (ANA)
ANCC. *See* American Nurses Credentialing Center (ANCC)
Anderson, Joan, 89
Anesthesiologists, 109
Anxiety, emotional support and alleviation, 202
AONE. *See* American Organization of Nurse Executives (AONE)
Ashley, Jo Ann, 81
  on change, 81
  on power, 82–83
Assertion cycle, 116
Assessment, focus on, 125
Assurance and advocacy, lack of, 210
Attending nurses, 77
Awareness, of patient's rights, 224

B

Baccalaureate nursing programs, 105–106
Bar coding, 4, 5
Barnard, C., 155
Barrett, Elizabeth, 81, 83–84
Beal, S., 189
Beck-Kritek, P., 163

Bedside project, transforming care, 7–9
Benchmark. *See* Metric
Benner, Patricia, 45
Berens, Michael, 48
Berkow, S., 99
Berwick, Donald, 117
Biomedicine, 71, 75
Birth of the Clinic: An Archeology of Medical Perception, The (Foucault), 90
Blouin, Ann, 9, 10
Blouin, Scott, 18
Board of Registration in Nursing, 49
Boise, Adam Michael, 148
Budget, 73

C

California Nurses Association (CNA), 10, 76, 79
CALNOC. *See* Collaborative Alliance for Nursing Outcomes (CALNOC)
Cardiopulmonary resuscitation (CPR), 140
Care coordinator, 200
Care environment, 201–202
Career options, 223–224
Caregiver burden, 203
Care team vitality, 103
Caring Behavior Inventory (CBI), 134
Carnegie Study of Nursing Education, 45
Case manager, 200
Cassandra Radical Nurses Network, 81
CBI. *See* Caring Behavior Inventory (CBI)
CCNE. *See* Commission on Collegiate Nursing Education (CCNE)
CDC. *See* Centers for Disease Control and Prevention (CDC)
C-diff. *See* Clostridium difficile (C-diff)
Center for Medicare and Medicaid Services (CMS), 64
Centers for Disease Control and Prevention (CDC), 18
Centers for Medicare and Medicaid (CMS), 42, 45
CFO. *See* Chief financial officer (CFO)
Challenges, 225
Change, 70–94, 244–245
  defined, 72
  methods of, 32–33
  models for, 33–34
  theoretical foundations, 72–73
  theories, 34–39
  understanding of, 78
Character, 242
Checklist Protocol, Central Venous Catheter Insertion, 218
Cheek, J., 90
Chenot, T. M., 17
Chief financial officer (CFO), 239
Chief nurse executive (CNE), 239